Sixth Edition

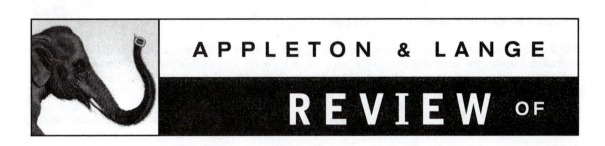

PEDIATRICS

Sara S. Viessman, MD
Medical Director
Center for Educational Development and Support
Lehigh Valley Hospital and Health Network
Allentown, Pennsylvania

Martin I. Lorin, MD
Professor of Pediatrics
Department of Pediatrics
Baylor College of Medicine
Houston, Texas

Appleton & Lange Reviews/McGraw-Hill
Medical Publishing Division

New York Chicago San Francisco Lisbon London Madrid Mexico City Milan
New Delhi San Juan Seoul Singapore Sydney Toronto

Appleton & Lange Review of Pediatrics, Sixth Edition

Copyright © 2004 by The **McGraw-Hill Companies**, Inc. All rights reserved. Printed in the United States of America. Except as permitted under the United States Copyright Act of 1976, no part of this publication may be reproduced or distributed in any form or by any means, or stored in a data base or retrieval system, without the prior written permission of the publisher.

Previous editions copyright © 1993, 1989 by Appleton & Lange; © 1981, by ARCO Publishing, Inc. under the title *Pediatrics Review.*

1 2 3 4 5 6 7 8 9 0 QPD/QPD 0 9 8 7 6 5 4

ISBN: 0-8385-0303-9

This book was set in Palatino by International Typesetting and Composition.
The editor was Catherine A. Johnson.
The production supervisor was Rick Ruzycka.
Project management was provided by International Typesetting and Composition.
Quebecor World was printer and binder.

This book is printed on acid-free paper.

Notice

Medicine is an ever-changing science. As new research and clinical experience broaden our knowledge, changes in treatment and drug therapy are required. The authors and the publisher of this work have checked with sources believed to be reliable in their efforts to provide information that is complete and generally in accord with the standards accepted at the time of publication. However, in view of the possibility of human error or changes in medical sciences, neither the authors nor the publisher nor any other party who has been involved in the preparation or publication of this work warrants that the information contained herein is in every respect accurate or complete, and they disclaim all responsibility for any errors or omissions or for the results obtained from use of the information contained in this work. Readers are encouraged to confirm the information contained herein with other sources. For example and in particular, readers are advised to check the product information sheet included in the package of each drug they plan to administer to be certain that the information contained in this work is accurate and that changes have not been made in the recommended dose or in the contraindications for administration. This recommendation is of particular importance in connection with new or infrequently used drugs.

Library of Congress Cataloging-in-Publication Data

Appleton & Lange review of pediatrics / [edited by] Sara S. Viessman. – 6th ed.
   p. ; cm.
  Rev. ed. of: Appleton & Lange's review of pediatrics / Martin I. Lorin. 5th ed. c1993.
  Includes bibliographical references and index.
  ISBN 0-8385-0303-9
  1. Pediatrics—Examinations, questions, etc. I. Title: Appleton and Lange review of pediatrics. II. Title: Review of pediatrics. III. Viessman, Sara S. IV. Lorin, Martin I. Appleton & Lange's review of pediatrics.
  [DNLM: 1. Pediatrics—Examination Questions. WS 18.2 A649 2004]
RJ48.2.A676 2004
618.92'00076—dc22

                                                      2003068639

Contents

Preface

Focusing on the health of children allows physicians to have a large impact on tomorrow's society. As Jonas Salk said, "Children are the message we send to a future we will never see." In order to play a role in the care of a child, medical students and physicians should commit themselves to excellence. One important aspect of this commitment is the ongoing acquisition of knowledge.

Though knowledge gained in conjunction with patient care remains the epitome of physician learning, other modalities are absolutely essential. This text is designed to supplement your education in pediatrics. Organized into 11 chapters of questions, answers, and corresponding explanations, it should be a source of information and understanding for you. Although in pediatrics a substantial fund of knowledge must be committed to memory, when possible, you should strive to understand rather than memorize information presented.

Chapter 1 is a warm-up practice examination that will also help you evaluate your test-taking skills. Chapters 2 through 9 are organized by topics and provide an opportunity to review and test your basic fund of pediatric knowledge. In Chapter 10, clinical cases followed by a series of questions are designed to test your ability to apply that knowledge to clinical problems. The Practice Test (Chapter 11) is a sample pediatric examination which covers a wide range of topic areas.

Occasionally, you will find a note in square brackets [*Note:*...]. These notes usually pertain to question construction and techniques for answering multiple-choice examination questions. Although there is no substitute for knowledge and understanding, it is recognized that exam-taking ability is a legitimate academic skill, and it is appropriate for you to strengthen your ability in this regard.

It is hoped that you will learn as much from using this book as the editors and authors did in preparing it, and that your reach exceeds your grasp.

Sara S. Viessman, MD

This edition is dedicated to all people striving to improve the lives of children.

I wish to thank my family Ron, Peter, Beth, and Hanna, who are synergistic sources of joy for me; my parents Jan and Tony, and my sisters Beth, Julie, and Jennie, whose support is constant and steadying; my nieces and nephews, whose choices I follow with pride; my friends, who make me laugh; my patients and their parents, who have provided me with an education in life; my students, residents, mentors, and colleagues, whose pursuit of excellence is inspirational; and each contributor whose accomplishments and friendship are equally appreciated.

I thank editors and others at McGraw-Hill and ITC, especially Catherine Johnson, Jack Farrell, Ben Kolstad, and Waseem Andrabi. Your support was professional and enjoyable! Thank you John VanBrakle, MD and Michael Consuelos, MD for your review of and insightful comments on Chapters 3 and 4.

Finally, I wish to thank Dr. Lorin, the original and sole author of the first five editions of this book, for giving me the opportunity and support to co-edit this edition. The intensity with which he pursues new information serves as an excellent model of self-learning and is adopted by many of his residents and students. As a result of the hundreds of students and residents with whom he has worked, his positive influence on the care provided for children is expansive. His joy for learning is exceeded only by his joy for life. Luckily, he is contagious.

Contributors

Joseph Y. Allen, MD
Instructor
Section of Emergency Medicine
Department of Pediatrics
Baylor College of Medicine
Houston, Texas

R. Blaine Easley, MD
Clinical Fellow
Division of Pediatric Anesthesiology and Critical Care
 Medicine
Department of Anesthesiology/Critical Care Medicine
The Johns Hopkins University
Baltimore, Maryland

Z. Leah Harris, MD
Assistant Professor
Fellowship Director, Pediatric Critical Care
Division of Pediatric Anesthesiology and Critical Care
 Medicine
Department of Anesthesiology/Critical Care Medicine
The Johns Hopkins University
Baltimore, Maryland

Mary Anne Jackson, MD
Professor of Pediatrics
University of Missouri—Kansas City School of
 Medicine
Kansas City, Missouri
Chief
Section of Pediatric Infectious Disease
Children's Mercy Hospital
Kansas City, Missouri

Catalina M. Kersten, MD
Assistant Professor of Pediatrics
Clerkship Director
Department of Child Health
University of Missouri—Columbia
Columbia, Missouri

Jeffrey G. Michael, DO
Assistant Professor of Pediatrics
University of Missouri—Kansas City School of
 Medicine
Kansas City, Missouri
Physician
Department of Emergency Medicine
Children's Mercy Hospital
Kansas City, Missouri

Timothy A. O'Connor, MD
Medical Director, Intensive Care Nursery
Boone Hospital Center
Columbia, Missouri

Shiv Someshwar, MD
Assistant Professor
Clinic Director, General Pediatrics
Department of Pediatrics
West Virginia University
Morgantown, West Virginia

Emily A. Thorell, MD
Assistant Professor of Pediatrics
University of Missouri—Kansas City School of
 Medicine
Attending Physician
Children's Mercy Hospital
Kansas City, Missouri

Joseph D. Tobias, MD
Vice Chair
Department of Anesthesiology
Chief
Division of Pediatric Anesthesiology/Pediatric
  Clinical Care
Russell and Mary Sheldon Chair of Pediatric Intensive
  Care Medicine
University of Missouri—Columbia
Columbia, Missouri

Mark A. Ward, MD
Assistant Professor of Pediatrics
Associate Director, Pediatric Housestaff Education
Baylor College of Medicine
Houston, Texas

CHAPTER 1

Warm-Up Questions and Exam-Taking Skills

Sara S. Viessman, MD

Most of the questions in this book contain explanations that begin with a letter representing the correct answer. However, in this chapter, several of the questions and some of the answers begin with a clue to help you analyze both the question and your approach to answering it. Case-management questions are scattered throughout as the questions proceed from easy to more difficult.

This chapter should be studied with no time constraints. Proceed at your own pace, taking as much time as needed for each question.

Questions

DIRECTIONS (Questions 1 through 28): Each of the numbered items or incomplete statements in this section is followed by answers or completions of the statement. Select the ONE lettered answer or completion that is BEST in each case.

Clue: Questions 1 and 2 are simple and straightforward, each with only one possible correct answer. For this type of question, you can actually answer the question before looking at the choices. Try it. Then read the choices to verify that your answer is there. Finally, review all the other choices to be sure that none is better than the one you selected.

1. You have just diagnosed a 3-year-old child as having cystic fibrosis. The parents are concerned about future pregnancies. You explain to them that the pattern of genetic transmission of cystic fibrosis is

   (A) autosomal dominant
   (B) autosomal recessive
   (C) X-linked recessive
   (D) X-linked dominant
   (E) autosomal recessive in some families and X-linked in others

2. Lyme disease is contracted by

   (A) ingestion of unripe fruit
   (B) ingestion of spoiled fruit
   (C) drinking of contaminated water
   (D) the bite of a tick
   (E) the bite of a mosquito

Clue: Unlike the preceding two questions, the answer to Question 3 cannot be anticipated before viewing the list of suggested answers, because there are many possible completions to the statement. Nevertheless, the question is simple and straightforward.

3. Minimal-change disease

   (A) is the most common cause of nephrotic syndrome in childhood
   (B) has a peak incidence in children between 10 and 15 years of age
   (C) usually results in end-stage renal disease in 5–10 years
   (D) is characterized by normal serum lipids and cholesterol
   (E) responds poorly to corticosteroids

Clue: Pay attention to key words when you read a question. Question 4 contains the key words "most likely."

4. You have just prescribed phenytoin (Dilantin) for a 12-year-old boy with new onset of epilepsy. Of the following side effects, which is most likely to occur in this patient?

   (A) lymphoma syndrome
   (B) Raynaud's phenomenon
   (C) acute hepatic failure
   (D) gingival hyperplasia
   (E) optic atrophy

5. Infants born to mothers who have been using crack cocaine are at increased risk of

   (A) anemia
   (B) cerebral infarction
   (C) hypercalcemia
   (D) macrosomia
   (E) postmaturity

6. You examine an 18-year-old male college student with a 5-day history of fever, sore throat, and fatigue. Physical examination reveals an exudative tonsillitis and bilateral enlarged and slightly tender posterior cervical lymph nodes. The spleen is palpable 3 cm below the rib cage. The agent most likely responsible for this patient's illness is

(A) group A beta-hemolytic *Streptococcus*
(B) adenovirus
(C) *Toxoplasma gondii*
(D) Epstein-Barr virus
(E) *Corynebacterium diphtheriae*

Clue: Questions 7 and 8 use a negative qualifier, "all . . . EXCEPT." This type of question has been eliminated from most standardized tests. Therefore, the rest of this book does not contain questions with negative qualifiers. These two questions are here only to enhance your awareness should you come across this type in an examination.

7. Intrauterine cytomegalovirus (CMV) infection has been associated with all of the following EXCEPT

(A) mental retardation
(B) deafness
(C) blindness
(D) jaundice
(E) intestinal obstruction

8. Chromosomal analysis on one of your patients reveals 47,XXY karyotype. You anticipate that the patient will have all of the following features EXCEPT

(A) small, defective testes
(B) gynecomastia
(C) tall stature, with disproportionately long legs
(D) subnormal intelligence
(E) microcephaly

9. Which of the following is a risk factor for meconium aspiration syndrome?

(A) neonatal meningitis
(B) congenital heart disease
(C) cystic fibrosis
(D) fetal distress
(E) tracheoesophageal fistula

10. A 12-year-old boy with juvenile diabetes mellitus has poorly controlled blood glucose levels. He is following an ADA diet and receiving one daily injection of a mixture of regular and NPH in the same syringe before breakfast. His blood glucose monitoring record reveals fairly normal glucose levels during the morning and early afternoon, somewhat low levels in the late afternoon, and very high levels after dinner. You decide to

(A) increase the dose of regular insulin
(B) increase the dose of NPH insulin
(C) administer the regular and the NPH insulins in separate syringes
(D) increase to two injections a day
(E) decrease the amount of carbohydrate in the evening meal

11. Which of the following statements regarding immunization against *Haemophilus influenzae* type b (Hib) is correct?

(A) It is indicated for high-risk children only.
(B) Currently available conjugated Hib vaccines can be administered effectively as early as 2 months of age.
(C) Children who have had allergic reactions to egg should not be given the Hib vaccine.
(D) It is recommended that the conjugated Hib vaccine not be administered to children with a history of reactions to DPT immunization.
(E) It is recommended that the conjugated Hib vaccine be given as a single dose without a booster.

12. The major advantage of the new acellular pertussis vaccine is that it

(A) is more immunogenic
(B) is less expensive
(C) has fewer side effects
(D) requires fewer doses
(E) can be combined with the varicella vaccine

13. It is recommended that young infants should sleep in the supine rather than in the prone position. This is based on data suggesting that the prone position is associated with an increased incidence of

    (A) delayed eruption of the first deciduous teeth
    (B) gastroesophageal reflux and aspiration
    (C) macrognathia
    (D) strabismus
    (E) sudden infant death

14. The feeding of honey to infants less than 6 months of age has been associated with

    (A) anaphylaxis
    (B) hypernatremia
    (C) infantile botulism
    (D) jaundice
    (E) listeriosis

15. The mother of a healthy 6-month-old infant is planning to return to work and stop breastfeeding within the next month and asks your advice about how she should proceed. The child had been fed on the breast only, without bottle supplementation and without solids. You advise her that she should

    (A) continue to breast-feed even if it means not returning to work
    (B) feed the infant a commercial infant formula
    (C) feed the infant unmodified whole cow's milk
    (D) feed the infant either formula or cow's milk by cup only, avoiding the use of a bottle
    (E) discontinue milk and introduce cereals followed by vegetables, fruits, meats, and then eggs

16. You have just examined a term, healthy, male newborn infant and found no abnormalities. In speaking to the mother, she asks you whether or not she should have the child circumcised. In your discussion with the mother, it would be most appropriate to explain that circumcision is associated with

    (A) a decreased incidence of urinary tract infection in infancy and a decreased incidence of penile cancer in adulthood
    (B) a decreased incidence of urinary tract infection in infancy and an increased incidence of penile cancer in adulthood
    (C) an increased incidence of urinary tract infection during infancy and a decreased incidence of penile cancer in adulthood
    (D) an increased incidence of urinary tract infection in childhood and an increased incidence of penile cancer in adulthood
    (E) no change in the incidence of either urinary tract infection or penile cancer

17. The mother listens carefully and appears to consider the information you have given. She then asks whether you, personally, would recommend circumcision for her infant. You should reply that routine neonatal circumcision is

    (A) medically indicated
    (B) medically indicated, but parents must be aware of the risks, which include bleeding, infection, and scarring
    (C) not medically indicated
    (D) not medically indicated and associated with certain risks, but in the final analysis the decision should be made by the parents on the basis of personal preference
    (E) not medically indicated, and you personally would advise against it

18. A 3-month-old infant presents with poor growth and inadequate weight gain. There is no history of vomiting or diarrhea. Except for the appearance of malnutrition and lack of subcutaneous fat, the physical examination is normal. The most likely cause of this child's failure to thrive is

    (A) renal disease
    (B) a metabolic disorder
    (C) tuberculosis
    (D) an endocrine disorder
    (E) a nonorganic cause

19. A 2-year-old child is being evaluated because the mother notes that her right eye has been turning in. Physical examination documents strabismus with a right esotropia. Attempts to visualize the fundi are unsuccessful, but it is noted that the red reflex is replaced by a yellow-white pupillary reflex in the right eye. This child most likely has

(A) retinitis pigmentosa
(B) retinoblastoma
(C) rhabdomyosarcoma
(D) severe hyperopia
(E) severe myopia

20. A 2-year-old child is admitted because of weakness and coma. According to the parents, he had been well until several hours prior to admission, when they noted diarrhea, cough, wheezing, and sweating. Physical examination reveals a comatose child with diffuse weakness and areflexia. Pupils are pinpoint and unresponsive. Examination of the chest reveals generalized wheezing. Oral secretions are copious. At this time you ought to administer a dose of

(A) adrenaline
(B) atropine
(C) cefotaxime
(D) methylprednisolone
(E) Tensilon (edrophonium)

21. A 3-week-old infant is admitted with vomiting of 5 days' duration. Physical examination reveals a rapid heart rate, evidence of dehydration, and ambiguous genitalia. Serum electrolytes are Na^+ 120 meq/L, K^+ 7.5 meq/L, HCO_3^- 12 meq/L, BUN 20 mg/dL. In addition to intravenous fluid replacement with normal saline, administration of which of the following would be most important?

(A) diuretics
(B) potassium exchange resin
(C) glucose and insulin
(D) antibiotics
(E) hydrocortisone

22. A previously well 12-year-old girl presents to clinic because of painful swellings on the front of the legs of about 3 days' duration. Examination reveals tender erythematous nodules, 1–2 cm in diameter, on the extensor surfaces of the lower legs. The remainder of the physical examination is unremarkable. Which of the following is most likely to confirm the cause of this condition?

(A) stool smear and culture
(B) urinalysis and BUN
(C) throat culture and ASO titer
(D) slit-lamp examination of the eye
(E) echocardiogram

23. An 18-year-old boy presents with cough, chest pain, and low grade nightly fevers of several weeks duration. He has a 4-year history of smoking two packs of cigarettes per day. Chest x-ray reveals a large mass in the mediastinum with extension into the right upper chest. Your leading diagnosis is

(A) adenocarcinoma
(B) squamous cell carcinoma
(C) small cell carcinoma
(D) lymphoma
(E) metastatic Wilms tumor

24. A 12-year-old child is seen because of a rash and severe headache. The skin lesion began as a red macule on the thigh, which gradually expanded over 1 week to reach approximately 15 cm in diameter with red borders and central clearing. The lesion was slightly painful. A few days after the onset of the skin manifestation, the child developed severe headache, stiff neck, myalgias, arthralgias, malaise, fatigue, lethargy, and generalized lymphadenopathy. Low-grade fever was present. The mother recalls that the child was bitten by a tick about 1 week prior to the onset of symptoms. This patient's disorder is probably best treated with

(A) corticosteroids
(B) diphenhydramine
(C) methotrexate
(D) nonsteroidal anti-inflammatory drugs
(E) doxycycline

25. An 8-year-old child is hospitalized because of paroxysms of severe colicky abdominal pain which does not radiate to the back or the groin. Physical examination is unremarkable except for generalized abdominal tenderness. An exploratory laparotomy reveals an edematous intestine without specific lesions. The appendix appears normal but is removed. Postoperatively the abdominal pain persists, and hematuria develops. BUN and creatinine are normal. On the second postoperative day, tender swelling of both ankles and knees is noted. This child should be observed closely for the development of

   (A) shock
   (B) meningitis
   (C) hepatitis
   (D) a purpuric rash
   (E) hemorrhagic pancreatitis

26. A 10-year-old boy has been having episodes of repetitive and semipurposeful movements of the face and shoulders. The parents believe these movements are worse when the child is under emotional stress. They also volunteer that they have never noted the movements while the patient is asleep. The movements have been present for more than 6 months. The parents are now especially concerned because the child has developed repetitive episodes of throat clearing and snorting. Physical and neurologic examinations are entirely normal. During the examination you note that the child has some blinking of the right eye, twitching of the right face and grimacing. You ask him to stop these movements, and he is temporarily successful in doing so, but the movements recur. The home situation, social history, and child's development and social adjustment appear normal. A head CT scan is normal. Of the following, which would be the most appropriate next step?

   (A) order an electroencephalogram
   (B) prescribe carbamazepine
   (C) prescribe corticosteroids
   (D) prescribe haloperidol
   (E) refer the child to a psychiatrist

27. A 3-month-old infant is hospitalized because of recurrent right focal seizures that progress to generalization. Birth and perinatal history are unremarkable. There is a flat, purplish-red hemangioma on the left side of the face extending onto the forehead. The remainder of the examination (neurologic and physical) is within normal limits. The results of a lumbar puncture are within normal limits. You order a CT scan of the head and anticipate seeing

   (A) agenesis of the corpus callosum
   (B) a porencephalic cyst
   (C) gyriform calcifications
   (D) hydrocephalus
   (E) normal findings

28. On routine examination of the children of a migrant farm worker, you notice that a 12-year-old child who has received little previous medical care is short and mentally retarded. Physical examination reveals that the liver is enlarged to 5 cm below the right rib cage, and the spleen is enlarged 6 cm below the left rib cage. Lumbodorsal kyphosis is prominent. The child has a peculiar facies with thick lips and a large tongue. Attempts to visualize the retina are unsuccessful because of clouding of the corneas. You expect that examination of this child's urine will reveal

   (A) dermatan and heparan sulfate
   (B) galactose
   (C) mannose
   (D) the odor of maple syrup
   (E) the odor of sweaty feet

DIRECTIONS (Questions 29 through 35): Each set of matching questions in this section consists of a list of several numbered items followed by 5–26 lettered options. For each numbered item select the ONE lettered option with which it is most closely associated. Each lettered option may be selected once, more than once, or not at all.

Selection of answers for questions 29 through 32

   (A) miliaria rubra
   (B) verrucae vulgaris
   (C) condyloma acuminatum

(D) molluscum contagiosum

(E) pityriasis rosea

29. Small (pinhead to 1 cm), pearly papules with translucent tops and waxy, whitish material inside, distributed on the face and anterior trunk. Some lesions are umbilicated

30. Soft, flesh-colored papular or pedunculated lesions around the genitalia and rectum

31. Oval, maculopapular lesions oriented with the long axis along skin tension lines

32. Characteristically pruritic

Selection of answers for questions 33 through 35

(A) ABO incompatibility

(B) Alpha$_1$-antitrypsin deficiency

(C) biliary atresia

(D) breastfeeding jaundice

(E) breast milk jaundice

(F) choledochal cyst

(G) cholelithiasis

(H) Crigler-Najjar syndrome

(I) cystic fibrosis

(J) Dubin-Johnson syndrome

(K) erythroblastosis (Rh incompatibility)

(L) galactosemia

(M) glucose-6-phosphate dehydrogenase deficiency

(N) hepatitis

(O) hereditary spherocytosis

(P) hypothyroidism

(Q) physiologic hyperbilirubinemia

(R) sepsis

33. A 3-day-old term, healthy infant is noted to be jaundiced. Physical examination is otherwise normal. Laboratory values: Hb 16.8 g/dL; reticulocytes 1.0%; bilirubin unconjugated 8.5 mg/dL, conjugated 0.8 mg/dL.

34. A 5-week-old infant has been jaundiced for about 2 weeks. He has been asymptomatic and physical examination is otherwise normal. Laboratory values: Hb 14.2 g/dL; reticulocytes 1.2%; bilirubin unconjugated 4.5 mg/dL, conjugated 5.5 mg/dL; ALT 25 IU/L, AST 75 IU/L. Abdominal ultrasound examination reveals a normal-size liver; a gallbladder is not visualized.

35. An otherwise well 4-week-old infant has remained jaundiced since day 3 of life despite two exchange transfusions and continuous phototherapy. Laboratory values: Hb 14 g/dL; reticulocytes 1.0%; bilirubin unconjugated 16 mg/dL, conjugated 0.2 mg/dL; ALT 15 IU/L, AST 40 IU/L. A Coombs test prior to the first exchange transfusion was negative. Ultrasound examination reveals a normal liver and gallbladder.

Answers and Explanations

For many of the questions below, the boldface letter indicating the correct answer appears within, or at the end of, the explanation rather than at the beginning. When this is the case, take care to not look ahead. Try to respond to the clues as you go along.

1. The correct answer is (**B**). Cystic fibrosis (CF) is an autosomal recessive disorder with a disease incidence in Whites of about 1:1500 and a corresponding carrier state of about 1:20. This is said to make CF the most common lethal genetic disease in the White population. The disease is much less common among Blacks and Asians. *(Oski:1490; Rudolph:1967)*

2. Like question 1, this question has only one possible correct answer, and you should have been able to come up with that answer before looking at the list of choices. The answer is (**D**), bite of a tick. *Borrelia burgdorferi,* the spirochete that causes Lyme disease, is transmitted to humans by the bite of a tick, most commonly *Ixodes* species, although in some geographic areas, other ticks such as *Ambylomma americanum* (the lone star tick) have been incriminated. *(Red Book:407–411)*

3. The correct answer is (**A**). This question is simple in that it deals with well-known and important clinical features of a common disease—minimal-change nephrotic syndrome (MCNS). It is straightforward in that not only is one of the listed choices (**A**) clearly the best, but the other four choices all are incorrect.

   Minimal-change disease is the most common cause of nephrotic syndrome in childhood, and accounts for more than all other causes combined. The peak incidence is between 2 and 5 years of age. The prognosis is very favorable, and the process rarely progresses to end-stage renal disease. Serum lipids and cholesterol are elevated, as they are with other causes of nephrotic syndrome. Finally, the disease characteristically responds well to treatment with corticosteroids, with only a small minority of patients failing to remit.

   If you answered this question incorrectly, try to determine why. Since the question is so straightforward, the most likely reason would be an incomplete fund of knowledge. *(Rudolph:1691–1693; Oski:1796–1797)*

4. The correct answer is (**D**). Optic atrophy is not a recognized complication of phenytoin (Dilantin) therapy. Acute hepatic failure, a lymphoma-like syndrome, and Raynaud's phenomenon all have been noted *rarely* with this drug. Gingival hyperplasia is a *common* and troublesome side effect, which often can be minimized by scrupulous dental hygiene.

   If the examinee knew that a lymphoma-like syndrome has been reported with phenytoin and focused in on that without carefully considering all subsequent choices, he or she might have selected (A). You can avoid such errors by carefully reading the question and asking yourself, "What are the common side effects of this drug?" even before looking at the choices. Knowing that gingival hypertrophy is a very common side effect of phenytoin would be sufficient knowledge to answer the question correctly. Another way to approach this question would be to ask yourself, "Of the following side effects, which is *most* frequent?" Obviously, that one would be the correct answer. *(Hay:740; Oski:2054)*

5. This is another straightforward, completely factual question. Only one choice is correct. As a matter of fact, two answers are not only incorrect, they are exact opposites of what actually happens with cocaine, so it should be easy to be confident that they are incorrect. Infants born to women using cocaine, especially crack cocaine, have an increased incidence of prematurity (not postmaturity) and low birth weight (not macrosomia). The vasoconstrictive action of cocaine not only impairs uterine and placental blood flow but also may result in cerebral infarction in the fetus or neonate and probably is a key factor in the increased incidence of necrotizing enterocolitis seen in these infants. The correct answer is (**B**). *(Rudolph:2023; Hay:21–22:1048)*

6. Although this question also is quite straightforward, it potentially is more difficult than the preceding questions because several of the agents listed can explain many of the features of this adolescent's illness. If you read the instructions carefully, you noted that you were asked to select *the one best answer,* which does not imply that all other choices are totally without merit. Consider which of the above choices best fits the clinical scenario, and therefore, which is most likely responsible for this patient's illness.

The correct answer is (**D**). The agent most likely responsible for this child's illness is the Epstein-Barr virus (EBV). The clinical picture is strongly suggestive of mononucleosis. Although this patient could be infected with group A *Streptococcus* or adenovirus, several features are much more characteristic of EBV infection than either of these. They include the fact that the child is a college student, the presence of splenomegaly, and the fact that the adenopathy is posterior rather than anterior and is only slightly tender. While these findings also could be explained by toxoplasmosis, this diagnosis is rarely confirmed as a cause of acute exudative tonsillitis and cervical adenitis in the United States. Although it is appropriate to think of diphtheria in patients with acute exudative tonsillitis, there is nothing specific in this case to suggest that diagnosis. Infectious mononucleosis is clearly *the most likely* diagnosis.

If you missed this question, was it because you didn't know enough about EBV or some of the other choices, or because you didn't make the right judgmental decision? *(Rudolph: 1035–1038; Hay:1123–1124)*

7. It generally is easier to be sure that two items are associated than it is to be sure that they are not. If the examinee knows of the association, then it probably exists. If the student doesn't know of an association, it may be because it doesn't exist or it may be that he or she just doesn't know about it. There are many recognized manifestations of cytomegaloviral infection in the neonate, including deafness, blindness, jaundice, petechiae, fever, convulsions, and mental retardation. Intestinal obstruction has not been noted.

Even if the student knew nothing about congenital CMV infection, a careful reading of the choices would suggest a best guess. Answer (**E**) is different from all the other choices in the sense that neonatal intestinal obstruction usually is caused by a discrete congenital abnormality such as intestinal atresia, malrotation, or annular pancreas. The other manifestations listed generally result from diffuse tissue damage or inflammation. Guessing, obviously, is a last resort, but it usually is possible to make an educated rather than a blind guess. Incidentally, since congenital CMV occurs as frequently as 1/100 live births, it is fortunate that most infections are asymptomatic. *(Rudolph:1031–1035)*

8. Several factors make this question difficult, even though it deals with the most common human sex chromosomal aberration, the 47,XXY karyotype. First, the name of the disorder (Klinefelter syndrome or seminiferous tubule dysgenesis) is not provided in either the question or the answer. Second, the use of "all . . . EXCEPT," as discussed above, adds to the complexity of the question.

Klinefelter syndrome is associated with small, defective testes, azoospermia, and sterility. Gynecomastia and other signs of eunuchoidism occur in about half the patients. Patients usually are long-legged and tall. Although mental deficiency, often severe, is common, microcephaly is not a feature. Therefore, the correct answer is (**E**). *(Rudolph: 2090–2091)*

9. **(D)** Fetal distress is the major risk factor for meconium aspiration. The mechanism involves the loss of anal sphincter tone, passage of meconium into the amniotic fluid, and aspiration by the distressed, gasping infant during the process of birth. The thick meconium obstructs the airways, causing tachypnea, retractions, and grunting.

   This is the type of question in which a little knowledge can go a long way. If you knew that meconium aspiration was a relatively *common* problem in the delivery room, you could eliminate (C) cystic fibrosis (a relatively *uncommon* disease) as its cause. (*Meconium ileus*, which is associated with cystic fibrosis, has nothing to do with meconium aspiration.) If you realized that aspiration of meconium can only occur before or during delivery, you also could eliminate (B) congenital heart disease and (A) neonatal meningitis, as neither of these usually causes distress during delivery. Finally, you should be able to figure out that a tracheoesophageal fistula, with or without associated esophageal atresia, would lead to aspiration of saliva, milk, or gastric contents after birth but would not predispose to aspiration of meconium. *(Hay:19)*

10. You should try to answer this question by selecting the one choice you consider best and then confirm it by verifying that the alternate choices are incorrect. A quick perusal of the possible answers reveals that the question is looking for a therapeutic not a diagnostic action. So, decide what you would do to manage this patient. The main problem appears to be the elevated blood glucose after dinner and in the evening. The best way to resolve this would be a second injection of regular insulin before dinner. Sure enough, a second injection is one of the options **(D)**.

    Now review each choice to see if any is better than your choice. What would happen if you increased the dose of regular insulin (A) in the morning injection? Because of the relatively short action of regular insulin, this would not help the evening hyperglycemia. Since the effect of NPH insulin peaks at 8–12 h and lasts about 24 h, increasing the dose of morning NPH (B) would help the evening hyperglycemia but would worsen the afternoon hypoglycemia. It is common practice to mix regular and NPH insulin in the same syringe and separating them (C) would accomplish nothing. Using two injections a day (D), each a mixture of regular and NPH, is standard practice to optimize control. The regular insulin in the before-dinner dose would correct the evening hyperglycemia, and moving some of the NPH from the morning to the evening injection would alleviate the afternoon hypoglycemia. Since there is nothing to suggest that the child is taking excess carbohydrates at dinner, it would be preferable to provide adequate insulin rather than to decrease the carbohydrate intake. Therefore, the best choice is **(D)**. *(Rudolph: 2125–2128)*

11. *Haemophilus influenzae* type b (Hib) infection is a major cause of morbidity and mortality in the young infant. The introduction of Hib immunization is relatively new. The Hib polysaccharide is not very immunogenic, and the first generation of vaccines was effective only when administered to children 2 years and older. Unfortunately, the greatest incidence of Hib meningitis is in the child less than 2 years. Just as information about the first vaccines was being incorporated into textbooks, a second generation of vaccines, which could be administered effectively at 18 months of age, was introduced into clinical use. Finally, conjugated vaccines were licensed. These vaccines are effective when administered as early as 2 months of age.

    The correct answer to this question, therefore, is **(B)**. It is now recommended that all infants be immunized with the conjugated Hib vaccine. Depending on the brand of vaccine used, infants should receive a series of two or three immunizations between 2 and 6 months of age, followed by one booster dose at 12–15 months of age. *(Red Book:24–25)*

12. Pertussis vaccine has been plagued by side effects, most minor but some devastating. The most common systemic reaction is fever, which may be very high and accompanied by a febrile seizure. The most important reaction is encephalopathy which, though rare, can result in permanent brain damage. The new acellular vaccine (DPaT) appears to be free of this devastating complication and that is its major advantage. The correct answer, therefore, is **(C)**.

The majority of questions in national examinations deal with basic material that is covered in standard textbooks, and therefore, standard texts are where examinees should spend the majority of their study time. A percentage of questions, however, deal with recent data, which although important and often well known, may not be found in textbooks 4 or 5 years old. Like the Hib vaccines in the previous question, the first strains of DPaT vaccine were released for use as boosters only. DPaT vaccines for primary immunization were not licensed in the United States until late 1996. *(Red Book:475–486)*

13. **(E)** Epidemiologic data suggests that there is an increased incidence of sudden infant death syndrome (SIDS) among infants sleeping prone as compared to those sleeping supine. Although the prone sleeping position was traditionally favored in the United States for many years, the American Academy of Pediatrics and others now recommend that infants routinely be put to bed in the supine position. However, since there appears to be less tendency to gastroesophageal reflux (GER) in the prone position, probably because the esophagus enters the stomach posteriorly, infants with GER are an exception and should be permitted to sleep in the prone position. Normal infants should sleep supine. *(Rudolph:1936)*

14. This is a straightforward but difficult question because it involves information not so widely known as the material in most of the preceding questions. Can you recall reading or hearing about honey being associated with a specific infection or disease? If not, can you eliminate any of the choices to improve your chances of a correct guess? You may have heard that *Listeria* is often spread through contaminated milk and cheese, but you have not heard that it is spread by honey. Jaundice is a common problem in the neonate, but the question refers to infants less than 6 months of age, not specifically to neonates.

The answer is **(C)**. Infants are especially vulnerable to infantile botulism. This disorder differs from the adult form of the disease in that it is indolent rather than acute and is characterized by progressive muscle weakness. The infantile form of botulism results from ingestion of *C. botulinum* spores, in contrast to the

adult form, which results from the ingestion of the preformed toxin in contaminated food. Honey has been incriminated as one source of *C. botulinum* spores. Therefore, honey is not recommended for infants younger than 6 months of age. *(Rudolph:918; Hathaway:1049)*

15. This question is very open ended, with many potentially correct completions. You must evaluate each choice, estimate its validity, and rank it against the other choices.

It would be inappropriate to advise the mother to continue breastfeeding at the cost of her job. Aside from the presumptuousness of such advice and the issues of personal life styles, there is little biological justification to push for breastfeeding beyond 6 months. So choice (A) is unacceptable.

While most 6-month-old infants will do well on unmodified cow's milk, infant formula has a closer resemblance to human milk and is preferable for many reasons, including better protein to carbohydrate ratio, better calcium to phosphorus ratio, and in some cases better casein to whey ratio than unmodified cow's milk. Therefore, **(B)** is a better answer than (C). Most 6-month-old infants are not developmentally ready to drink from a cup, so (D) is incorrect. Discontinuing all milk at this early age (E) would be ill advised in regard to nutritional balance, digestive capabilities and developmental readiness. **(B)** is the correct answer. *(Rudolph:27–30)*

16. Although the topic of this question, circumcision, is a controversial and often emotional issue, the question is straightforward and deals only with facts. There are now several studies indicating a decreased incidence of urinary tract infection among circumcised as compared to noncircumcised males during infancy and the preschool years. The effect is most pronounced in the first few months of life. If you were aware of these data, you would be able to exclude answers (C), (D), and (E), giving yourself a 50% chance of guessing the correct answer. If you also knew that data show a decreased incidence of penile cancer among circumcised males in late adulthood, you would have selected **(A)** as the correct answer. *(J Pediatr 128:23–27, 1996; Am J Dis Child 134:484–486, 1980; Pediatrics 103:686–693, 1999)*

17. In contrast to the preceding question, this is a subjective question and therefore difficult and often frustrating for the examinee. The question looks not only for your fund of knowledge but also for how you would use that knowledge in dealing with a specific situation. When faced with such questions, you should try to answer in accordance with what you know or believe to be closest to standard medical practice or the majority opinion, even if you personally disagree. Most authorities suggest that the brief decrease in prevalence of urinary tract infections and the decrease in penile cancer in late adulthood are not sufficient benefits to medically justify a routine recommendation for the surgical procedure of circumcision. In the final analysis, the decision must be made by the parents on the basis of personal preference. The correct answer, therefore, is (D), which is logical in regard to the available data and also is in accordance with the recommendations of the American Academy of Pediatrics. (*Pediatrics 103:686–693, 1999; Rudolph:105–106*)

18. (E) Failure to thrive (FTT) is a common pediatric problem characterized by poor growth, especially in regard to weight gain. Today, in the United States, nonorganic causes of FTT account for 30% to more than 50% of the cases in most series and are responsible for more cases than any other etiology. Nonorganic causes encompass a diverse spectrum extending from poverty and lack of food, through poor parenting skills and misguided feeding to frank neglect or abuse. If you missed this question, why? Were you unaware of the importance and frequency of nonorganic causes of FTT? Did you think that one of the other choices was more common? If so, that reflects a lack of information rather than uncertainty between close items, because none of the other choices listed accounts for more than 5 or 10% of cases. If gastrointestinal problems had been a choice, the question would have been more difficult, because gastrointestinal disorders account for up to 25% of cases of FTT in most series. (*Oski:1048–1049*)

19. (B) Retinoblastoma is the most likely cause of this child's strabismus and white pupillary reflex (leukokoria, *cat's eye reflex*). Although rhabdomyosarcoma may involve the orbit, it is extrinsic to the globe and doesn't cause a white pupillary reflex. Other causes of leukokoria include visceral lava migrans (*Toxocara canis* infection) and retrolental fibroplasia. Although retinoblastoma is rare, the association with leukokoria is a classic and important pediatric entity with which all students as well as pediatric house officers should be familiar. (*Rudolph: 2395; Hay:913–915*)

20. This format is common on national medical examinations. It makes the question difficult because it requires recall rather than recognition. The question asks you to identify a disease or condition but does not provide a list of diagnoses from which to choose; instead, it provides a list of associated findings, in this case, treatments. To answer the question correctly you must analyze the clinical findings and recall the disease rather than selecting (recognizing) it from a list.

The sudden onset of neurologic signs or symptoms in a previously well toddler always ought to raise suspicion of a toxin or poisoning. Review the question. Can you think of any toxins that might explain the findings in this case?

The correct answer is (B). This child is a victim of organophosphate poisoning. Organophosphate and carbamate insecticides are widely used throughout the United States and are important causes of poisoning in children. These drugs produce both muscarinic effects (rhinorrhea, wheezing, pulmonary edema, salivation, vomiting, cramps, bradycardia, and pinpoint pupils) as well as nicotinic effects (twitching, weakness and paralysis, convulsions, coma, and respiratory failure). These children often ingest the toxic substance unobserved, and the diagnosis must be suspected on the basis of the clinical picture even when there is no history of ingestion or exposure. Atropine will reverse the muscarinic effects of these agents and is a useful part of treatment.

Edrophonium is a short and rapidly acting cholinergic drug used diagnostically to reverse the muscle weakness of myasthenia gravis. Myasthenia, however, would not explain the pinpoint pupils, salivation, wheezing, bradycardia, or convulsions. (*Rudolph:373–374; Hay:351*)

21. (E) The child described probably has congenital adrenal hyperplasia (CAH), an inborn metabolic

error of the adrenal cortex. The acidosis (HCO_3^- 12 meq/L) helps to rule out pyloric stenosis as the cause of the emesis, as most infants with pyloric stenosis have a metabolic alkalosis. The enzyme deficiency in CAH results in decreased production of cortisol and other adrenal cortical hormones and secondary hypertrophy of the adrenal gland. Accumulation of androgen-like precursors of cortisol during fetal development leads to masculinization of the female fetus and ambiguous genitalia, which is an important clue in this case. The low serum sodium and high serum potassium levels are classic findings in this condition, reflecting the lack of mineralocorticoids. In addition to the use of saline, administration of a mineralocorticoid such as cortisone or hydrocortisone is critical. The elevated serum potassium level usually responds rapidly to administration of saline and steroids, and specific therapy with exchange resins or glucose and insulin usually is unnecessary.

As did the preceding question, this question tests the examinee's ability of recall rather than recognition, a more difficult but clinically more relevant skill. Instead of providing a list of diseases or syndromes as possible answers, it provides a list of additional features or findings, one of which is associated with the disorder in question. In this case, as in the preceding question, the feature to be selected is the appropriate therapy. The question tests more than the examinee's ability to recite the treatment of hyperkalemia. It tests his or her ability to analyze the clinical situation, make a correct diagnosis, set priorities, and tailor therapy to the specific pathophysiology involved. *(Rudolph: 2032–2041; Hay: 969–972)*

22. Again, this question requires recall rather than recognition. The stem of the question gives no information except the age and sex of the patient and a description of the skin lesions—tender erythematous nodules on the extensor surfaces of the legs. On the basis of these data you must decide what disease the patient most likely has. Which of the following best fits the skin lesions described: erythema nodosum, rheumatic nodules, subcutaneous fat necrosis, hematomas, septic emboli, or Henoch-Schoenlein purpura?

The correct answer is (**C**). To answer this question you must not only identify the rash as erythema nodosum (an uncommon but not rare disease) but you must also know that group A beta-hemolytic streptococcal infection is a common cause. Erythema nodosum is a reactive phenomenon characterized by tender, erythematous nodules 1–2 cm in diameter. The lesions usually are on the extensor surfaces of the extremities and are more common on the legs. This rash is seen in a variety of infections including histoplasmosis, tuberculosis, coccidioidomycosis, and group A streptococcal infection. Today, the most common cause in an otherwise well child in the United States is group A streptococcal infection. *(Oski:911)*

23. The differences between adults and children frequently are emphasized in medical training. The differences between adults and adolescents should also be recognized. The differential diagnosis for many conditions, such as an intrathoracic mass seen in this case, is age dependent. While carcinoma of the lung is a leading cause of intrathoracic mass in adults, it is very rare in adolescents, even those who have a significant smoking history. That eliminates choices (A), (B), and (C). While it is true that Wilms tumor frequently metastasizes to the lung, this malignancy almost always presents in the first few years of age and would be unheard of in an 18-year-old. That leaves lymphoma as the only remaining choice and the most likely diagnosis. (**D**) is the correct answer. Other causes, such as tuberculosis, histoplasmosis, and sarcoid need to be considered but were not listed as choices. *(Hay:901–906)*

24. Here again, you are required to make a diagnosis but are not given a list of diseases from which to choose. You should analyze the data, identify the important features, and generate a list of most likely diagnoses. The major problems appear to be fever, a localized rash, and meningeal inflammation (headache and stiff neck). The malaise, fatigue, lethargy, generalized lymphadenopathy, and arthralgia are less specific. Of note is the fact that the child was bitten by a tick a week prior to the onset of the illness. If the tick bite is related to the illness, it

would suggest an infectious etiology. The systemic findings, the central clearing of the rash, and the time course permit us to rule out a simple cellulitis. What are the common infections carried by ticks? Rocky Mountain spotted fever, Lyme disease, Q fever, tularemia, relapsing fever, and Colorado tick fever are all spread by ticks, but only Lyme disease fits with the localized rash described—erythema migrans. This disease is caused by the spirochete *Borrelia burgdorferi*. The organism is sensitive to a number of antibiotics, including doxycycline, which generally is the treatment of choice. The correct answer is (**E**). *(Oski:1171–1173; Rudolph:Color Plate 22:1212–1213)*

25. This question also challenges you to identify a disease without providing a list of diagnoses from which to choose. What disease do you believe this child most likely has: juvenile rheumatoid arthritis, inflammatory bowel disease, cystic fibrosis, Henoch-Schonlein purpura (HSP), *Salmonella* infection?

    The correct answer is (**D**). This child has anaphylactoid purpura, also known as HSP. This is an important and not rare pediatric entity, well known to pediatricians and pediatric residents but not so well known by students. The question is difficult because the scenario given is infrequent although well recognized in this disorder. The major features of this disease are colicky abdominal pain, nephritis, arthritis, and a characteristic purpuric rash limited to the area below the waist. The purpuric rash listed as a possible answer does not specify location or distribution, but is still the best answer. If you missed this question, was it because you weren't familiar with HSP or because you didn't recognize it from this presentation? The only atypical feature in this case is that the child was taken to the operating room. When abdominal pain is the first complaint, diagnosis is virtually impossible until other features appear. *(Rudolph:Color Plate 12:1212–1213; Hay:878–879)*

26. What disorder do you believe this child probably has: psychomotor seizures, Tourette syndrome, drug abuse, brain tumor, or psychologic disorder?

The child most likely has Tourette syndrome, a disorder characterized by blinking, twitching, grimacing, and jerking movements that often have a repetitive and semipurposeful character. Like simple habit tics, the movements usually can be voluntarily suppressed momentarily, disappear during sleep, and are made worse by emotional tension. These features could mislead the examinee to assume a psychologic etiology. Ultimately, the muscles of respiration and swallowing become involved so that throat clearing, coughing, snorting, hiccups, and other noises are common. Coprolalia, echolalia, and spitting are classic features but are not always present.

The correct answer is (**D**). Haloperidol is the drug of choice for Tourette syndrome, although not all patients require therapy. *(Hay:768)*

27. This question deals with a rare but dramatic pediatric syndrome. What is the significance of the hemangioma on one side of the face? If you can identify the disease, can you then anticipate the findings on CT scan? Do you think this child has congenital toxoplasmosis, holoprosencephaly, Sturge-Weber disease, subdural effusions, porencephalic cyst? Providing a list of diagnoses would have changed the question from one of recall to one of recognition.

    The association of a unilateral facial hemangioma, particularly in the distribution of the trigeminal nerve, and focal seizures suggests Sturge-Weber disease, also referred to as Sturge-Weber-Dmitri syndrome and encephalotrigeminal angiomatosis. Incidentally, national examinations often use eponyms for diseases and syndromes even when other specific names exist. Examples include Down syndrome rather than trisomy 21 and Werdnig-Hoffmann disease for spinomuscular atrophy. Sturge-Weber disease is characterized by a port-wine capillary nevus on the face (classically in the distribution of the first division of the trigeminal nerve), focal seizures on the contralateral side, and intracranial calcifications on the ipsilateral side. Therefore, the correct answer to question 28 is (**C**), gyriform calcifications. The intracranial pathology is caused by hemangiomatous changes of the meninges. This is a congenital disorder, probably of nongenetic basis. The seizures often are very difficult to control. Other common features include mental deficiency and a contralateral hemiparesis.

Pay attention to all information. Although there is always the possibility that some incidental information, unrelated to the diagnosis, has been included, you need to consider the potential significance of each piece of data, such as the hemangioma.

If you missed the question initially but were able to choose the correct diagnosis after seeing the list of diseases in the answer section, it suggests that your fund of knowledge in this area is adequate but that your ability to recall what you know needs strengthening. If you were unable to identify the correct answer even with the list above, you are unfamiliar with this syndrome. This question is very difficult because the subject matter (Sturge-Weber disease) is rare and because the question requires recall rather than recognition, a double dose of difficulty. *(Hay:758)*

28. This question is exceedingly difficult, so don't be discouraged. Do you know what disease or condition this child has, and if so, what would be found in the urine? Your first task is to establish a probable diagnosis. If you were not able to deduce the diagnosis from the question, how about from the list of answers? Do you know for what condition each finding is suggestive or diagnostic? Think about each one.

Urinary Finding	Disease
Dermatan and heparan sulfate	Hurler syndrome
Galactose	Galactosemia
Mannose	Mannosidosis
Odor of maple syrup	Branched-chain aminoacidemia
Odor of sweaty feet	Isovaleryl CoA dehydrogenase deficiency

The correct answer is (**A**). The child described has Hurler syndrome, a form of mucopolysaccharidosis. This rare, autosomal recessive disorder is characterized by growth retardation that generally starts after the first

year of life. Classically, facial features become coarse and eventually appear gargoyle-like. Hepatosplenomegaly results from the accumulation of mucopolysaccharide and often is striking. Bone and joint involvement with kyphosis and joint contractures is frequent. Corneal clouding results from the deposition of mucopolysaccharide in that organ. The accumulation of mucopolysaccharide within the brain leads to mental retardation.

If you were not familiar with Hurler syndrome and did not know that it is characterized by dermatan and heparan sulfate in the urine, you would not be able to answer the question. On the other hand, you might know that information and still not be able to answer the question if you could not successfully recall the disease and match the features to the patient in the question. Exploring each potential answer and trying to recall the conditions with which it is associated could help. *(Rudolph:2329; Hay:1005)*

29. (**D**) In a matching question with six or fewer choices it is practical to read and briefly think about each lettered choice before attempting to answer the numbered questions.

The lesions of molluscum contagiosum are typically quite small, from pinhead size to 5 or 10 mm in diameter. Larger lesions do occur but are infrequent. The lesions usually have an easily recognized appearance: round, dome-shaped papules with a translucent top and a waxy, whitish material inside. Umbilication is common, especially of larger lesions. The condition is caused by a DNA pox virus and is spread by direct contact with an infected individual. Lesions may occur anywhere but are most common on the arms and trunk. *(Oski:831)*

30. (**C**) Condyloma acuminatum are soft, fleshy, papular, or pedunculated lesions occurring around the genitalia and/or rectum. Although these lesions are caused by the human papillomavirus and are sexually transmitted in adolescents and older children, it is now believed that most cases in infants and very young children are not sexually acquired but rather are acquired during passage through the birth canal. *(Rudolph:938)*

31. (E) The typical lesion of pityriasis rosea is an ovoid, pink papule or plaque with fine scales. Lesions typically follow tension lines on the skin, giving the appearance of the branches of a pine tree or a Christmas tree on the patient's back. A single lesion appearing a week or two before other lesions is a common occurrence and is referred to as a herald patch. *(Rudolph:1181)*

32. (E) Of the five conditions listed, only pityriasis rosea is typically pruritic. Itching in this condition is often intense and prolonged. *(Rudolph:1181; Oski:831–832)*

33. In this type of matching question, up to 26 options are presented for each item. When the list of options is long (more than six), it becomes inefficient and time consuming to evaluate each possible lettered choice for each numbered item. However, it is helpful to scan or preview the list of options. Then, for each numbered item, decide what the best answer would be and look for it in the list of possible choices.

It is clear that the 3-day-old term infant in this question has unconjugated hyperbilirubinemia but is otherwise well and has no evidence of hemolysis. The most likely cause of these findings would be physiologic jaundice, a generally benign condition of neonates associated with hepatic immaturity and a peak bilirubin level of less than 13 mg/dL on day of life 3 or 4 for a term infant and 15 mg/dL or less on day 5–7 for a preterm infant. Since physiologic jaundice is one of the options listed (**Q**), the examinee need look no further. However, if time permits, scanning the list for other potential answers would be a wise safety measure. Although it is true that some of the other conditions listed, such as breast milk jaundice or Crigler-Najjar syndrome, could cause similar findings, we are not told that the infant is being breast-fed, and Crigler-Najjar syndrome is exceedingly rare. Physiologic jaundice is clearly the most likely cause and therefore the best choice. *(Oski:199–200)*

34. (C) This 5-week-old infant has persistent mixed hyperbilirubinemia, suggesting a hepatic disorder. The normal liver enzymes indicate an obstructive rather than an inflammatory condi-

tion. Finally, the inability to visualize a gallbladder on ultrasound examination makes biliary atresia the only plausible diagnosis. *(Rudolph:1506–1507; Oski:199–200)*

35. (H) This infant has had severe, persistent unconjugated hyperbilirubinemia for 4 weeks but is otherwise well. The normal serum levels of conjugated bilirubin and hepatic enzymes rule out most forms of liver disease (obstructive or inflammatory), and there is no evidence of hemolysis. The Coombs test was negative, and the hyperbilirubinemia is too severe and prolonged for either a blood group incompatibility or breast milk jaundice. Such a course for neonatal jaundice is very rare, and therefore one must consider rare causes. Crigler-Najjar syndrome, a congenital deficiency of hepatic enzymes involved in conjugation of bilirubin, is the only disorder that could explain this patient's findings. If the examinee were unable to recall the entity of Crigler-Najjar syndrome, a quick scan of the list might "ring a bell." If this fails, make the best guess possible and return to the question, if time permits, after completing the test booklet to evaluate each option for the best fit. *(Rudolph:166,1489)*

BIBLIOGRAPHY

AAP, Circumcision policy statement. *Pediatrics* 1999; 103:686–693.

American Academy of Pediatrics. *2003 Red Book, Report of the Committee on Infectious Diseases,* 26th ed. Elk Grove, IL: American Academy of Pediatrics, 2003.

Craig JC, Knight JF, et al. Effect of circumcision of urinary tract infection in preschool boys. *J Pediatr* 1996; 128:23–27.

Hay WW, Hayward AR, Levin MJ, Sondheimer JM. *Current Pediatric Diagnosis & Treatment,* 16th ed. New York, NY: McGraw-Hill, 2003.

Kochen M, McCurdy S. Circumcision and the risk of cancer of the penis. *Am J Dis Child* 1980;134:484–486.

McMillan JA, DeAngelis CD, Feigin RD, Warshaw JB. *Oski's Pediatrics, Principles & Practice,* 3rd ed. Philadelphia, PA: JB Lippincott, 1999.

Rudolph CD, Rudolph AM, Hostetter MK, et al. *Rudolph's Pediatrics,* 21st ed. New York, NY: McGraw-Hill, 2003.

CHAPTER 2

The Neonate

Timothy A. O'Connor, MD

Acquiring an education in neonatology, the study of the newborn infant, is an important component of pediatric training. Most youngsters go through childhood without ever having a cardiac, neurologic, or renal problem, but all children are originally neonates. Newborns with their unique physiology can develop severe organic disease with unique pathophysiology. Most children are hospitalized because of diseases unrelated to their age (e.g., asthma, sickle cell disease, trauma, osteomyelitis). The newborn, in contrast, is most often sick as the result of a problem directly related to his age—respiratory distress syndrome, pneumonia, meningitis and sepsis, intestinal obstruction, congenital malformations, etc. In the last decade, intensive technology was developed to assist in the management of these disorders. The examinee will be expected to understand this unique physiology and pathophysiology as well as to have knowledge of the diseases and management technology associated with this period of life. The examinee will also be expected to know that the norms for many laboratory values (e.g., Hb, CSF protein) are quite different for the neonate than for the older infant or child.

The neonatal period is formally defined as the first 30 days of life. However, very premature, small, or sick newborns may remain in the neonatal intensive care unit for several months. For the neonate, congenital malformations, congenital diseases, and genetic diseases should always be considered, for even what appear to be acute symptoms. Finally, the student must always remember that the normal neonate is not immunologically mature and is vulnerable to severe infection by "unusual" organisms.

Questions

DIRECTIONS (Questions 1 through 88): Each of the numbered items or incomplete statements in this section is followed by answers or by completions of the statement. Select the ONE lettered answer or completion that is BEST in each case.

1. An infant is diagnosed with a given disorder below. Which of these poses the greatest recurrence risk for this patient's future siblings?

   (A) Hirschsprung disease
   (B) cystic fibrosis
   (C) ventricular septal defect
   (D) trisomy 21
   (E) trisomy 13

2. The most common permanent complications of congenital cytomegalovirus infection involve the

   (A) central nervous system
   (B) heart
   (C) hematopoietic system
   (D) immune system
   (E) liver

3. Among the following, the most common cause of acquired sensorineural hearing loss in infancy is

   (A) hyperbilirubinemia
   (B) congenital infection
   (C) ototoxic drug exposure
   (D) neuroblastoma
   (E) late onset group B streptococcal meningitis

4. Which of the following congenital defects of the gastrointestinal tract has the highest incidence of associated cardiac defects?

   (A) omphalocele
   (B) congenital volvulus
   (C) Hirschsprung disease
   (D) gastroschisis
   (E) pyloric stenosis

5. The most common manifestation of cystic fibrosis in the newborn infant is

   (A) pneumonia
   (B) intrauterine growth retardation
   (C) meconium ileus
   (D) wheezing
   (E) hypochloremic alkalosis

6. Of the following, which physical finding is most indicative of a full-term infant?

   (A) veins and tributaries are seen over the abdomen
   (B) long lanugo is present on the back
   (C) palpable breast tissue of 8.0 mm
   (D) pitting edema over the tibia
   (E) incurving of the upper pinnae of the ears only

7. Oral candidiasis (thrush) in a 1-week-old term newborn infant usually

   (A) responds well to topical therapy with mycostatin
   (B) requires systemic therapy with amphotericin B

(C) requires both topical (mycostatin) and systemic (amphotericin) therapy

(D) requires investigation to rule out DiGeorge syndrome

(E) is associated with cleft palate

8. During a normal term newborn resuscitation, which of the following should be performed first?

(A) The infant should be dried and the wet towel removed from beneath the infant's body.

(B) The heart rate should be auscultated.

(C) Breath sounds should be auscultated.

(D) The nose and oropharynx should be suctioned.

(E) Color assessment should be performed and oxygen administered if necessary.

9. The major route for excretion of bilirubin in the fetus in utero is

(A) via the kidney

(B) transplacental passage

(C) degradation to biliverdin

(D) reincorporation into hemoglobin

(E) hepatic secretion and storage in the intestinal lumen

10. The breakdown of 1 g of hemoglobin yields about

(A) 0.035 mg of bilirubin

(B) 0.35 mg of bilirubin

(C) 3.5 mg of bilirubin

(D) 35 mg of bilirubin

(E) 350 mg of bilirubin

11. Which of the following would most likely be an indication for intrauterine transfusion of the fetus?

(A) erythroblastosis fetalis

(B) sickle cell anemia

(C) spherocytosis

(D) fetal distress and bradycardia

(E) congenital heart disease

12. Among the following, the most common complication of intrauterine transfusion is

(A) a transfusion reaction (mismatch)

(B) graft-versus-host reaction

(C) premature onset of labor

(D) acquired immunodeficiency syndrome (AIDS)

(E) renal failure

13. Kernicterus is most closely related to the serum level of

(A) total bilirubin

(B) conjugated bilirubin

(C) unconjugated bilirubin

(D) haptoglobin

(E) hemoglobin

14. Over the first week of life, a typical term newborn will

(A) gain approximately 30 g per day

(B) gain approximately 60 g per day

(C) neither gain nor lose weight

(D) lose approximately 5–10% of its birth weight

(E) lose approximately 15% of its birth weight

15. In most cases of ABO isoimmune hemolytic disease of the newborn, the mother is

(A) type A and the infant is type B

(B) type A and the infant is type AB

(C) type O and the infant is type A

(D) type O and the infant is type AB

(E) type O and the infant is type B

16. The most common serious late clinical manifestation of ABO isoimmune hemolytic disease is

(A) kernicterus

(B) congestive heart failure

(C) gallstones

(D) bilirubinuria

(E) iron deficiency

17. Small amounts of unconjugated bilirubin in the plasma generally do not enter the brain because

    (A) unconjugated bilirubin is not lipid soluble
    (B) unconjugated bilirubin is tightly bound to albumin
    (C) unconjugated bilirubin is tightly bound to hemoglobin
    (D) the blood-brain barrier is impermeable to unconjugated bilirubin
    (E) unconjugated bilirubin is rapidly metabolized by cerebrospinal fluid

18. Which of the following is most closely associated with the development of neonatal respiratory distress syndrome (hyaline membrane disease)?

    (A) gestational age
    (B) birth weight
    (C) cesarean section delivery
    (D) maternal diabetes
    (E) meconium in the amniotic fluid

19. Among infants of comparable weight and gestational age in the U.S.

    (A) there is no difference in mortality rates between males and females and African Americans and Whites
    (B) males have a higher mortality rate than females, and African Americans have a higher mortality rate than Whites
    (C) males have a lower mortality rate than females, and African Americans have a lower mortality rate than Whites
    (D) males have a higher mortality rate than females, and African Americans have a lower mortality rate than Whites
    (E) males have a lower mortality rate than females, and African Americans have a higher mortality rate than Whites

20. Pulmonary surfactant is a complex compound composed primarily of

    (A) surfactant protein A
    (B) surfactant protein B

    (C) neutral lipids
    (D) water
    (E) phospholipids

21. Mortality rates in newborn infants

    (A) decrease with increasing gestational age from 30 weeks through 43 completed weeks of gestation
    (B) are not related to birth weight
    (C) are not related to race
    (D) are higher than the mortality rates of adolescents
    (E) have not changed significantly since the 1950s

22. Which of the following is true of surfactant production?

    (A) Surfactant is synthesized and stored in the type I alveolar cells.
    (B) Surfactant is synthesized and stored in the type II alveolar cells.
    (C) Surfactant is produced by the pulmonary alveolar macrophages.
    (D) Surfactant is stored in the interstitial spaces in the lungs.
    (E) Surfactant is not produced until after labor ensues.

23. The average birth weight of a 30-week gestation infant is about

    (A) 500 g
    (B) 1000 g
    (C) 1500 g
    (D) 2000 g
    (E) 2500 g

24. Which of the following maternal conditions most predisposes her fetus to congenital heart disease?

    (A) hypertension
    (B) diabetes mellitus
    (C) atherosclerotic coronary vascular disease
    (D) anemia
    (E) rheumatoid arthritis

25. Which of the following statements is true of the foramen ovale in the *fetus*?

    (A) Blood flows through the foramen ovale from the right ventricle to the left ventricle.

    (B) Blood flows through the foramen ovale from the left ventricle to the right ventricle.

    (C) Blood flows through the foramen ovale from the left atrium to the right atrium.

    (D) Blood flows through the foramen ovale from the right atrium to the left atrium.

    (E) Blood must pass through the foramen ovale for blood to enter the right atrium from the umbilical vein.

26. Erythema toxicum is

    (A) more common among term than premature infants

    (B) usually associated with fever and a general toxic state

    (C) uncommon before the fifth day of life

    (D) usually associated with an elevated peripheral white blood cell count

    (E) manifested in less than 10% of newborns

27. The lecithin–sphingomyelin ratio of amniotic fluid is a useful indicator of the maturity of the fetal

    (A) central nervous system

    (B) lungs

    (C) liver

    (D) kidneys

    (E) immunologic system

28. Bronchopulmonary dysplasia is most commonly associated with

    (A) an inflammatory insult to the lungs late in fetal development

    (B) failure of development of pulmonary arterioles during early fetal life

    (C) failure of development of the bronchial buds during early fetal life

    (D) intrauterine viral infection

    (E) the use of oxygen and positive-pressure breathing in the treatment of respiratory distress syndrome

29. Surfactant replacement therapy for respiratory distress syndrome

    (A) is considered experimental

    (B) is only useful in infants <1500 g birth weight

    (C) has no known complications

    (D) has not been shown to reduce mortality in very low birth weight infants

    (E) requires tracheal intubation to administer

30. The characteristic roentgenographic findings of infantile respiratory distress syndrome are

    (A) lobar atelectasis and interstitial edema

    (B) bilateral patchy densities and pneumothorax

    (C) diffuse reticulogranular changes and air bronchograms

    (D) diffuse hyperaeration and cardiomegaly

    (E) cardiomegaly and interstitial edema

31. The major goal of continuous positive airway pressure in the treatment of infants with respiratory distress syndrome is to

    (A) prevent infection

    (B) prevent pneumothorax

    (C) improve cardiac output

    (D) raise arterial PO_2

    (E) lower arterial PCO_2

32. The major danger associated with an arterial PO$_2$ greater than 100 mmHg in a premature infant receiving oxygen for respiratory distress syndrome is

    (A) alveolar proteinosis
    (B) atelectasis
    (C) fire or explosion
    (D) kernicterus
    (E) retinopathy of prematurity

33. The pathophysiology of infantile respiratory distress syndrome in the premature infant appears to involve

    (A) increased production of pulmonary surfactant
    (B) decreased production of pulmonary surfactant
    (C) increased metabolism of pulmonary surfactant
    (D) decreased metabolism of pulmonary surfactant
    (E) rerouting of pulmonary surfactant to the systemic circulation

34. A healthy term infant is circumcised and experiences excessive blood loss eventually requiring transfusion. Among the following, the most likely diagnosis is

    (A) factor IX deficiency
    (B) factor VIII deficiency
    (C) von Willebrand disease
    (D) disseminated intravascular coagulopathy
    (E) protein C deficiency

35. Which of the following is most likely to be associated with a cataract in the newborn?

    (A) maple syrup urine disease
    (B) glucose-6-phosphate dehydrogenase deficiency
    (C) phenylketonuria
    (D) galactosemia
    (E) propionic acidemia

36. Which of the following is true of pigmented lesions known as mongolian spots?

    (A) They never occur in White infants.
    (B) They are identified in over 40% of African American infants.
    (C) They consist of small well demarcated lesions approximately 2 mm in diameter.
    (D) Malignant degeneration is common.
    (E) The most common site of occurrence is the nape of the neck.

37. A newborn infant is noted to be cyanotic and tachypneic. He is placed in 50% oxygen and the cyanosis clears completely. The infant most likely has

    (A) cyanotic congenital heart disease
    (B) lung disease
    (C) central nervous system disease
    (D) liver disease
    (E) methemoglobinemia

38. A 35-week gestation infant is delivered weighing 3.9 kg, with an omphalocele and a large tongue. No other abnormalities are detected. The most likely diagnosis is

    (A) congenital hypothyroidism
    (B) trisomy 18
    (C) trisomy 13
    (D) fetal alcohol syndrome
    (E) Beckwith-Wiedemann syndrome

39. A 3-week-old infant is noted to have microcephaly, cerebral calcifications on skull roentgenogram, and blindness. Which of the following is the most likely cause of these findings?

    (A) bilateral subdural hemorrhages
    (B) cerebral agenesis
    (C) cytomegalovirus infection
    (D) erythroblastosis
    (E) primary microcephaly

40. A 5-day-old infant with white, cheesy patches on the tongue and buccal mucosa, with mild inflammation of the mucosa. Which of the following organisms is most likely the cause of these oral lesions?

   (A) *Candida albicans*
   (B) *Listeria monocytogenes*
   (C) *Escherichia coli*
   (D) group A *Streptococcus*
   (E) group B *Streptococcus*

41. You are examining a newborn and elicit a family history of seizures. Cutaneous findings which most likely would be associated with this include

   (A) hypopigmented patch
   (B) harlequin color change
   (C) salmon patch on the nasal glabella
   (D) hemangioma of the thigh
   (E) pustular melanosis

42. A term otherwise healthy neonate has isolated premature synostosis of the sagittal suture. This condition usually is associated with

   (A) scaphocephaly
   (B) increased intracranial pressure
   (C) microcephaly
   (D) hydrocephalus
   (E) subdural effusions

43. A newborn is noted to have numerous 3 mm vesicles on the chest and neck, along with several similar sized hyperpigmented lesions in the same distribution. The most likely diagnosis is

   (A) mucocutaneous herpes simplex infection
   (B) acne neonatorum
   (C) erythema toxicum
   (D) incontinentia pigmenti
   (E) transient pustular melanosis

44. Which of the following tracheoesophageal anomalies is most common?

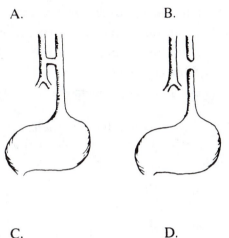

A.   B.

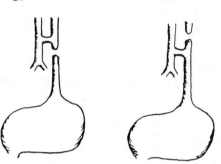

C.   D.

45. A cephalhematoma is best differentiated from caput succedaneum by

   (A) absence of a history of prolonged or difficult labor
   (B) limitation of swelling to the area over one bone
   (C) a normal neurologic examination
   (D) a prolonged prothrombin time
   (E) a normal lumbar puncture

46. Advancing maternal age most affects the incidence of

   (A) autosomal recessive disorders
   (B) nondisjunction chromosome disorders
   (C) autosomal dominant disorders
   (D) X-linked disorders
   (E) inborn errors of metabolism

47. Advancing paternal age most affects the incidence of

    (A) autosomal recessive disorders
    (B) nondisjunction chromosome disorders
    (C) autosomal dominant disorders
    (D) X-linked disorders
    (E) inborn errors of metabolism

48. Hypoglycemia in a term infant less than 48 h old usually is defined as a blood glucose level below

    (A) 10 mg/dL
    (B) 20 mg/dL
    (C) 40 mg/dL
    (D) 60 mg/dL
    (E) 80 mg/dL

49. Congenital clubfoot is most commonly associated with disorders of which of the following systems?

    (A) the central nervous system
    (B) the hematopoietic system
    (C) the gastrointestinal system
    (D) the cardiovascular system
    (E) the respiratory system

50. The most urgent problem in infants with the Pierre Robin syndrome is

    (A) heart failure
    (B) seizures
    (C) intestinal obstruction
    (D) metabolic acidosis
    (E) upper airway obstruction

51. Which of the following problems in a newborn infant might respond to a pharmacologic dose of pyridoxine?

    (A) blindness
    (B) seizures
    (C) jaundice
    (D) rash
    (E) urinary retention

52. Which of the following is true of mitochondrial inheritance?

    (A) These disorders follow a paternal line of inheritance only.
    (B) These disorders have not been identified in humans thus far.
    (C) Only females are affected.
    (D) Organ systems with low energy demands are the most affected.
    (E) These disorders follow a maternal line of inheritance only.

53. Of the following, which correlates best with subsequent neurologic abnormalities?

    (A) fetal bradycardia
    (B) failure to breathe at birth
    (C) a low 1-min Apgar score
    (D) a low 5-min Apgar score
    (E) seizures in the first 36 h of life

54. An 8-day-old infant develops papules, pustules, and comedones on the forehead, nose, and malar areas of the face. The child is otherwise well, and the remainder of the physical examination is normal. The most likely diagnosis is

    (A) congenital syphilis
    (B) impetigo
    (C) neonatal acne
    (D) staphylococcal pustulosis
    (E) tuberous sclerosis

55. The maternal serum alpha-fetoprotein test is most useful in diagnosing

    (A) duodenal atresia
    (B) club foot
    (C) cleft lip and palate
    (D) myelomeningocele
    (E) alveolar proteinosis

56. A newborn with trisomy 21 develops repeated emesis on the first day of life. An abdominal x-ray reveals a dilated stomach. Which of the following is the most likely diagnosis?

    (A) annular pancreas
    (B) duodenal atresia

(C) gastric volvulus

(D) pyloric stenosis

(E) lactobezoar

57. A 1700-g infant was asphyxiated at birth and, after successful resuscitation, had numerous apneic episodes. On the third day of life, the infant began to vomit, and abdominal distention and bloody stools were noted. The most likely diagnosis is

(A) aganglionosis

(B) intussusception

(C) necrotizing enterocolitis

(D) Shigella enteritis

(E) volvulus

58. The natural history of the elevated capillary or cavernous hemangioma is best described by which of the following statements?

(A) no significant change in size after birth

(B) an increase in size during the first few years after birth and then regression

(C) an increase in size during the first decade of life and then no further change

(D) a slow but progressive increase in size throughout life

(E) a slow but progressive decrease in size starting shortly after birth

59. Scalded skin syndrome (toxic epidermal necrolysis) of the newborn is associated with

(A) maternal diabetes

(B) staphylococcal infection or colonization

(C) thiamine deficiency

(D) an immunologic defect or deficiency

(E) excessive vitamin K administration

60. A Wright's stain of the contents from a lesion of erythema toxicum usually will reveal

(A) basophils

(B) eosinophils

(C) lymphocytes

(D) immature lymphocytes

(E) polymorphonuclear leukocytes

61. An infant born to a mother with hyperparathyroidism is likely to develop

(A) hypercalcemia

(B) hypocalcemia

(C) parathyroid carcinoma

(D) hyperthyroidism

(E) hyperparathyroidism

62. Which of the following is associated with conjugated hyperbilirubinemia?

(A) sequestrated blood

(B) tyrosinemia

(C) hereditary spherocytosis

(D) Rh incompatibility

(E) physiologic jaundice

63. An infant with ambiguous genitalia and salt-losing congenital adrenal hyperplasia has a chromosome analysis result of 46,XY. The enzymatic defect probably is

(A) complete 21-hydroxylase

(B) partial 21-hydroxylase

(C) 3-β-hydroxysteroid dehydrogenase

(D) 11-hydroxylase

(E) 17-hydroxylase

64. Thyrotoxicosis in the first day of life most likely occurs in an infant born to a mother

(A) with untreated hypothyroidism

(B) with untreated Graves disease

(C) with Graves disease being treated with antithyroid medications

(D) with euthyroid goiter

(E) receiving iodides as therapy for chronic bronchitis

65. The most common site of initial lesions in HSV II cutaneous infections in a 5-day-old would be the

(A) mouth

(B) scalp

(C) eyes

(D) buttocks

(E) chest

66. Which of the following is true of serum calcium levels in the newborn?

    (A) High PTH levels suppress the serum calcium.

    (B) The serum calcium promptly decreases after delivery.

    (C) The serum calcium remains essentially unchanged over the first 3 days.

    (D) The serum calcium is usually higher on day 2 than day 1.

    (E) Infants of diabetic mothers have an accentuated PTH response resulting in hypercalcemia.

67. One should be concerned about a term infant who has not passed a meconium stool

    (A) during the process of birth

    (B) within a few minutes of birth

    (C) by 1–2 h of life

    (D) by 6–12 h of life

    (E) by 24 h of life

68. On the fifth day of life, an infant is noted to have a violaceous, circumscribed, subcutaneous nodule immediately beneath fading forceps marks on one cheek. The most likely diagnosis is

    (A) an abscess

    (B) a hemangioma

    (C) a pericytoma

    (D) periorbital cellulitis caused by *Haemophilus influenzae*

    (E) subcutaneous fat necrosis

69. Which of the following is true of congenital hypothyroidism?

    (A) Affected infants are usually clinically apparent by the third day of life.

    (B) Affected infants have unusually small fontanelles.

    (C) Affected infants appear thin.

    (D) Prolonged hyperbilirubinemia is common.

    (E) Usually have a goiter present at birth.

70. Which of the following infants is at greatest risk of developing an early iron deficiency anemia?

    (A) A premature infant

    (B) An infant with ABO incompatibility

    (C) An infant with physiologic hyperbilirubinemia

    (D) A postmature infant

    (E) An infant with polycythemia

71. Fetal hemoglobin has an increased affinity for oxygen as compared with adult hemoglobin. This difference results from

    (A) an increased mass of fetal hemoglobin

    (B) thinness of the red cell membrane in the fetus

    (C) the presence of unconjugated bilirubin in the red cell

    (D) decreased binding with 2,3-diphosphoglycerate (2,3-DPG)

    (E) intracellular alkalosis

72. The mass shown below is most likely a

    (A) scalp abscess

    (B) posterior hydrocephalus

    (C) encephalocele

    (D) diastematomyelia

    (E) hydrocele

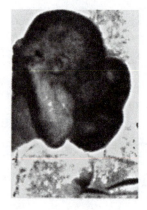

73. An infant born with malformed forearms is noted to develop severe hemorrhagic manifestations. A roentgenogram of the arm is shown below. Which of the following would be the most likely cause of the bleeding problem?

    (A) leukemia
    (B) hypoprothrombinemia
    (C) thrombocytopenia
    (D) hypersplenism
    (E) hemophilia

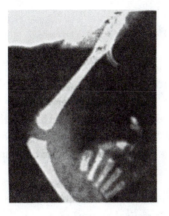

74. "Physiologic jaundice" of the newborn

    (A) is an unconjugated hyperbilirubinemia
    (B) usually appears within the first 12 h of life
    (C) is more common in term than in preterm infants
    (D) is generally associated with moderate anemia and reticulocytosis
    (E) is uncommon in Black infants

75. Which of the following is the most common complication found in infants of diabetic mothers?

    (A) birth asphyxia
    (B) sacral agenesis
    (C) hypocalcemia
    (D) hypoglycemia
    (E) cardiac septal hypertrophy

76. Infantile glaucoma

    (A) is best treated with medical management
    (B) is frequently seen with trisomy 21
    (C) presents with the white pupil sign

    (D) rarely is diagnosed before 6 months of age
    (E) is associated with congenital rubella and neurofibromatosis

77. Which of the following is an uncommon finding in respiratory distress syndrome (hyaline membrane disease)?

    (A) tachypnea
    (B) grunting
    (C) cyanosis
    (D) wheezing
    (E) retractions

78. A high-risk labor is being followed by electronic fetal heart rate monitoring (EFM). Which of the following most commonly would be seen in a healthy baby?

    (A) heart rate 60–80/min
    (B) accelerations of the heart rate
    (C) heart rate below 60/min
    (D) decreased beat-to-beat variability in heart rate
    (E) fixed heart rate

79. Which of the following clinical signs most likely represent those seen in a newborn with tension pneumothorax?

    (A) cyanosis, apnea, and bradycardia
    (B) apnea, hypotension, and bradycardia
    (C) tachypnea, cyanosis, and bradycardia
    (D) wheezing, tachycardia, and hypertension
    (E) wheezing, hypotension, and apnea

80. An infant born at 39 weeks gestation weighing 2000 g should be classified as

    (A) low birth weight
    (B) premature
    (C) small for gestational age
    (D) low birth weight and small for gestational age
    (E) premature and small for gestational age

81. Which of the following is more common among term rather than premature infants?

    (A) intraventricular hemorrhage
    (B) hemorrhagic disease of the newborn
    (C) sepsis
    (D) subdural hemorrhage
    (E) congenital infection

82. A term neonate begins vomiting during the first few days of life, and develops a distended abdomen. The family history is positive for cystic fibrosis. Which of the following conditions, if found, would most likely be related to the family history?

    (A) annular pancreas
    (B) duodenal atresia
    (C) hypertrophic pyloric stenosis
    (D) meconium ileus
    (E) volvulus

83. Which of the following is most suggestive of early congenital syphilis?

    (A) disseminated intravascular coagulation
    (B) bullous lesions of the palms and soles
    (C) hepatitis
    (D) dermal erythropoiesis
    (E) pneumonia

84. Which of the following roentgenographic findings in a newborn infant is most suggestive of hypothyroidism?

    (A) epiphyseal dysgenesis
    (B) absence of ossification of the hamate bone
    (C) prominent thymic shadow
    (D) osteoporosis
    (E) cardiomegaly

85. A 5-day-old average for gestational age male presents with tachypnea, poor feeding, and lethargy. On examination, the neonate appears in shock with hypotension, pallor, and poor capillary refill. Among the following, which is the most likely diagnosis?

    (A) tetralogy of Fallot
    (B) tricuspid atresia
    (C) transposition of the great vessels
    (D) truncus arteriosis
    (E) hypoplastic left heart syndrome

86. The initial lesions of incontinentia pigmenti are

    (A) deeply pigmented
    (B) scaly
    (C) waxy papules
    (D) inflammatory bullae
    (E) small vesicles

87. A newborn infant is noted to have a peculiar face with low-set ears and folded helices. The chin is small, and the nose is flat. Oligohydramnios was noted prior to delivery. Examination of the placental membranes reveals amnion nodosum. One should suspect the possibility of

    (A) bilateral renal agenesis
    (B) congenital toxoplasmosis
    (C) esophageal atresia
    (D) group B streptococcal infection
    (E) transposition of the great vessels

88. Hydrocephalus, chorioretinitis, and diffuse cerebral calcifications are present in a newborn male. Of the following pets, which is the most likely to be the source of this zoonotic congenital infection?

    (A) dog
    (B) cat
    (C) horse
    (D) rabbit
    (E) gerbil

DIRECTIONS (Questions 89 through 109): Each set of questions in this section is followed by the possible lettered answers. For each numbered question or item select the ONE lettered option with which it is most closely associated. Each lettered option may be selected once, more than once, or not at all.

Questions 89 through 93

(A) respiratory distress syndrome (hyaline membrane disease)

(B) meconium aspiration syndrome

(C) transient tachypnea of the newborn

(D) congenital pneumonia

(E) pulmonary hypoplasia

89. Postterm delivery is a risk factor

90. Most likely to be associated with renal anomalies

91. Hyperexpansion is common on chest x-ray

92. Often resolves without therapy

93. Most closely associated with cesarean delivery

Questions 94 through 98

(A) cephalhematoma

(B) caput succedaneum

(C) cephalhematoma and caput succedaneum

(D) subgaleal hematoma

(E) cephalhematoma, caput succedaneum, and subgaleal hematoma

94. Can lead to substantial elevations of serum bilirubin

95. Most likely to induce acute hypovolemic shock

96. Drainage is contraindicated

97. Generally resolves by 48 h of age

98. Associated with an underlying fracture of the skull in 5–10% of cases

Questions 99 through 103

(A) trisomy 13 (Patau syndrome)

(B) trisomy 18 (Edwards syndrome)

(C) 5p deletion (cri du chat syndrome)

(D) trisomy 21 (Down syndrome)

(E) 45,X or XO (Turner syndrome)

99. Low-set ears, nail hypoplasia, "rocker-bottom" feet, growth retardation, severe mental retardation

100. Holoprosencephaly, microphthalmia or anophthalmia, cleft lip and palate, polydactyly, severe mental retardation

101. Hypotonia and hyperextensible joints, clinodactyly, Brushfield's spots, duodenal atresia, flattening of the occiput

102. Microcephaly, mental retardation, hypertelorism, and cat-like (mewing) cry in infancy

103. Redundant skin at nape of neck, low posterior hairline, edema of dorsum of feet in newborn period, cardiac, and renal anomalies

Questions 104 through 109

(A) Rh disease

(B) ABO hemolytic disease

(C) Rh and ABO hemolytic disease

104. More severe in pregnancies subsequent to an affected pregnancy

105. Prenatal abnormalities can be seen by ultrasound in some cases

106. A naturally occurring antibody is thought to be responsible for the disorder

107. Exchange transfusion may be required to control hyperbilirubinemia

108. The disorder is mediated by IgG antibodies

109. Examination of the peripheral blood smear in affected infants reveals numerous microspherocytes

DIRECTIONS (Questions 110 through 120): Each of the numbered items or incomplete statements in this section is followed by answers or by completions of the statement. Select the ONE lettered answer or completion that is BEST in each case.

110. A 42-week gestation neonate is born by cesarean delivery following repeated fetal heart rate decelerations. At rupture of membranes, thick meconium was noted. The infant has no respiratory effort but slight movement and a heart rate of 90 beats per minute. Of the following, you would first

    (A) pass an umbilical artery catheter to measure pH and PO$_2$
    (B) start bag-and-mask ventilation with 100% oxygen
    (C) suction the oropharynx, then suction the trachea with an endotracheal tube to remove the meconium
    (D) intubate the trachea and begin ventilation with 100% oxygen
    (E) establish monitoring with ECG and pulse oximeter

111. An ultrasound at 33 weeks gestation reveals a small for gestational age fetus with no other abnormalities. At birth at 39 weeks, the 1.6-kg neonate requires no resuscitation. On examination, the infant is noted to have a generalized rash consisting of dozens of blue-purple macules. His abdominal examination reveals hepatosplenomegaly. The most likely diagnosis is

    (A) group B streptococcal septicemia
    (B) isoimmune thrombocytopenia
    (C) congenital cytomegalovirus infection
    (D) congenital toxoplasmosis
    (E) congenital *Listeria monocytogenes* infection

112. A term infant at 12 h of age is normal except for jaundice. Initial laboratory values reveal a total bilirubin of 12 mg/dL and several spherocytes on the peripheral blood smear. Among the following, the most likely diagnosis is

    (A) hereditary elliptocytosis
    (B) hereditary spherocytosis
    (C) pyruvate kinase deficiency
    (D) disseminated intravascular coagulopathy
    (E) ABO isoimmune hemolytic disease

113. A 3.5-kg term male delivered by uncomplicated vaginal delivery has a normal physical examination. On the day of discharge the mother tells you that an older sibling has just broken out with chickenpox. Which of the following is true?

    (A) All newborns are very susceptible to varicella upon exposure.
    (B) This infant is likely already infected because of the maternal exposure to the sick sibling.
    (C) Varicella immune globulin should be administered to all infants in this situation.
    (D) If the mother had varicella in the past, the infant is likely protected with passively acquired antibody from the mother.
    (E) The infant will not develop a typical varicella infection, but will likely develop varicella zoster.

114. A previously healthy term infant is brought to clinic by his mother at 2 weeks of age because of rapid breathing, poor breastfeeding, and excessive sleeping. He is afebrile. The most common arrhythmia at this age which may account for these symptoms is

    (A) supraventricular tachycardia
    (B) atrial flutter
    (C) atrial fibrillation
    (D) complete atrioventricular block
    (E) ventricular tachycardia

115. A 1-hour-old 33-week gestation male neonate develops tachypnea, grunting respirations, and deep intercostal retractions. A chest x-ray reveals a homogeneously grainy appearance to both lung fields. An arterial blood would most likely reveal

   (A) respiratory alkalosis
   (B) metabolic alkalosis
   (C) respiratory acidosis
   (D) respiratory and metabolic alkalosis
   (E) metabolic acidosis

116. A college student delivers an infant in the campus housing area after denying her pregnancy and experiencing 6 h of abdominal pain. Paramedics arrive and find an infant they estimate to be 3–4 lbs in weight, crying but slightly dusky. They administer oxygen. The newborn's temperature is 94°F. Hypothermia most likely will complicate the infant's course by causing

   (A) apnea
   (B) hypocalcemia
   (C) an increased oxygen requirement
   (D) tachycardia
   (E) metabolic alkalosis

117. A 24-day-old former 24 weeks gestation 730 g neonate had a difficult initial respiratory course complicated by a tension pneumothorax. She had serial head ultrasound evaluations during the first weeks of life. All previous studies revealed a normal immature brain. Now, the head ultrasound reveals an abnormality. Among the following, which is most likely?

   (A) grade II intraventricular hemorrhage
   (B) grade IV intraventricular hemorrhage
   (C) aqueductal stenosis
   (D) periventricular leukomalacia
   (E) vein of Galen aneurysm

118. A newborn infant has signs of congestive heart failure. Physical examination does not reveal a significant cardiac murmur. Auscultation of the head reveals a loud cranial bruit. The most likely diagnosis is

   (A) polycythemia
   (B) hyperthyroidism
   (C) ruptured cerebral aneurysm
   (D) transposition of the great vessels
   (E) arteriovenous malformation of the great vein of Galen

119. A term 4.3-kg infant is delivered vaginally to a 33-year-old woman with juvenile onset diabetes. The delivery was complicated by severe shoulder dystocia and the infant experienced a brachial plexus injury with limited movement of the right arm. At 72 h of age the infant is noted to be tachypneic but he is pink and well perfused. The most likely explanation for his symptom is

   (A) infantile respiratory distress syndrome (RDS)
   (B) diaphragmatic paralysis
   (C) pulmonary hemorrhage
   (D) pneumothorax
   (E) cystic adenomatoid malformation of the lung

120. A term infant is delivered vaginally to an 18-year-old primagravida after an uncomplicated pregnancy. The delivery was complicated by a low-grade fever which resolved after the delivery. At 30 h of age the infant is mottled, not feeding well, and cries when handled. A lumbar puncture is performed and the spinal fluid reveals 660 WBC/mm^3 and a CSF protein of 290 mg/dL. The most likely agent causing this infant's infection is

   (A) group B *Streptococcus*
   (B) *Escherichia coli*
   (C) *Listeria monocytogenes*
   (D) *Haemophilus influenzae*
   (E) *Streptococcus pneumoniae*

Answers and Explanations

1. **(B)** Cystic fibrosis (CF) is inherited in an autosomal recessive fashion, creating a 25% recurrence risk for subsequent pregnancies. Hirschsprung disease usually is inherited in a multifactorial manner with a risk of about 7% to siblings of an affected case. There are rare families with Hirschsprung disease transmitted as an autosomal dominant trait. Ventricular septal defects are also multifactorial in inheritance. Trisomies are most typically sporadic events and recurrence varies depending on the mother's age. A small proportion of trisomies are transmitted by a parent as part of a balanced translocation with higher recurrence risks in those families. *(Rudolph:727, 1967)*

2. **(A)** Although the majority (90–95%) of newborn infants infected with cytomegalovirus are asymptomatic at birth, up to 20% eventually demonstrate central nervous system abnormalities. More than 75% of those infants who are symptomatic at birth are left with permanent neurologic sequelae including microcephaly, sensorineural hearing loss, and impaired intellect or development. The liver frequently is involved, but permanent hepatic damage is rare. *(Feigin:866–869; Rudolph:1033)*

3. **(B)** Approximately 50% of sensorineural hearing loss is hereditary. Of acquired forms, congenital infection (particularly involving cytomegalovirus) accounts for the largest group. Hyperbilirubinemia and asphyxia account for a smaller proportion. Ototoxic medications such as aminoglycocides pose a small risk for hearing impairment. Late onset group B streptococcal meningitis has a strong association with hearing

impairment but is not a common disorder. *(Rudolph:486)*

4. **(A)** Cardiovascular anomalies occur in 15–25% of infants with omphaloceles. In addition, omphaloceles also are frequently associated with chromosomal anomalies and the Beckwith-Wiedemann syndrome (omphalocele, severe hypoglycemia, macrosomia, and macroglossia). The other obstructive lesions typically are not associated with other anomalies. *(Rudolph:1399; Klaus:306)*

5. **(C)** The newborn with cystic fibrosis generally is asymptomatic. The most common manifestation, meconium ileus, occurs in 10–20% of CF patients. The hyperviscous intestinal mucus leads to inspissation of the meconium with resultant intestinal obstruction. While sweat chloride testing of suspected CF cases has always been troublesome in the newborn period, DNA testing is now available and diagnostic in approximately 90% of cases. *(Rudolph:1407)*

6. **(C)** Generous palpable breast tissue is characteristic of full-term infants. Long lanugo, translucent skin, edema, and only partial ear overfolding are each more indicative of prematurity. The Ballard scoring system uses physical findings such as these to determine the gestational age of the newborn. *(Hay:3; Klaus:104)*

7. **(A)** Oral candidiasis is a common problem and typically does not indicate a serious underlying problem. It is seen frequently in the first few weeks of life and sometimes results from

maternal transmission via breastfeeding. As an isolated finding in an otherwise asymptomatic neonate, it requires no immunologic investigation and usually responds rapidly to topical therapy with mycostatin suspension. Although thrush generally is not painful to babies, the resultant diaper dermatitis may be quite irritating. Cases that fail to respond to therapy or that recur should make one think of immunodeficiency diseases such as DiGeorge syndrome. In the sick, premature infant, especially those with central lines or other invasive devices, oral thrush is more serious and may herald systemic infection. *(Rudolph:1080, 1088)*

8. **(A)** Resuscitation of the newborn is a systematic procedure with a logical progression of events which best ensures a successful outcome. Drying the infant initially not only is stimulating for the infant to initiate spontaneous respirations, but more importantly, prevents heat loss through evaporation. Heat loss dramatically increases the oxygen requirement, making further resuscitative steps more complicated. The smaller or sicker the infant, the more important this step becomes. *(Klaus:48)*

9. **(B)** Unconjugated bilirubin passes easily across the placenta, and this is the major mechanism for fetal elimination of bilirubin. Intestinal degradation of bilirubin to biliverdin is accomplished primarily by the intestinal bacterial flora, which obviously are not present in utero. The inability of the fetus to conjugate bilirubin, therefore, is clearly advantageous during intrauterine life. *(McMillan:197)*

10. **(D)** Breakdown and metabolism of 1 g of hemoglobin yields about 34 mg of bilirubin. This is important because it explains why very little hemolysis is required for the development of hyperbilirubinemia in the presence of impaired hepatic ability to conjugate or excrete bilirubin, such as occurs in the newborn (and especially the premature) infant. [*Note:* The exact number is unimportant to the clinician and the average reader. The individual values listed as choices, however, are sufficiently spread out so that answering the question really only requires knowledge of the concept

that in the newborn a little bit of hemoglobin goes a long way toward hyperbilirubinemia.] *(Hay:12)*

11. **(A)** Erythroblastosis fetalis, usually a result of Rh incompatibility, is the major indication for intrauterine transfusion. The transfusion is accomplished by injection of donor blood (packed red cells) into the fetal abdominal cavity or the vessels of the umbilical cord under ultrasound guidance. This reasonably safe but highly specialized technique generally is available only in high-risk obstetric centers. Were a fetus with erythroblastosis to develop severe hydrops fetalis (essentially the result of congestive heart failure), it would be too late for transfusion, and delivery would be the only option likely to save the infant. Although spherocytosis can cause neonatal jaundice, neither spherocytosis nor sickle cell disease causes serious intrauterine problems. *(Arias:114; McMillan:203)*

12. **(C)** Current technology, including the use of ultrasound monitoring during the procedure, has made intrauterine transfusion relatively safe. Premature onset of labor is the major complication. Graft-versus-host reaction has been reported but is rare. Testing of donor blood for human immunodeficiency virus (HIV) antibody is routine and usually will prevent transfusion transmission of AIDS. Transfusion reactions have not been reported to be a problem. *(Clin Obstet Gynecol 18:1–23, 1975; Br J Hosp Med 34:141, 1985)*

13. **(C)** Kernicterus is a condition of neurologic damage that is the direct result of the toxic effects of bilirubin on the central nervous system. Since unconjugated bilirubin crosses the blood-brain barrier, whereas conjugated bilirubin does not, the risk of kernicterus is most closely related to the serum level of unconjugated bilirubin. The basal ganglia are particularly susceptible to damage with high levels of unconjugated bilirubin. *(McMillan:199–200)*

14. **(D)** Infants are born in a state of relative extravascular fluid expansion. Through the first week of life dilute urine and relatively low

intake of fluid result in a loss of 5–10% of their birth weight. In a term baby this physiologic diuresis that occurs during the first 3 days of life usually amounts to 1–2 oz (30–60 g) of weight lost each day. *(Klaus:147–148)*

15. **(C)** Blood type A is more common in the population than type B. In most cases of ABO isoimmune hemolytic disease of the newborn, the mother is type O and the infant is type A. Anti-A antibodies produced by the mother cross the placenta and cause hemolysis of fetal erythrocytes. And remember, the placenta efficiently removes bilirubin from the fetus, thus the infant typically does not exhibit jaundice at birth. *(McMillan:361–362)*

16. **(B)** Late onset chronic anemia in ABO isoimmune hemolytic disease is the most common late complication and usually presents as high output congestive heart failure. The symptoms of CHF in neonates are usually tachypnea and failure to feed. The hemoglobin will reach its nadir at the sixth to twelfth week of life. Kernicterus and gallstones are uncommon. Bilirubinuria is benign. *(Klaus:82:470)*

17. **(B)** Unconjugated bilirubin in the serum is tightly bound to albumin. The unconjugated bilirubin molecule is lipid soluble, and that which is not bound to albumin enters the brain readily. This is why kernicterus usually occurs only at serum levels of unconjugated bilirubin exceeding 20 mg/dL (the approximate limit of albumin binding). Factors that are associated with low serum albumin levels (e.g., prematurity) and factors that impair bilirubin binding to albumin (e.g., acidosis) can result in kernicterus at lower serum bilirubin levels. *(McMillan:198)*

18. **(A)** Prematurity is the strongest predisposing factor to surfactant deficiency disease or respiratory distress syndrome. While low birth weight infants are also at risk, the risk is more associated with the gestational age. Maternal diabetes also somewhat predisposes newborns to RDS by causing delayed surfactant release compared to infants of comparable gestational age. Cesarean delivery predisposes more to a condition known as transient tachypnea of the

newborn, related to excessive fluid retention within the lungs. *(Rudolph:127–134)*

19. **(D)** Males have a higher neonatal mortality rate than females, both overall and when corrected for weight and gestational age. African Americans have a higher rate of prematurity and low birth weight and therefore have an overall higher neonatal mortality rate than Whites. Among infants of comparable weight and gestational age, however, African American infants have a lower mortality than do White infants. *(Rudolph:57–61)*

20. **(E)** Pulmonary surfactant is a hydrophobic substance composed mostly (65%) of phosphatidylcholine. The total protein contribution is about 10% and 10% neutral lipids. Other phospholipids account for most of the rest of the surfactant structure. The proteins appear to be important in structural lipid organization and, to some degree, for regulation of surfactant production. *(Klaus:253)*

21. **(D)** The mortality rates in the newborn are the highest of any period in childhood averaging about 10/1000 live births. While mortality decreases as maturity and birth weight increase, infants who are delivered after 42 weeks gestation have an increased mortality rate compared to their term counterparts. African American newborns still have nearly twice the infant mortality of White infants, mostly from complications of preterm delivery. Improvements in prenatal care and postnatal nutrition since the 1950s have decreased infant mortality more than 50%. *(Rudolph: 57–61; Klaus:597)*

22. **(B)** Pulmonary surfactant is produced in a complex set of structuring steps involving the endoplasmic reticulum and Golgi apparatus of the type II alveolar cells of the lung. It is stored within these cells in structures known as lamellar bodies. Surfactant production is sufficient to prevent respiratory distress syndrome only after 30–32 weeks gestation. *(Fanaroff:981–982)*

23. **(C)** The normally grown 30-week gestation infant weighs 1300–1700 g. Intrauterine weight gain is nearly linear from 30 to 38 weeks at a

rate of about of 200 g per week. (*Klaus:172–174, 588*)

24. **(B)** Maternal diabetes mellitus during cardio-genesis results in an approximately threefold increase in the incidence of structural anomalies of the heart. In late gestation, poor glucose control also predisposes to ventricular septal hypertrophy which can lead to aortic outflow obstruction. Maternal diabetes also predisposes the fetus to CNS and lower spine abnormalities. (*Fanaroff:282; Rudolph:126*)

25. **(D)** Blood returning to the fetus via the umbilical vein courses through the ductus venosus and into the right atrium. This blood with higher oxygen saturation than that returning via the superior vena cava, crosses the foramen ovale into the left atrium and is pumped into the aorta by the left ventricle. After delivery of the baby, umbilical venous flow ceases resulting in decreased right atrial pressure. Simultaneously, left atrial pressure increases as a result of increased pulmonary vascular flow and hence greater flow to the left side of the heart. These events result in a physiologic cessation of flow across the foramen ovale. (*Klaus:396; Rudolph:1751*)

26. **(A)** Erythema toxicum is a benign condition seen in 30–70% of normal, term infants. It is much less common among premature infants. The skin lesions usually appear within the first 3 days of life and are not associated with any systemic signs or symptoms. Infants are afebrile, and the peripheral white blood cell counts are normal. The rash presents with one or more of three types of skin lesions including erythematous macules, wheals, and vesiculopustules on an erythematous base. (*Rudolph:1169*)

27. **(B)** The lecithin–sphingomyelin ratio of amniotic fluid specimens reflects the composition of fetal lung fluid which is effluxed from the lungs into the amniotic sac. It is a useful indicator of lung maturity and risk of development of respiratory distress syndrome or hyaline membrane disease. (*Rudolph:131*)

28. **(E)** Some infants with severe respiratory distress syndrome who require therapy with positive-pressure respirators and high concentrations of oxygen develop chronic pulmonary changes known as bronchopulmonary dysplasia (BPD). (*Rudolph:1964*)

29. **(E)** Surfactant replacement therapy is delivered directly into the lungs via an endotracheal tube. Multiple studies have documented the improvement in survival of infants with respiratory distress syndrome who receive surfactant replacement after delivery. Common complications include transient hypoxemia from endotracheal tube occlusion and air leak syndromes from undetected rapid improvement in pulmonary compliance. (*Rudolph:134*)

30. **(C)** The characteristic roentgenographic findings in infants with respiratory distress syndrome are a diffuse reticulogranular pattern and air bronchograms. These changes are presumed to represent diffuse alveolar atelectasis. Lobar densities are infrequent and lung volume usually is diminished rather than increased. Pneumothorax does occur, but generally as a complication of treatment rather than as a feature of the disease itself. (*Rudolph:130*)

31. **(D)** The purpose of continuous positive airway pressure is to prevent alveolar collapse, increase mean airway pressure, and thereby improve oxygenation. Such therapy usually does not improve arterial PCO_2 or cardiac output; in fact, these parameters may worsen. Pneumothorax is one of the complications of treatment with continuous positive airway pressure. There is no evidence that continuous positive airway pressure prevents infection. To the contrary, the invasive technology (e.g., endotracheal tube) often required can predispose to infection. (*Rudolph:208*)

32. **(E)** Retinopathy of prematurity (ROP) is the major danger of hyperoxemia and is the reason that the arterial oxygenation should be closely monitored in the premature infant. It is clear that oxygen alone is not the only predisposing factor. Acidosis, apnea of prematurity, and alterations in cerebral perfusion all appear to

play a role in some infants. However, premature infants appear to be uniquely sensitive to retinal damage from oxygen. *(Klaus:248–249)*

33. **(B)** A decrease in production of pulmonary surfactant by alveolar cells has been demonstrated in the lungs of infants and experimental animals with respiratory distress syndrome. The biologic function of surfactant is to lower the surface tension of the alveolar lining and thereby stabilize the alveoli. Absence of surfactant leads to alveolar collapse (atelectasis), which in turn causes the pathophysiologic, clinical, and roentgenographic changes characteristic of this disorder. *(Rudolph:130)*

34. **(B)** Among bleeding disorders in the healthy term male infant, hemophilia A (factor VIII deficiency) is five times more common than factor IX deficiency. DIC is unlikely in a healthy infant. von Willebrand factor is high just after birth making symptoms uncommon in the newborn. [*Note*: It is mandatory to ask for a family history of bleeding problems prior to any newborn circumcision. Once bleeding has begun after a fresh circumcision in a patient with factor VIII deficiency, bleeding is very difficult to control.] *(Rudolph:1570–1572)*

35. **(D)** Inborn errors of metabolism that regularly produce cataracts in the newborn are disorders involving carbohydrate metabolism (for example, galactosemia) and lysosomal storage disorders (such as G_{M1}-gangliosidosis). Cataracts have also been reported in some cases of peroxisomal defects such as adrenoleukodystrophy. *(Rudolph:2389)*

36. **(B)** Mongolian spots (dermal melanosis) occur most commonly on the buttock or back and are present in 50–70% of African American newborns. They are benign lesions but can be mistaken for bruising later in infancy. Thus, their presence and location should be documented. They are produced by the persistence of migrating melanocytes in the lower dermis and are thus more frequent in populations with darker skin pigmentation. *(Rudolph:1192)*

37. **(B)** The rapid and complete resolution of cyanosis speaks strongly against the presence of cyanotic congenital heart disease. By far the most common cause of tachypnea and cyanosis in the newborn is pulmonary disease. Methemoglobinemia should not resolve with oxygen administration. *(Klaus:82, 416)*

38. **(E)** Beckwith-Wiedemann syndrome encompasses abdominal wall defects (especially omphalocele), macroglossia, and macrosomia. Its recognition is critical in the immediate newborn period as they also have severe hyperinsulinemia. This results in severe hypoglycemia which can lead to brain injury. It is inherited in an autosomal dominant manner. Thus, one of the parents may be large and often overweight. This disorder should be considered in all macrosomic infants and any infants with abdominal wall defects, even umbilical hernias. Patients with this disorder also have an alarmingly high incidence of abdominal tumors during childhood. *(Rudolph:1399, 1614)*

39. **(C)** The combination of microcephaly, cerebral calcifications, and blindness is typical of the damage caused to neural tissues by intrauterine infection with either cytomegalovirus or toxoplasmosis. Subdural bleeding results in enlargement of the head. Cerebral agenesis is not associated with calcifications, and erythroblastosis would not explain any of the findings listed. Primary microcephaly is not associated with either cerebral calcifications or blindness. *(Hay:52:1120–1123)*

40. **(A)** The findings described are typical of thrush (oral infection with *Candida albicans*), which is common in young infants. Although *E. coli*, *Listeria monocytogenes*, and group B *Streptococcus* all are important pathogens in the neonatal period, they typically are not associated with pharyngeal infection or oral exudate. Group A *Streptococcus* is a common cause of exudative tonsillitis in the older child but is an extremely rare pathogen in the newborn infant. Additionally, the exudate noted with group A streptococcal infection would be in the area of the tonsils rather than on the buccal mucosa. *(Hay:1241–1243)*

41. **(A)** Hypopigmented patches observed in the newborn period may be a sign of tuberous sclerosis or neurofibromatosis and would raise great suspicion if seen on the body of an infant with a family history of seizures. Neurofibromatosis is more likely to have pigmented cafe-au-lait spots develop over time as well. Salmon patches and pustular melanosis are normal variants. The harlequin color change, while striking, typically is harmless. *(Hay:404, 756)*

42. **(A)** The cranium of the child grows at right angles to several sutures, primarily the sagittal, coronal, lambdoidal, and temporal. Isolated premature closure (craniosynostosis) of the sagittal suture results in a long and narrow skull (scaphocephaly) with a slightly greater than normal total circumference. With early fusion of a single suture there usually are no signs of increased intracranial pressure, and the problem is chiefly cosmetic. Craniosynostosis of multiple sutures, however, often is associated with increased intracranial pressure. *(Rudolph:11–12)*

43. **(E)** Transient pustular melanosis is a common normal variant characterized by vesicles which leave behind a 3–4 mm hyperpigmented oval lesion, usually many in number, on the face and head. They are somewhat more common in infants with greater amounts of skin pigment. *(Hay:5, 403)*

44. **(D)** The most common congenital defect of the esophagus is atresia of the proximal segment with a fistula between the distal segment and the trachea. This type of esophageal atresia accounts for 80–90% of all cases. The clinical significance of this configuration is that attempts to feed the infant will result in regurgitation and that even prior to feeding, aspiration of gastric secretions may occur through the distal fistula. It is important to diagnose this condition as quickly as possible to prevent the development of aspiration pneumonia. *(Rudolph:1386)*

45. **(B)** Both cephalhematoma and caput are associated with prolonged and difficult labors, and both are associated with a normal neurologic examination unless there has been concomittant intracranial trauma. Caput, however, is diffuse and poorly demarcated edema of the scalp, whereas a cephalhematoma is a subperiosteal collection of blood. Therefore, a cephalhematoma is sharply demarcated and limited to a single bone. Cephalhematomas may be bilateral, but each is separate and sharply demarcated. [*Note*: The student might wish to argue that response (B) is incorrect in that cephalhematomas can be bilateral and therefore are not limited to the area over one bone. Each swelling, however, is limited to the area over one bone. Since all other choices are totally incorrect, (B) is the best choice.] *(Rudolph: 186–187)*

46. **(B)** There is a clear association between advancing maternal age and nondisjunction chromosome disorders. The rate of chromosome abnormalities in infants delivered to women increases from approximately 1/400 at age 25 to more than 1/100 by age 40. While the risk is substantially increased with advancing maternal age, most infants with errors of chromosome number are born to women less than 35. Obviously this is because a tremendous proportion of all births occurs in women less than 35. *(Rudolph:733)*

47. **(C)** While the association of maternal age and chromosome problems is well known, a lesser discussed phenomenon is the clear relationship of autosomal dominant disorders and paternal age at conception. The paternal age in disorders such as achondroplasia and Marfan syndrome, for example, is substantially higher than the general population. It is thought that the accumulation of DNA replicative errors is responsible for this phenomenon. *(Fanaroff:81)*

48. **(C)** Term infants usually maintain their blood glucose levels above 30 mg/dL, and 20 mg/dL appears to be the lower level ordinarily encountered for premature and low birth weight infants. It is believed, however, that these levels, although frequent, are unphysiologic and may cause symptoms. It has been suggested that

40 mg/dL be considered the lower limit of normal for all newborns. *(Klaus:304)*

49. **(A)** Club foot is a common and usually isolated congenital anomaly. When associated with another disorder, the central nervous system is most commonly involved. This may result from primary brain abnormalities, chronic intoxication from maternal drug use or spina bifida leading to decreased movement. Genitourinary disorders resulting in low amniotic fluid volumes and resultant club foot abnormalities are also common. *(Rudolph:2425)*

50. **(E)** The most consistent features of Pierre Robin syndrome are micrognathia, glossoptosis, and cleft palate. The underlying embryologic defect is poor growth of the mandible causing upward deviation of the tongue, blocking medial fusion of the palatine ridges. The posterior displacement of the tongue can cause significant airway obstruction, which is the most urgent problem encountered in these infants. While substantial spontaneous growth of the mandible occurs in many of these patients, temporary tracheostomy often is required. Prone positioning may also be helpful in less severe cases. *(McMillan:393)*

51. **(B)** So-called pyridoxine dependency is a group of rare, inborn metabolic errors that cause severe neonatal seizures that respond to pharmacologic (as opposed to physiologic) doses of pyridoxine. Although the disorder is extremely rare, it has given rise to the practice of sometimes empirically administering an intravenous dose of pyridoxine to infants with unexplained and otherwise uncontrollable seizures. *(Fanaroff:896–897)*

52. **(E)** Genes on chromosomes follow Mendelian patterns of inheritance. However, DNA is also found in mitochondria. A newborn's functional mitochondria are acquired from the cytoplasm of the oocyte, thus a maternal line of inheritance is seen in these disorders. As would be anticipated, disorders of energy metabolism predominate in this group of disorders. The more common are hereditary disorders of eye muscle weakness, hypertrophic cardiomyopathy, and some disorders of the CNS. *(Rudolph:598)*

53. **(E)** Most infants who experience fetal bradycardia during labor are not severely asphyxiated at birth and ultimately have a good neurologic outcome. Likewise, most infants who fail to breathe initially or are cyanotic at birth and have a low 1-min Apgar score recover promptly and do well neurologically. Although a low 5-min Apgar score generally indicates more prolonged oxygen problems and correlates somewhat better with outcome than does the 1-min score, most of these infants also will be normal. In contrast, a substantial population of newborns with low Apgar scores and seizures in the first 36 h of life will show neurologic abnormalities on long-term follow-up. *(Rudolph:2270)*

54. **(C)** The lesions described are typical for neonatal acne (acne neonatorum), a skin eruption occurring during the first few weeks of life, probably secondary to transplacental passage of maternal hormones. Adenoma sebaceum, one of the several cutaneous manifestations of tuberous sclerosis, typically is not present in the neonatal period. The distribution of the rash in this patient and the presence of comedones are not typical of congenital syphilis, impetigo, or pustulosis. *(McMillan:684, 714–715)*

55. **(D)** The maternal serum alpha-fetoprotein (MSAFP) test relies on the diffusion of fetal proteins in the amniotic sac into the maternal circulation to identify open neural tube defects. The excessive seepage of fetal proteins into the amniotic fluid raises the maternal serum level of these proteins as well. Amniocentesis can further clarify abnormal results. High MSAFP levels are seen in some abdominal wall defects as well. Low MSAFP levels have been linked with nondisjunction chromosome errors and are used to fine tune risk assessments for these disorders. *(Klaus:11–12, 21, 38)*

56. **(B)** While all of the listed disorders may cause gastric distension and vomiting, duodenal atresia alone is responsible for approximately 50% of all congenital duodenal obstructions. Thirty

percent of infants with duodenal atresia have Down syndrome. *(McMillan:312)*

57. **(C)** Necrotizing enterocolitis (NEC) occurs especially frequently among low birth weight infants who have had repeated episodes of hypoxia or poor perfusion. The usual signs of NEC are abdominal distention, bloody stools, vomiting, hypothermia, and lethargy. Intussusception is rare in the neonatal period. Volvulus and aganglionosis are unrelated to low birth weight or to hypoxia and usually are associated with failure to pass stool. Shigella infection is very uncommon in the nursery. *(McMillan:325–332)*

58. **(B)** Most capillary or cavernous hemangiomas are small or even invisible at birth. During the first weeks or months of life, they begin to grow and may become very large before finally starting to regress after a few years. Spontaneous regression usually (but not invariably) is complete or nearly so. Recognition of the natural history of this lesion permits reassurance of parents and avoidance of unnecessary therapy. The best cosmetic results are achieved by natural regression. Active intervention (surgery or laser therapy) should be advised only when a complication such as trapping of platelets (Kassabach-Merritt syndrome), erosion of tissue, or impairment of vision is a problem. *(Rudolph:1205)*

59. **(B)** Scalded skin syndrome (toxic epidermal necrolysis) is caused by a circulating toxin released by certain strains of *Staphylococcus aureus*. The staphylococci frequently are not growing in the involved areas of skin but may have infected or colonized the pharynx or umbilicus. The disease is most frequent in young infants but is not restricted to neonates. Infants with scalded skin syndrome have no discernible immunologic abnormality. The rash of scalded skin syndrome occasionally may be confused with the rash of Leiners disease, which is characterized by a more chronic, seborrheic dermatitis. Patients with Leiners disease have a defect in the fifth component of complement. *(Rudolph:86)*

60. **(B)** Characteristically, the lesions of erythema toxicum (erythematous macules and papules) are loaded with eosinophils. The cause of this transient disorder of term newborns is unknown, and the lesions resolve spontaneously within a few days. Cultures of the lesions are sterile. It is important not to confuse this totally benign condition with the rash of serious disorders such as staphylococcal pustulosis or disseminated viral infection. *(Rudolph:86)*

61. **(B)** Infants born to mothers with hyperparathyroidism often develop transient hypoparathyroidism, resulting in hypocacemia and tetany. The mechanism, presumably, is suppression of the fetal parathyroid glands by excessive transplacental maternal parathyroid hormone. Occasionally, the mother's condition may be undiagnosed, and otherwise unexplained hypocalcemia in an infant can lead to the diagnosis of hyperparathyroidism in the mother. *(Klaus:313–314)*

62. **(B)** Hereditary tyrosinemia is an aminoacidopathy that results in progressive hepatocellular dysfunction by the buildup of toxic metabolites (fumarylacetoacetate to be specific). The hepatic dysfunction frequently presents as conjugated hyperbilirubinemia, also known as direct hyperbilirubinemia. The other problems listed cause indirect (or unconjugated) hyperbilirubinemia. *(McMillan:198–201)*

63. **(C)** Ambiguous genitalia in association with congenital adrenal hyperplasia usually indicates a female pseudohermaphrodite, since most of the defects result in masculinization of the fetus. The patient described, however, is genetically an XY male. The rare defect of 3-β–hydroxysteroid dehydrogenase results in the inability to synthesize testicular androgen and, therefore, failure of normal masculinization of the male fetus, as in this patient. Although the 17-hydroxylase defect also can cause feminization, it is not associated with salt loss. [*Note:* To answer the question correctly, the reader first must note that the patient is XY and then reason that the ambiguous genitalia, therefore, must result from feminization rather than masculinization.] *(Fanaroff:1453–1454)*

64. **(B)** Infants born to women with active and untreated Graves disease may be hyperthyroid at birth, presumably as a result of transplacental passage of long-acting thyroid stimulator (LATS) or a similar substance. If the mother is receiving antithyroid medication, this also crosses the placenta, and the infant generally will be euthyroid or even hypothyroid at birth. Yet because the plasma half-lives of these agents are much shorter than that of LATS, thyrotoxicosis may begin a week or so after birth. Iodides administered to the mother during pregnancy can cross the placenta and block the function of the fetal thyroid. Such infants have been born with huge goiters, but they are either euthyroid or hypothyroid rather than hyperthyroid. *(Rudolph:2076)*

65. **(B)** As inoculation at the time of delivery is the most common route of acquiring the organism, it follows that the presenting part, namely the head, is the most common site of initial lesions. This is particularly true when the scalp is disrupted by fetal scalp monitor leads. *(McMillan:434)*

66. **(B)** After delivery, the infant is cut off from its continuous calcium supply prompting a precipitous fall in serum calcium over the first 1–2 days. In the normal circumstance, this stimulates PTH causing a gradual return to higher serum calcium levels. PTH secretion is inhibited in infants of diabetic mothers. Therefore, hypocalcemia is a common problem in infants of diabetic mothers. *(Klaus:310)*

67. **(E)** More than 95% of term infants will have passed their first meconium stool by the age of 24 h and 99.8% by 48 h. In a term infant, failure to pass meconium by 24–48 h should suggest problems such as intestinal obstruction, Hirschsprung disease, or hypothyroidism. In contrast, as many as 20% of infants less than 1500 g at birth may fail to pass meconium by 48 h of life. *(Pediatrics 60:457–459, 1977)*

68. **(E)** The description and location of the lesion (*beneath fading forceps marks*) are typical of subcutaneous fat necrosis, which may follow trauma (forceps) or cold exposure. Buccal cellulitis caused by *H. influenzae* frequently has a violaceous color but is exceedingly rare in the newborn period. *(Rudolph:185)*

69. **(D)** If congenital hypothyroidism is not detected by neonatal screening tests, it generally becomes apparent over several weeks. The infants usually are edematous, have large anterior fontanelles, and have a history of prolonged jaundice. *(Rudolph:2068–2070)*

70. **(A)** Premature infants are born with a smaller total hemoglobin mass than the term infant. Since most of the iron stores at birth are contained in the circulating hemoglobin, the premature infant starts life at a serious disadvantage in regard to iron stores. In cases of hemolysis (as with ABO incompatibility), the liberated iron is not lost from the body, so the risk of iron deficiency is not increased. The same is true of physiologic hyperbilirubinemia. *(Rudolph:198, 1525)*

71. **(D)** Fetal hemoglobin binds poorly to 2,3-DPG. Because 2,3-DPG binding decreases the affinity of hemoglobin for oxygen, fetal hemoglobin, unbound to 2,3-DPG, has an increased affinity for oxygen. Prenatally this works to the advantage of the fetus in obtaining oxygen from the maternal blood (across the placenta), but postnatally it is to the infant's disadvantage in releasing oxygen at the tissue level. *(Fanaroff: 1186–1187)*

72. **(C)** The mass shown is a typical example of an encephalocele. These lesions, which consist of herniation of the meninges, with or without brain tissue, through a defect in the skull, occur most commonly in the occipital region. The mass is far too large to be an abscess. There is no such entity as posterior hydrocephalus. Hydroceles are limited to the scrotum. Diastematomyelia is a defect in the spinal cord that leads to neurologic signs but is unassociated with an external mass. *(Rudolph:88, 2179)*

73. **(C)** The roentgenogram reveals absence of the radius and suggests the thrombocytopenia absent radii (TAR) syndrome. In this disorder, thrombocytopenia and bleeding occur early.

In Fanconis syndrome (absent radii and pancytopenia), the hematologic abnormalities usually become manifest after the first or second birthday rather than immediately in the newborn period. *(Rudolph:737)*

74. **(A)** Physiologic jaundice results from an increase in unconjugated bilirubin. Although there are many factors contributing to physiologic jaundice, the most important is hepatic immaturity, which is more pronounced in premature than in term infants. Physiologic jaundice does not appear in the first 24 h of life. It is not associated with hemolysis and, therefore, is not associated with anemia or reticulocytosis. It is a common problem in infants of all races. *(Rudolph:168–169)*

75. **(D)** Infants of diabetic mothers present with a variety of problems. The most common is hypoglycemia resulting from hyperinsulinism. This usually can be prevented with early and frequent feeds but close monitoring is required. A variety of birth defects, including sacral agenesis, are attributable to prenatal hyperglycemia. Large birth weights are common among infants of diabetic mothers. This predisposes the babies to birth trauma and asphyxia. *(Hay:17–18)*

76. **(E)** Infantile glaucoma typically presents in infants less than 6 months of age, and requires surgical treatment. Signs and symptoms include enlargement and clouding of the cornea, tearing, blepharospasm, and photophobia. It is associated with many other conditions including Marfan syndrome, neurofibromatosis 1, and congenital rubella. The white pupil sign is suggestive of a congenital cataract. *(McMillan:674)*

77. **(D)** Tachypnea, retractions, cyanosis, and grunting are common findings in the neonatal respiratory distress syndrome. Wheezing is not a feature of RDS. The clinical findings relate to the pathogenesis of the disease which primarily is atelectasis. *(Rudolph:128–131)*

78. **(B)** EFM can be helpful in assessing the oxygenation status of the fetus in utero. The fetal heart rate is usually over 100/min with considerable beat-to-beat variation. A rate less than 100/min is unusual and worrisome. A fixed heart rate or decreased beat-to-beat variability often indicates fetal hypoxia (fetal distress). Accelerations of the rate are normal and not usually of concern. Decelerations may be of no consequence or may be ominous depending on their temporal relationship to uterine contractions. Early decelerations are usually benign, whereas late or variable decelerations can indicate fetal distress. *(Rudolph:70–71, 75)*

79. **(C)** Infants with a tension pneumothorax typically are tachypneic, with apnea being an uncommon sign. Cyanosis and bradycardia are common features. Hypotension develops from sequestration of blood in the collapsed lung vasculature combined with pressure on the pliable venous great vessels. Prompt diagnosis and treatment is optimal. *(Rudolph:148–150)*

80. **(D)** Since the infant in question was more than 38 weeks gestational age, she is not premature. She is, however, of low birth weight (<2500 g), and is small for gestational age. This can be confirmed by the use of standard intrauterine growth charts. [*Note*: Answers (C) and (D) are correct, but (D) is the BEST answer.] *(Hay:1–5)*

81. **(D)** Subdural hemorrhage over the cerebral cortex is uncommon in premature infants, who, because of their small size, are less likely than term infants to have trauma to, or molding of, the skull during the birth process. Intraventricular hemorrhages occur primarily in premature infants. Hemorrhagic disease of the newborn can occur in either premature or term infants who do not receive vitamin K prophylaxis but is not more common in term infants. Both congenital infection and neonatal sepsis are more common in premature than term infants. *(Hay:57)*

82. **(D)** Meconium ileus results from thick inspissated meconium (putty-like consistency) packed into the terminal ileum. Progressive abdominal distention and bilious vomiting are the hallmarks of the clinical presentation. Nearly all neonates presenting with meconium ileus have cystic fibrosis. Of neonates with

cystic fibrosis, 10% will present with meconium ileus. Though this patient had a family history of cystic fibrosis, in only 10% of newly diagnosed cases of CF is the family history positive. *(Rudolph:203–204)*

83. **(B)** Neither DIC nor dermal erythropoiesis is a recognized manifestation of congenital syphilis. There are a variety of highly characteristic skin manifestations, including bullous lesions on the palms and soles and a diffuse copper-colored maculopapular rash, most intense on the face, palms, and soles. Pneumonia and hepatitis may occur but also are seen in many other neonatal infections. *(Rudolph:1004–1005)*

84. **(A)** Epiphyseal dysgenesis with irregular or stippled ossification centers is characteristic of hypothyroidism (although it also is seen in some other conditions). The development of ossification centers is retarded in hypothyroidism, but since the ossification center of the hamate does not normally appear until the age of 4 months, x-ray examination of the wrist is of no value in the newborn period. Roentgenographic demonstration of absence of the distal femoral epiphyses (normally evident at 34–36 weeks of gestation) in a term infant would be suggestive of hypothyroidism. Although cardiomegaly from myxedema of the heart can be seen, there are so many other, much more common causes of cardiomegaly in the newborn that an enlarged heart would not be suggestive of hypothyroidism. *(Rudolph:2021; Fanaroff:1408)*

85. **(E)** Hypoplastic left heart syndrome typically presents within the first weeks of life with tachypnea, lethargy, and poor feeding. The condition of the neonate worsens dramatically with closing of the PDA. The other choices represent cyanotic congenital heart diseases. This patient did not present with cyanosis. *(Tobias: 155–161)*

86. **(D)** The initial lesions of incontinentia pigmenti are inflammatory bullae that eventually evolve into pigmented lesions. The majority of affected patients are female. Mental retardation and seizures are common. The disease also involves the heart, eyes, and skeletal system. *(Rudolph:1186)*

87. **(A)** Amnion nodosum suggests oligohydramnios, which, in conjunction with the "Potter's facies" described, is characteristic of bilateral renal agenesis. Esophageal atresia often is associated with polyhydramnios, not oligohydramnios. None of the features of this case are suggestive of congenital heart disease or infection. *(Rudolph:1704)*

88. **(B)** Cats are the definitive host for *Toxoplasma gondii*, an intracellular parasite that can be transmitted from mother to fetus through the placenta (transplacental transmission). Typically, this is the result of a primary infection in the mother. The most severely infected fetuses aquire the infection during the first trimester of pregnancy. [*Note:* The table of clinical findings of infants with congenital infections found in McMillan on page 430 is worth reviewing!] *(McMillan:430, 444–446)*

89. **(B)** Meconium aspiration syndrome (MAS) is much more likely than the other diagnoses to occur in a postterm infant. This likely is due to placental insufficiency leading to the passage of meconium. MAS is distinctly unusual in the premature infant, even when severely stressed in utero. *(Hay:19)*

90. **(E)** Pulmonary hypoplasia is caused most frequently by severe oligohydramnios. Common causes include renal agenesis (Potter syndrome) and early rupture of membranes. *(Hay:697, 1029)*

91. **(B)** Hyperexpansion is a characteristic of meconium aspiration syndrome and predisposes these infants to pneumothoraces. The other disorders primarily are characterized by underexpansion. *(Hay:17–18)*

92. **(C)** Transient tachypnea of the newborn (suggested by its name) usually is a self-limited disorder which manifests as mild to moderate respiratory distress. Its etiologic mechanism is thought to be a delay in resorption of fetal lung fluid. *(Hay:18–19)*

93. **(C)** Transient tachypnea occurs more frequently after cesarean deliveries, particularly those performed before the onset of labor. The symptoms overlap with pneumonia and lead to a significant newborn ICU admission rate. *(Rudolph:179–181)*

94. **(E)** Sequestrated blood in each of these lesions can cause an acute indirect hyperbilirubinemia requiring phototherapy. *(Rudolph:186–187)*

95. **(D)** Subgaleal hemorrhages associated with birth are much less common than caput succedaneum and cephalhematoma. However, they have the potential to hold the largest blood volume and can hold enough of the infant's circulating volume to cause symptoms of hypovolemia. A 3-kg infant has a circulating blood volume of 250–300 mL. A subgaleal hematoma which causes a 1 cm increase in the infant's head circumference would hold approximately 38 mL of blood. This would be a loss of 10% of the infant's circulating blood volume and could induce acute symptoms. Symptomatic infants require fluid administration and occasionally transfusion. *(Rudolph:187)*

96. **(E)** Sequestrated blood from a cephalhematoma, subgaleal hematoma or caput is best left alone. Open drainage promotes the onset of infection. The pressure from the lesions will provide a tamponade effect in the vast majority of cases. *(Rudolph:186–187)*

97. **(B)** The caput succedaneum usually resolves in the first 48 h of life. A cephalhematoma rarely resolves before 2 weeks and frequently is noticeable months after delivery as calcified masses. *(Rudolph:187)*

98. **(A)** Underlying skull fractures are a common complication of cephalhematomas. Roentgenographic examination of these lesions as a regular practice is debated however, as regular surgical intervention for mildly depressed fractures has not proven to be efficacious. *(Rudolph:187)*

99. **(B)** Trisomy 18 (Edwards syndrome) is characterized by severe retardation of growth and mental development. Most of the patients die in early infancy. Characteristic abnormalities include low-set and malformed ears, nail hypoplasia, abnormal fisting with index finger overlying third finger, and rocker-bottom feet. The abnormalities of the hands and feet are clinically distinctive features. Congenital heart disease is usual, most commonly a ventricular septal defect or a patent ductus arteriosus. The face is round with a narrow forehead, frontal bossing, hypertelorism, micrognathia, and antimongoloid palpebral fissures. *(McMillan:2230)*

100. **(A)** The cardinal features of trisomy 13 (Patau syndrome) include cleft lip and palate, holoprosencephaly, and severe mental retardation. Holoprosencephaly is an incomplete development of the forebrain, often associated with absence of the corpus callosum, fusion of the frontal lobes, and a single ventricle. Other features of trisomy 13 include ocular abnormalities, congenital heart disease, and cutaneous defects of the scalp (cutis aplasia), which can be diagnostic. *(McMillan:2229)*

101. **(D)** Among live births, Down syndrome is the most common chromosomal abnormality. It occurs in about 1 in 770 live births. Fewer than 5% of patients have a translocation rather than an extra (47) chromosome. Hypotonia and hyperextensible joints are characteristic. Mental retardation is present in all patients but is less severe than in other trisomy syndromes (i.e., trisomies 13 and 18). Clinodactyly, especially of the fifth finger, a single plamar crease, an increased distance between the first and second toes, upward slanting palpebral fissures, epicanthal folds, flat nasal bridge, and flat occiput are some of the physical findings associated with this syndrome. Many of these patients have serious congenital malformations such as congenital heart disease or duodenal atresia. Brushfield spots (tiny white spots that form a ring in the midzone of the iris) are present in the majority of Down syndrome children but also are present in up to 25% of normal individuals, especially those with blue eyes. *(McMillan:2230)*

102. **(C)** The cri du chat (cry of the cat) syndrome is so named because of the characteristic cry, which is reminiscent of a mewing cat. This characteristic cry is present in infancy but disappears as the child grows and usually is gone by the age of 1 or 2 years. The cry is high pitched and distinctive and results from a small, narrow, hypoplastic larynx. These patients also have microcephaly, severe mental retardation, epicanthal folds, hypertelorism, and low-set ears. The syndrome is associated with a deletion of the short arm of chromosome 5. [*Note:* The student who understands French has an obvious advantage in answering this question.] *(McMillan:2232)*

103. **(E)** Features of Turner syndrome, 45,X or XO, in the older child include short stature, lack of development of sexual characteristics, primary amenorrhea, webbing of the neck, cubitus valgus (wide-carrying angle of the arms), and short fourth metacarpals. Pathologically, there is ovarian dysgenesis. In the newborn period, redundant skin at the nape of the neck, a low posterior hair line, and edema of the dorsum of the feet are characteristic. Cardiac defects (especially coarctation of the aorta) and renal anomalies are common. Intelligence usually is normal, but perceptual difficulties are frequent and can be severe. *(McMillan:2231)*

104. **(A)** Repeated sensitization only affects the outcome in Rh disease. In ABO hemolytic disease, severity is unrelated to previous pregnancies. Consequently, a newborn can have severe ABO hemolytic disease with the first pregnancy which is rare in Rh disease. *(McMillan:202–203)*

105. **(A)** Moderate or severe Rh disease can cause symptoms of congestive heart failure which can be identified on prenatal ultrasound. Such severity is not seen with ABO hemolytic disease. *(McMillan:202–203)*

106. **(B)** It is thought that anti-A and anti-B antibodies are raised against substances which occur in foods or bacteria. In Rh disease, on the other hand, exposure of the Rh negative mother to Rh positive cells is required for sensitization. *(Oki:202–204)*

107. **(C)** Exchange transfusion can be required in both disorders. While Rh disease generally is more severe and a given case more likely to require exchange transfusion, ABO hemolytic disease is so much more common in the population that about as many exchange transfusions are performed annually for ABO hemolytic disease as for Rh disease. High dose immune globulin shortly after birth, by not yet understood mechanisms, delays the rapid rise of serum bilirubin seen after birth in affected infants for both ABO and Rh disease. This decreases the number of exchange transfusions necessary. *(McMillan:202–204)*

108. **(C)** Both disorders are mediated by transplacentally acquired IgG antibodies. *(McMillan: 202–204)*

109. **(C)** Both disorders cause extravascular hemolysis. Thus, the most common finding on the peripheral blood smear is microspherocytes. *(Fanaroff:1213)*

110. **(C)** Some infants born with meconium staining have meconium below the vocal cords. If it is not removed, the meconium can be aspirated with potentially dire pulmonary complications. If the meconium is thick or particulate (*pea soup*), and the infant is not vigorous, removal by tracheal intubation and suctioning directly through the endotracheal tube should be accomplished before initiating ventilation. Intubation and suctioning of vigorously breathing meconium stained infants is not indicated. *(Klaus:260–261; Pediatrics 105:1–7, 2000)*

111. **(C)** While most infants with cytomegalovirus infection are asymptomatic at delivery, the combination of growth impairment, hepatosplenomegaly and the "blueberry muffin" rash of extramedullary hematopoiesis (specifically dermal erythropoiesis) are characteristic of CMV infection. *(McMillan:430–431)*

112. **(E)** Jaundice in the first day of life nearly always is a pathologic process in term infants. Hereditary spherocytosis has an incidence of approximately 1/5000 in populations of northern European origin, less in most other ethnic groups. ABO isoimmune hemolytic anemia occurs much more frequently, in about 3% of pregnancies, and is also associated with early onset jaundice and spherocytes on the blood smear. The spherocytes are generated as splenic disruption of the red cell membrane occurs. Disseminated intravascular coagulopathy usually results in numerous other abnormalities of the peripheral blood smear. (McMillan: 201–204, 361)

113. (D) Varicella infections in the newborn are frequently life threatening. Fortunately maternal antibody IgG is protective for weeks after delivery. Certainly infants who face exposure *without* maternal antibody protection acquire the infection at a high rate with serious morbidity, mainly from varicella pneumonia. Varicella immune globulin is useful in preventing acquisition of infection in susceptible infants, but is not required in most term infants who have natural antibody protection. (McMillan: 436–437)

114. (A) Supraventricular tachycardia is the most common neonatal arrhythmia to require treatment. It can develop as reentry or increased automaticity tachycardias. Often predisposing conditions are identified such as Wolff-Parkinson-White syndrome or structural abnormalities of the heart. The presenting complaints in neonates usually are tachypnea and poor feeding. (McMillan:290–291)

115. (C) Infants with severe respiratory distress syndrome (hyaline membrane disease) commonly develop hypercapnia and respiratory acidosis, with PCO_2 levels in the 50–70 torr range. This hypercapnia results from diffuse atelectasis and ventilation/perfusion mismatching. (McMillan:254–255)

116. (C) Homeothermic hypermetabolism in response to cold stress can dramatically increase the oxygen requirement of the newborn. The large surface area to mass ratio of the newborn predisposes to this problem. When cold stress is manifest in a child who has underlying pulmonary disease, such as the premature infant with respiratory distress syndrome, the increase

in oxygen requirement may surpass the lung's capacity to deliver oxygen and rapidly lead to metabolic acidosis. (Fanaroff:524–526)

117. (D) Periventricular leukomalacia usually is visualized as cystic lesions surrounding the lateral ventricles. These lesions are thought to be due to ischemic infarct in this watershed area of white matter. While the injury likely occurs early on, the ultrasonographic findings usually are delayed several weeks. Congenital anomalies of the brain and intraventricular hemorrhage usually are readily apparent on imaging in the first days of life. (Fanaroff:882)

118. (E) Congestive heart failure is a common complication of large intracranial arteriovenous fistulas, and a cranial bruit usually is readily audible in these patients. The great vein of Galen is a frequent location for such arteriovenous malformations. Hyperthyroidism and polycythemia cause congestive heart failure only rarely; transposition of the great vessels usually is associated with a cardiac murmur and not with a cranial bruit. Ruptured cerebral aneurysms are exceedingly rare in the newborn period and present with neurologic findings rather than heart failure or cranial bruits. (McMillan:1934)

119. (B) Brachial plexus injury may be associated with phrenic nerve injury on the same side because of the proximity of the involved spinal nerve roots. The phrenic nerve injury results in diaphragmatic paralysis, which can lead to progressive respiratory difficulty. The fact that this is a large infant strengthens the supposition of brachial plexus injury during birth. Respiratory distress syndrome is uncommon in term infants and almost always presents initially in the first 24 h of life. Pulmonary hemorrhage, pneumothorax, and cystic adenomatoid malformation can cause cyanosis and respiratory distress but have no association with brachial plexus injury. (McMillan:2122; Fanaroff:475)

120. (A) The most common cause of neonatal meningitis in most hospitals today is group B *Streptococcus*. *E. coli* generally is the second leading cause. *Listeria* is less frequent but not

uncommon. *Haemophilus influenzae* and *Streptococcus pneumoniae* are uncommon causes of meningitis during the first month of life. While the group B *Streptococcus* is usually vertically transmitted from the mother before or at delivery, 10% of all neonates in a typical nursery are colonized, making the potential for horizontal transmission via healthcare workers a real threat to the noncolonized infants. (*McMillan:413–416, 422*)

BIBLIOGRAPHY

Arias F. *Practical Guide to High-Risk Pregnancy and Delivery*, 2nd ed. St. Louis, MO: Mosby, 1993.

Clark DA. Times of first void and first stool in 500 newborns. *Pediatrics* 1977;60:457–459.

Fanaroff AA, Martin RJ. *Neonatal-Perinatal Medicine*, 7th ed. St. Louis, MO: Mosby, 2001.

Feigin RD, Cherry JD. *Textbook of Pediatric Infectious Diseases*, 4th ed. Philadelphia, PA: W.B. Saunders, 1998.

Hay WW, Hayward AR, Levin MJ, Sondheimer JM. *Current Pediatric Diagnosis & Treatment*, 16th ed. New York, NY: McGraw-Hill, 2003.

Hon EH, Petrie RH. Clinical value of fetal heart rate monitoring. *Clin Obstet Gynecol* 1975;18(4):1–23.

Klaus MH, Fanaroff AA. *Care of the High Risk Neonate*, 5th ed. Philadelphia, PA: W.B. Saunders, 2001.

Nicolaides KH, Rodeck CH. Rhesus disease: the model for fetal therapy. *Br J Hosp Med* 1985;34:141–148.

McMillan JA, DeAngelis CD, Feigin RD, Warshaw JB. *Oski's Pediatrics, Principles & Practice*, 3rd ed. Philadelphia, PA: JB Lippincott, 1999.

Rudolph CD, Rudolph AM, Hostetter MK, et al. *Rudolph's Pediatrics*, 21st ed. New York, NY: McGraw-Hill, 2003.

Tobias JD. *Pediatric Critical Care: The Essentials*. Armonk, NY: Futura Publishing Co., 1999.

Wiswell TE, Gannon CM, Jacob J, et al. Delivery room management of the apparently meconium-stained neonate: results of the multicenter, international collaborative trial. *Pediatrics* 2000;105:1–7.

CHAPTER 3

Injuries, Poisoning, and Substance Abuse

Sara S. Viessman, MD

"Childhood injury: it's no accident." This statement used by the American Academy of Pediatrics in injury prevention programs is representative of cultural and social progress in the safety of children and adolescents. That is, attempts have been made to heighten awareness of the fact that nearly every single *accident* is preventable. The word itself seems to indicate a random, unavoidable event. Therefore, the words unintentional injury are used instead.

Unintentional injuries and homicide remain the leading and second-leading causes of death for children aged 1–19 years. Among unintentional injuries, motor vehicle "accidents," drownings, and poisonings remain common causes of morbidity and mortality in the pediatric population. The rates of firearm-related injuries and deaths are manyfold higher in the United States than in other developed countries. Poisonings, substance abuse, and child abuse often lead to lifelong medical and social consequences.

Prevention is the most important treatment for injuries, poisonings, and substance abuse. After all, "it's no accident."

Questions

DIRECTIONS (Questions 1 through 42): Each of the numbered items or incomplete statements in this section is followed by answers or by completions of the statement. Select the ONE lettered answer or completion that is BEST in each case.

1. Most deaths related to ecstasy have been linked to

   (A) cerebrovascular accident
   (B) myocardial infarction
   (C) hyponatremia or hyperthermia
   (D) metabolic alkalosis with compensatory respiratory acidosis
   (E) hyperkalemia or hypothermia

2. The major cause of morbidity and mortality in acute poisoning with acetaminophen is

   (A) hepatic injury
   (B) gastric bleeding
   (C) metabolic acidosis
   (D) methemoglobinemia
   (E) hypoglycemia

3. Following closed head injury, which of the following would be most ominous?

   (A) irritability
   (B) vomiting
   (C) dilated, fixed pupils
   (D) amnesia for the event
   (E) drowsiness

4. Yearly, over 20,000 children and adolescents younger than 21 years sustain traumatic head injuries while bicycling. Helmet use while bicycling prevents what percent of serious brain injury?

   (A) <10%
   (B) 20–25%
   (C) 50%
   (D) 80–90%
   (E) 99%

5. During a well-child visit, you note blue and yellow bruising over the buttocks and thighs of an 18-month-old boy. Parents deny any history of bleeding or bruising other than what you see. They state they have been disciplining him with "spanking" while attempting to toilet train him. Laboratory studies including a urinalysis, platelet count, bleeding time, and PT/PTT reveal normal values. The most likely explanation for this scenario is as follows:

   A) This child has von Willebrand disease.
   (B) The parents' expectations of toilet training at this age are appropriate.
   (C) Toddlers commonly sustain diffuse bruising of buttocks at this age due to frequent falls.
   (D) This child has idiopathic thrombocytopenic purpura.
   (E) This represents child abuse.

6. Most cases of serious physical child abuse involve children

   (A) less than 1 month old
   (B) between 1 month and 4 years old
   (C) between 5 and 12 years old

(D) between 13 and 16 years old

(E) who are neurologically impaired

7. Most pediatric cases of symptomatic lead poisoning in the United States occur in children

(A) less than 6 months old

(B) between 6 and 12 months old

(C) between 1 and 3 years old

(D) between 3 and 5 years old

(E) between 10 and 15 years old

8. Which of the following combinations of signs and symptoms is most suggestive of chronic lead poisoning?

(A) ataxia, fever, diarrhea, and polycythemia

(B) lethargy, vomiting, hallucinations, and vesicular rash

(C) anemia, leukopenia, thrombocytopenia, and hepatomegaly

(D) lethargy, abdominal cramps, constipation, and anemia

(E) hypertension, rash, cough, and leukocytosis

9. A 3-year-old child is brought to the emergency room with a history of playing with an open kerosene bottle. The parents state the child seemed fine initially, but within an hour developed transient difficulty breathing. They immediately brought the child to you for evaluation. The child's examination is completely normal. What is the most appropriate action at this time?

(A) discharge to home, advise parents to return if they note any problems

(B) obtain a chest x-ray

(C) observe child in emergency room for 1 h

(D) induce emesis with syrup of ipecac

(E) admit to the hospital for 24 h of observation

10. A 4-year-old child is brought to the urgent care by parents who were concerned because the child suddenly developed unusual posture and movements. Examination reveals an alert child who holds the head in a tilted position and has uncontrolled, writhing movements of the hands and arms. The examination is otherwise normal. When questioned regarding medications at home, parents state they do have routine cold medicine, acetaminophen, and some kind of antiemetic medication in an unlocked medicine cabinet. At this time you should

(A) perform a head computerized tomography (CT) scan

(B) perform a lumbar puncture

(C) obtain an electroencephalogram

(D) administer naloxone intravenously

(E) administer diphenhydramine intravenously

11. A 4-year-old boy was found playing with an open bottle of ammonia-containing cleaner about 1 h ago. His mother reports that he now refuses to drink and talk but appears otherwise well. You should advise the mother to

(A) administer syrup of ipecac

(B) closely observe the child and bring to the emergency room if condition worsens

(C) administer milk of magnesia

(D) give the child cold frozen fruit popsicles

(E) immediately bring the child to the emergency room for evaluation

12. Shellfish poisoning, which is caused by eating shellfish that have ingested toxic dinoflagellates (*red tide*), is characterized by

(A) blindness

(B) vomiting and diarrhea

(C) seizures and coma

(D) weakness and paralysis

(E) rash and fever

13. A toddler presents with a known ingestion of iron tablets. By parental count of pills remaining in the bottle it appears he ingested more than 20 mg/kg of elemental iron. Upon admission to the pediatric intensive care unit he is vomiting. Which of the following chelating agents should be administered?

   (A) deferoxamine mesylate
   (B) ethylene diamine tetraacetic acid (EDTA)
   (C) British anti-lewisite (BAL)
   (D) hemoglobin
   (E) penicillamine

14. A 3-year-old child who is unresponsive presents with weaknesses, excessive salivation, bradycardia, and constricted pupils. The parents are so distraught, it is difficult to get information. However, an astute emergency room physician realizes the most likely drug or toxin to cause these signs is

   (A) diphenhydramine
   (B) phenobarbital
   (C) ethyl alcohol
   (D) a hydrocarbon
   (E) an organophosphate

15. Following stabilization of the patient in the above question, the emergency room physician administers a test dose of a drug. To the parents' amazement, the child's pupils dilate and the child temporarily appears to respond to the parents. What drug did this physician most likely administer?

   (A) naloxone
   (B) diphenhydramine
   (C) atropine
   (D) N-acetylcysteine
   (E) phenobarbital

16. Among 18-year-old males, approximately what percent have used anabolic steroids as performance enhancers?

   (A) 1%
   (B) 2–5%
   (C) 5–10%

   (D) 15–20%
   (E) 30–40%

17. Three symptomatic adolescents with a history of ingesting seeds of jimsonweed are arriving via ambulance from a referring hospital emergency room. Which of the following best describes the expected signs and symptoms of jimsonweed poisoning?

   (A) agitation/hallucinations, dilated pupils
   (B) coma, pinpoint pupils
   (C) hallucinations, bradycardia
   (D) coma, bradycardia
   (E) pallor, pinpoint pupils

18. Ingestion of LSD will most likely result in

   (A) convulsions
   (B) euphoria
   (C) hallucinations
   (D) sedation
   (E) tremors

19. A youngster who sniffs spot remover and then engages in stressful physical activity is at risk for

   (A) convulsions
   (B) hypertension
   (C) rhabdomyolysis
   (D) severe headache
   (E) sudden death

20. The most commonly used "date-rape" drugs are

   (A) amphetamines and LSD
   (B) gamma-hydroxybutyrate and flunitrazepam
   (C) cocaine and phenobarbital
   (D) ephedra and codeine
   (E) phenobarbital and gamma-hydroxybutryate

21. After being lifted up by one hand, a young toddler refuses to use that arm and holds it against her trunk flexed at the elbow with the forearm midway between pronation and supination. The child most likely has

(A) a shoulder dislocation

(B) a radial head subluxation

(C) a fracture of a carpal bone

(D) avulsion of the ulnar nerve

(E) a fracture of the radius

22. A 4-year-old child falls on an outstretched arm. The child is likely to sustain a

(A) fracture displacement of the radial epiphysis

(B) Colles' fracture

(C) comminuted radial and ulnar fracture

(D) shoulder dislocation

(E) humeral fracture

23. Which of the following sets of blood gas values is most compatible with acute aspirin poisoning in a 16-month-old child?

(A) pH 7.60, PCO_2 40, HCO_3 40

(B) pH 7.5, PCO_2 40, HCO_3 30

(C) pH 7.25, PCO_2 20, HCO_3 8

(D) pH 7.20, PCO_2 45, HCO_3 20

(E) pH 7.00, PCO_2 35, HCO_3 8

24. Hyperventilation due to salicylate poisoning

(A) is apparent on physical examination within minutes of ingestion

(B) is characterized by an increase in rate and depth of ventilation

(C) is characterized by an increase in depth of ventilation only

(D) is characterized by an increase in rate of ventilation only

(E) does not occur in young children

25. Which of the following findings would be most suggestive of the form of child abuse referred to as the shaken baby syndrome?

(A) ecchymosis over the mastoid area

(B) retinal hemorrhages

(C) ecchymoses and petechiae over the upper arms and upper trunk

(D) circumferential ecchymosis on extremities

(E) cervical spine dislocation

26. A 9-year-old is injured while sledding. On admission, the child appears in shock and is complaining of pain in the left shoulder. Of immediate concern is the likely diagnosis of

(A) rupture of the descending aorta

(B) dislocation of the left shoulder

(C) rupture of the spleen

(D) rupture of the left diaphragm

(E) fracture of the humerus

27. Most unintentional fatal injuries to children 1–19 years of age involve

(A) motor vehicles

(B) swimming pools

(C) firearms

(D) bicycles

(E) fireworks

28. A 1-year-old child is brought to the emergency room because of a swollen left thigh. The parents, who appear very concerned, state they left the child in the care of a newly hired housekeeper early that morning, and when they returned home in the evening they noted the swelling. Other than tender swelling of the thigh, physical examination is entirely normal. X-ray examination discloses a displaced fracture of the shaft of the femur; skeletal survey reveals no other fractures or abnormalities. The grandparents, who live with the parents and who had accompanied them on their trip, corroborate the parents' story. The most appropriate action for you to take at this time would be to admit the child for treatment of the fracture and

(A) order a computerized tomography (CT) scan of the head

(B) ask the parents to send in the housekeeper so that you can question her

(C) instruct the parents to discharge the housekeeper

(D) ask the parents if they wish to press charges against the housekeeper

(E) report the incident to a child protection agency

29. Syrup of ipecac should be administered in the home to which of the following children?

   (A) 3-year-old child who ingested lye (sodium hydroxide) 5 min prior
   (B) 4-year-old child found obtunded, suspected of narcotic poisoning
   (C) 2-year-old child who is having brief seizures, suspected of ingesting sibling's phenytoin
   (D) 2-year-old child who ingested toilet bowl cleaner
   (E) none of the above

30. A 4-year-old child is playing in the basement. The child suddenly comes upstairs, screaming of being bitten by a spider. There is a red weal-like lesion on the child's face. Over the next few hours the lesion becomes larger, more painful, and darker, until it is violaceous. The most likely complication in this child would be

   (A) necrosis at the site of the bite
   (B) renal failure
   (C) hepatic failure
   (D) muscle cramps and seizures
   (E) convulsions

31. Management with multiple-dose activated charcoal may be indicated in the overdose of

   (A) iron
   (B) cyanide
   (C) tricyclic antidepressants
   (D) ethanol
   (E) methanol

32. A 2-year-old child is retrieved from a near-drowning episode in a pool. The child is apneic on retrieval, but is quickly and successfully resuscitated. On arrival in the emergency room, abnormalities which are likely to be present and require immediate attention would include

   (A) hyponatremia and hypokalemia
   (B) hyponatremia and hyperkalemia
   (C) hyperkalemia and acidosis

   (D) acidosis and hypoxemia
   (E) hypoxemia and hemolysis

33. Manifestations of the first stage of severe acute iron poisoning include

   (A) lethargy and coma
   (B) metabolic alkalosis and hypertension
   (C) hemolysis and neutropenia
   (D) renal, hepatic, and cardiac failure
   (E) hypoglycemia and hepatic injury

34. Which of the following statements regarding automobile safety for children is correct?

   (A) Children, beyond the age of 1 year, or 20 lbs, may ride either facing the front or rear of the car.
   (B) Children over 25 lbs may use adult-type restraints
   (C) A 1-year-old child held in the lap of a seat-belted adult is almost as safe as in an infant restraint device.
   (D) Safety restraints are not needed for infants less than 3 months of age or 10 lbs of body weight.
   (E) Infants under the age of 1 year should ride in restraint devices facing the rear of the car.

35. Which of the following statements regarding drowning and near-drowning is correct?

   (A) Four-sided fencing around pools has not decreased the incidence of drownings.
   (B) Children under the age of 5 years who drown in home pools most often enter the pool by climbing over a fence.
   (C) The incidence of drowning peaks in elementary school-aged children.
   (D) For every child who drowns, four are hospitalized for near-drowning.
   (E) Among children who survive, neurologic impairment is uncommon.

36. Concerning child sexual abuse, which of the following is correct?

    (A) Boys and girls are at equal risk.
    (B) In the majority of cases, the abuser is well known to the child.
    (C) Physical contact is necessary to fulfill diagnostic criteria for child sexual abuse.
    (D) An estimated 10% of children are sexually abused each year in the United States.
    (E) There must be evidence of sexual intercourse for successful prosecution.

37. Which of the following statements regarding firearm-related injuries in children less than 19 years of age is correct?

    (A) Unintentional firearm-related injuries outnumber intentional firearm-related injuries.
    (B) Fewer than 10% of firearm-related deaths are the result of suicide.
    (C) Firearms account for 20–23% of all injury deaths in this age group.
    (D) Firearm-related injuries result in more deaths than do motor vehicle accidents each year.
    (E) Most firearm-related deaths occur after prolonged hospital course.

38. Which of the following is most suggestive of unintentional (nonabuse) injuries in children?

    (A) hand print bruise on the face of a child
    (B) belt marks on the buttocks of a 3-year-old child
    (C) bruises on upper thighs reported to result from "spanking"
    (D) fractured femur of a 1-month-old baby from rolling off the bed
    (E) multicolored bruises along the shins of a 4-year-old child

39. Injuries remain the leading cause of death among all children of age 1–19 years. For those 15–19 years of age, which of the following lists the categories of injuries from most common to least common?

    (A) suicide, homicide, motor vehicle accidents (MVA)
    (B) homicide, suicide, MVA
    (C) MVA, suicide, homicide
    (D) MVA, homicide, suicide
    (E) homicide, MVA, suicide

40. Overdose of which of the following is most likely to be complicated by hypoglycemia?

    (A) salicylates
    (B) lead
    (C) tricyclic antidepressants
    (D) opioids
    (E) organophosphates

41. What percentage of high school students have smoked ≥1 cigarette per day for 30 days?

    (A) <3%
    (B) 5–10%
    (C) 20%
    (D) 25–30%
    (E) 40%

42. A 12-month-old infant who has been walking well for 3–4 weeks, now limps on the right leg. No specific injury can be recalled by the parents. The child is afebrile. Examination reveals tenderness with gentle twisting of the lower right leg. An x-ray reveals an oblique nondisplaced fracture of the distal tibia. This condition is referred to as

    (A) toddler's fracture
    (B) Monteggia fracture
    (C) nursemaid's ankle
    (D) Cozen fracture
    (E) Osgood-Schlatter disease

DIRECTIONS (Questions 43 through 52): For each numbered substance select the ONE lettered option which most commonly is recognized as an antidote for an overdose of the numbered substance. Each lettered option may be selected once, more than once, or not at all.

Questions 43 through 52

    (A) naloxone
    (B) flumazenil
    (C) oxygen
    (D) ethanol or 4-methylpyrazole
    (E) deferoxamine
    (F) sodium bicarbonate
    (G) atropine
    (H) sodium nitrite/sodium thiosulfate
    (I) methylene blue

43. Organophosphates

44. Cyanide

45. Cyclic antidepressants

46. Benzodiazepines

47. Ethylene glycol

48. Carbon monoxide

49. Methemoglobinemic agents

50. Opioids

51. Methanol

52. Iron

Answers and Explanations

1. **(C)** Raves, or underground all-night parties, typically are attended by adolescents and young adults. Probably the most popular club drug used at raves is ecstasy, or methlyene-dioxymethamphetamine (MDMA). The use of ecstasy, an amphetamine with hallucinogenic and stimulant properties, results in CNS agitation, tachycardia, hypertension, and diaphoresis. Serotonergic effects of ecstasy also include enhanced sensual perceptions and blunted perceptions of hunger and thirst. Most ecstasy-related deaths have been linked to hyperthermia (increased physical activity in enclosed space) or hyponatremia (water intoxication or SIADH). *(Pediatr Emerg Care 18:216–218, 2002; www.usdoj.gov/ndic)*

2. **(A)** Ingestion of acetaminophen in therapeutic doses typically does not result in side effects. However, ingestion of potentially toxic doses (>7.5 g in adults and >150 mg/kg in children) may result in hepatotoxicity. When present, hepatotoxicity peaks 48–96 h after ingestion. The use of antidotal therapy with *N*-acetylcysteine is guided by the serum acetaminophen level drawn no less than 4 h following ingestion. *(Rudolph's Fundamentals: 409–411)*

3. **(C)** Following head trauma, eye changes such as fixed, dilated pupils usually are indicative of increasing intracranial pressure or focal neurologic damage. A history of unconsciousness, irritability and lethargy, amnesia for the event, and/or vomiting are seen commonly in the absence of major intracranial injury. *(Rudolph CD:348, 2244; Pediatrics 62:819, 1978)*

4. **(D)** An astounding 88% of serious brain injury sustained while bicycling is prevented with helmet use. Additionally, helmet use prevents an estimated 65% of injuries to the mid and upper face. Two factors have been identified as having a strong association with bicycle helmet use by young children. These are helmet use by an accompanying parent and a state mandatory helmet use law or local ordinance. Communities have successfully raised the rate of helmet use with a variety of programs. (Do you have a toddler? Along with his or her first riding toy, such as a tricycle or scooter, purchase for them an appropriate helmet!) *(Pediatrics 108:1030–1032, 2001)*

5. **(E)** Two problems are evident in this scenario. One is the parents' expectation that this toddler is ready for toilet training, and the other is their aggressive "discipline" to accomplish this skill. The average age of successful toilet training is 29 months (bowel) and 32 months (bladder). Boys generally acquire this skill at an older age than girls. Successful toilet training involves realistic parental expectations, patience, consistency, and positive reinforcements. Despite the availability of alternate forms of discipline, corporal punishment is still used by some parents. Although there is state to state variability, injury resulting from discipline generally is considered child abuse. *(Rudolph's Fundamentals: 416; Levine:46–47, 244)*

6. **(B)** Most cases of physical child abuse and almost all deaths from abuse occur in the age group less than 4 years, especially less than 2 or 3 years, before the child can communicate effectively with others. In approximately 10%

of all emergency room visits for injuries in children younger than 5 years, abuse is the etiology of those injuries. Although neurologically im-paired children are at increased risk for abuse, most victims are neurologically normal. (Behrman:111)

7. (C) Cases of lead poisoning in the United States are seen chiefly in the toddler age group. This is understandable, considering the mechanism of poisoning. The major source of lead poisoning in children living in urban areas is old, flaking lead paint, found in pre-1950 buildings. Some children will chronically ingest the paint flakes. Although it is no longer legal to use lead paints indoors, old buildings still may have layers of paint with high lead content beneath the more recent coats of "lead-free" paint. Children become exposed to lead as older homes are renovated. As severe, overt lead poisoning has become less common, there has been an increased concern about the long-term neurodevelopmental effects of subclinical lead poisoning, and guidelines for lead screening are issued by the CDC. (McMillan:599–632)

8. (D) Common signs of lead poisoning include lethargy, abdominal cramps, constipation, and anemia. Vomiting also is common. Ataxia is seen occasionally. The other items listed—fever, diarrhea, rash, hallucinations, hypertension, thrombocytopenia, and cough—are not associated with lead poisoning. [Note: In answering this type of question, it is helpful to examine each answer for a clearly false item. Diarrhea and polycythemia rule out choice (A) since the opposites, constipation, and anemia, are associated with lead poisoning. Rash is not a feature of plumbism, so choices (B) and (E) can be excluded. Choice (C) contains three incorrect items—leukopenia, thrombocytopenia, and hepatomegaly.] (McMillan:632)

9. (B) Up to 28,000 children (usually <5 years of age) ingest hydrocarbons each year. Most children will remain asymptomatic. Those who develop respiratory symptoms, even if transient, should be evaluated by a physician. A CXR should be part of initial evaluation of all those children who developed respiratory symptoms, such as wheezing, coughing, gagging, or dyspnea, even if symptoms were transient. If symptoms then recur, or if abnormalities are noted on CXR, or if new symptoms develop, the child should be admitted to the hospital for observation and possibly further evaluation. (Fleisher:914–915)

10. (E) The child described has developed extrapyramidal symptoms typical of phenothiazine toxicity. These findings may occur with therapeutic as well as excessive dosage and are common in children. Akinesia, trismus, opisthotonos, torticollis, chorea, dystonia, and oculogyric crises may be seen. These symptoms usually respond dramatically to intravenous diphenhydramine (Benadryl) or benztropine mesylate, although relapses are frequent. The clinical picture is so classic that it can be suspected even in the absence of a history of ingestion. Aside from managing this ingestion and screening for other medications this child may have ingested, you must work with these parents to prevent future episodes of ingestion. (Pediatr Clin North Am 33:299, 1986; Gunn:40)

11. (E) This child should be evaluated immediately by a physician. Ingestion of caustic agents, alkaline or acidic, results in dermal and mucosal injury from contact. Refusal to drink may indicate tissue damage and an assessment should be performed to determine the extent of this damage. The physical examination should include close examination of the oropharynx. Clinical or radiographic evaluation can demonstrate signs of esophageal or tracheal perforation. This includes subcutaneous air and crepitus, pneumothorax, pneumomediastinum or pneumoperitoneum. If endoscopic evaluation is indicated, it should be performed within the first 24 h because of increased risk of iatrogenic perforation with this procedure after 48 h following ingestion. Long-term effects of caustic ingestions include esophageal stricture formation. (Tobias:423–424)

12. (D) Shellfish poisoning is characterized by paresthesia and numbness of the mouth and face, generalized weakness, and paralysis. The incubation period is brief, minutes to hours.

In severe cases, mechanical ventilatory assistance may be required. Presumably the flagellates ingested by the shellfish produce a neurotoxin, which is, in turn, ingested when the shellfish are eaten, accounting for the symptoms. Larger numbers of dinoflagellates in the water where the shellfish are harvested can impart a red or reddish-brown color to the water, the so-called red tide. *(N Engl J Med 295:1117, 1976)*

13. **(A)** Deferoxamine is the chelating agent of choice for iron poisoning. It combines with iron to form ferrioxamine, which is excreted in the urine. Parenteral administration (intravenous) is reserved for children with severe poisoning, as the iron ferrioxamine complexes are potentially toxic. *(Tobias:430–431)*

14. **(E)** The signs described—coma, weakness, excessive salivation, bradycardia, and constricted pupils—are classic for organophosphate poisoning. Organophosphates are potent and persistent inhibitors of acetylcholinesterase. Excessive salivation is not seen in phenobarbital, diphenhydramine, ethyl alcohol, or hydrocarbon poisoning. *(Rudolph CD:373–374)*

15. **(C)** Atropine is the major antidote in the treatment of organophosphate poisoning. Administered intravenously, it can result in rapid improvement in signs and symptoms. This improvement, however, typically is short-lived, necessitating repeat dosing. *(Gunn:39)*

16. **(C)** Surveys of graduating high school students reveal up to 5–11% of males and 2.5% of females have used anabolic steroids for performance or appearance enhancement. The use of ergogenic aids or performance-enhancing substances (PES) is widespread among adolescents. Generally, these substances are classified as supplements (such as caffeine, creatine, or androstenedione), or prescription drugs (such as anabolic steroids, beta-blockers, or diuretics). Some have been banned by governing boards or made illegal by law. These are classified as illicit or banned substances and include, among others, narcotics, human growth hormone, anabolic steroids, and gamma-hydroxybutyrate. *(Pediatrics 99, 1997; Pediatr Rev 23:310–317, 2002)*

17. **(A)** Jimsonweed seeds are abused because of their profound hallucinogenic effect. This, as named, is a weed with widespread growth through the continental United States and many other countries. Though some data suggest the use of this substance by adolescents is declining, fatalities associated with ingestion of jimsonweed continue to be reported. Typically patients present as agitated adolescents with signs of anticholinergic toxicity such as tachycardia, dilated pupils, and flushed skin. Convulsions are infrequent, and can be severe and difficult to control. *(Fleisher:924; www.usdoj.gov/ndic; Tobias:416)*

18. **(C)** Hallucinations, especially visual, are the most common and most striking effect of LSD. Sensations are magnified and distorted. The patient may imagine seeing odors or hearing colors. The emotional response can be either positive and pleasurable or negative and frightening. *(Fleisher:934)*

19. **(E)** Sudden death is not infrequent in youngsters who sniff organic solvents. The risk appears to be especially great if the inhalation involves a halogenated hydrocarbon (frequently used as solvents or spot removers) and is followed by exercise or other vigorous physical activity. It has been postulated that this may be related to sensitization of the myocardium by the volatile hydrocarbons. A lethal arrhythmia then is precipitated by the catecholamine release occasioned by the exercise. *(Pediatr Clin North Am 34:335, 337, 1987)*

20. **(B)** Both flunitrazepam (Rophynol; street names: roachies, roofies, the forget pill, roofenol) and gamma-hydroxybutyrate (GHB; street names: easy lay, grievous body harm) are used as agents in date-rape. Flunitrazepam (Rophynol), a benzodiazepine not licensed for use in the United States but readily available from dealers for less than $5 per tablet, quickly dissolves in liquids as a colorless and odorless sedative/hypnotic agent. Symptoms of dizziness, disorientation and/or nausea begin within

15–20 min following ingestion, and peak with unconsciousness within 1–2 h. These, along with the amnestic properties of flunitrazepam, have enabled sexual predators to render their victims helpless, and have made prosecution for sexual assault crimes even more challenging. GHB, commonly used as a euphoriant or aphrodisiac at parties or raves, also can be unknowingly ingested by a victim who is subsequently sexually assaulted or raped. This compound can be obtained in small quantities at large parties or in liter bottles from Canadian web sites. GHB also is popular among body builders because it is reputed to increase the production of growth hormone which increases muscle mass. (Fliesher:939; www.rapecrisiscenter.com; Pediatr Emerg Care 18:53–59, 2002)

21. (B) When a young child is lifted off the ground, dragged, or swung by one arm, the youngster's radius may partly escape from the annular ligament at the elbow. This subluxation of the radial head is a common injury, the so-called nursemaid's injury or nursemaid's elbow. The child holds the injured arm flexed at the elbow and refuses to move it. The subluxation usually is easily reduced by supination of the arm. Recurrent radial head subluxations are seen in 33% of patients. Therefore, caretakers should be informed of this risk and of preventive measures. (Rudolph CD:2448; Fleisher:1600–1601)

22. (A) Epiphyseal separations are common childhood injuries. The growth plate or epiphysis is generally the weakest part of a child's bone, weaker even than surrounding ligaments. Trauma which would result in a tear of the ligament in an adult, often results in an epiphyseal fracture in a child. A fall onto an outstretched arm, which might result in a Colles' fracture in an adult, is likely to cause a separation fracture of the distal radial epiphysis in a child. (Rudolph CD:1436)

23. (C) Aspirin poisoning results in a mixed disturbance of metabolic acidosis and respiratory alkalosis. In adolescents and adults, the predominant abnormality usually is the respiratory alkalosis. Before the age of 2 years, however, metabolic acidosis is the predominant process and the net change in arterial pH generally is a decrease. (Rudolph CD:375–376; Pediatrics 70:566, 1982)

24. (B) Salicylate poisoning results in an increase in both rate and depth of ventilation. The latter usually is especially striking. Generally, neither tachypnea nor deep respirations are clinically apparent until several hours after ingestion. Even young infants show this response. (Rudolph CD:375–376; Pediatrics 70:566, 1982)

25. (B) Retinal hemorrhages and cerebral hemorrhages are characteristic of the shaken baby syndrome. Often, there are no external signs of trauma. This type of child abuse occurs most commonly in children less than 1 year of age and is associated with high morbidity and mortality. Of children who survive this injury, 35% will be blind or visually impaired. Increasingly, this syndrome is referred to by other names such as shaken baby/impact syndrome, non accidental head trauma, and abusive head trauma. (Fleisher:1677; Rudolph CD:2415; Pediatrics 54:396, 1974)

26. (C) The child described most likely has sustained an injury to the spleen. Splenic trauma, with or without rupture, is a common sledding injury. Shock can occur rapidly, or some time later. Pain in the left shoulder is common and reflects irritation to the left diaphragm by subphrenic blood. The current approach to management is conservative, with every attempt to salvage, rather than remove, the spleen. (Fleisher:1365)

27. (A) Unintentional injuries remain the leading cause of death among children aged 1–19 years. Of these fatal unintentional injuries, two-thirds involve motor vehicles. (McMillan:9; Pediatrics 110:1037–1052, 2002)

28. (E) All states have laws requiring any person having reason to suspect child abuse or neglect to report the case to the proper child protective authority. Proof is not a prerequisite for reporting. In a case of suspected abuse, physicians must identify and treat physical injuries and must insure the child's immediate safety.

Detailed recording of exact history given, including history in the child's own words if he/she is old enough to speak, and physical findings (photographs or videos) can be extremely useful to the child protective team. (*Rudolph's Fundamentals:415–418*)

29. **(E)** In November 2003, the American Academy of Pediatrics (AAP) issued a policy statement, *Poison Treatment in the Home*, which stated syrup of ipecac should no longer be used routinely as a home treatment strategy. Further, it recommends safe disposal of all ipecac from homes. Caregivers of a child who may have ingested a toxic substance should consult with local poison control centers by telephoning 800-222-1222. (*Pediatrics:112:1182–1185*)

30. **(A)** The most likely villain in this case is the brown recluse spider (fiddler spider, *Loxoseles reclusa*). Envenomation is characterized by severe local reaction, often leading to local tissue necrosis. Severe systemic symptoms and painful muscle cramps are characteristic of black widow spider (*Latrodectus mactans*) bite, in which case there is little local reaction, although local pain is common. (*Rudolph CD:1152*)

31. **(C)** Activated charcoal administered orally or via nasogastric tube adsorbs certain substances onto its surface thereby decreasing the amount available for absorption from the gastrointestinal tract. Additionally, clearance of specific toxins, such as aspirin, tricyclic antidepressants, phenobarbital, and phenothiazines is enhanced by "gastrointestinal dialysis" with multiple-dose use of charcoal. Specific substances which are not effectively adsorbed by activated charcoal include alcohols (ethanol, methanol, ethylene glycol), hydrocarbons, acids/alkalis, iron, cyanide, and lithium. (*McMillan:618–619; Fleisher: 894–895*)

32. **(D)** The most immediate concern in patients successfully resuscitated from a near-drowning episode is correction of hypoxemia and acidosis. The consequences of cerebral hypoxia with acute brain swelling are the major causes of morbidity and mortality. Aspiration pneumonia is common. Life-threatening electrolyte disturbances are quite rare in patients who survive to the emergency room. Most victims of near-drowning aspirate relatively late in the immersion episode, after they have become severely hypoxic secondary to apnea. Aspiration of large quantities of fluid, therefore, is rare. [*Note*: A key to answering this question correctly is attention to the phrase "require immediate attention."] (*Fleisher:944–945*)

33. **(A)** The clinical manifestations of iron poisoning have been organized into four stages. The first stage is characterized by gastrointestinal (vomiting, diarrhea, abdominal pain, and gastrointestinal bleeding) and neurologic (lethargy or coma) signs. This is followed by a second stage of deceptive quiescence, of up to 48 h, and then a third stage characterized by shock and metabolic acidosis, with or without evidence of hepatic injury. Leukocytosis is common. Late sequelae (stage 4) include pyloric or antral stenosis and hepatic cirrhosis. (*Tobias:430–431; Rudolph's Fundamentals:411–413*)

34. **(E)** The head of an infant is relatively larger (compared to total body size or weight) than the older child or adult. For this reason, the neck is subjected to proportionally increased force during a crash. Having the infant face backward diffuses the blow (deceleration) over the entire back. Infants under the age of 1 should ride facing the rear of the car. All older children should ride properly restrained, facing forward. It has been shown that the force generated by a 1-year-old infant in a front-end crash far exceeds the ability of an adult to hold a child in the lap. The child will be propelled against the interior of the automobile or outside the automobile. (*Rudolph CD:38*)

35. **(D)** Drowning is defined as death from suffocation within 24 h of submersion in water. Near-drowning victims survive at least 24 h. Therefore, near-drowning victims may survive or die from complications of the submersion. As with many injuries and poisonings, there are peaks in occurrence of drownings in toddlers and in teenagers. Of children and adolescents who survive near-drowning, an estimated 35% will have significant neurologic

impairment. Prevention is of utmost importance. Installation of four-sided fences around pools decreases the number of pool immersion injuries by more than 50% in children aged 1–4 years. As with all injuries, brief lapses in appropriate supervision may result in tragedies. *(Fleisher:943–944; Pediatrics 92:292–294, 1993)*

36. **(B)** Childhood sexual abuse is defined as "the engaging of dependent, developmentally immature children in sexual activities that they do not fully comprehend and to which they cannot give consent or activities that violate the laws and taboos of a society." The abusers frequently are relatives or others well known to the child. Impotence and low self-esteem are often seen in abusers. It is estimated that about 1% of children are sexually abused each year in the United States. Girls are six times more likely than boys to be victims of sexual abuse. *(Rudolph's Fundamentals:418–419; Hay:215–220)*

37. **(C)** Firearm-related deaths in children aged 1–19 years are overwhelmingly intentional, with fewer than 8% unintentional. Most of these deaths occur prior to arrival at the hospital. In 1997, 30% of all firearm-related deaths in this age group were the result of suicide with highest rates among African American males. Though the rates of motor vehicle accident deaths have declined over the past two decades, they remain the leading cause of injury-related deaths in this age group. *(Pediatrics105:888–895, 2000)*

38. **(E)** It is extremely important to recognize patterns of abuse to prevent escalating abuse or additional injury and also to prevent unnecessary family anxiety with unwarranted referrals to child protective authorities. Trends found in cases of child abuse include a history not consistent with the injury or the developmental stage of the child (*he rolled off the bed and broke his leg*, said by the parent of the 1-month-old baby), the presence of a pattern of injuries known not to occur except with abuse (handprint bruise on the face), a pattern of injury that reflects injury with an instrument in a manner that would not occur in play or natural injury (hanger or loop cord marks on buttocks), delay in seeking medical attention, a history that changes during the course of

the evaluation, and a history of recurrent injuries. On the other hand, bruises along the anterior lower leg, where children often bump into objects and where the bone is close to the skin, are characteristic of active preschoolers. *(Pediatrics 110:644–645, 2002; Rudolph CD:464–465; Pediatr Clin North Am 32:41–60, 1985)*

39. **(D)** Motor vehicle accidents, homicide, and suicide account for approximately 70% of all deaths in this age group. Deaths from motor vehicle accidents have decreased by over 40% in the past 25 years, and deaths from suicide have remained fairly constant. Deaths from homicide, however, continue to increase in this age group. *(McMillan:9; Pediatrics 110:1037–1052, 2002)*

40. **(A)** Ingestion of an overdose of salicylates, ethanol, or oral hypoglycemic agent may result in symptomatic hypoglycemia. Close monitoring and aggressive therapy with dextrose is appropriate. *(Fleisher:895)*

41. **(C)** Nationwide, 64% of high school students have ever tried cigarette smoking. Over 35% of high school seniors smoke cigarettes once a month. Most astounding, 20% of all high school students have smoked ≥1 cigarette every day for 30 days (lifetime daily cigarette use). Overall, smoking rates of White and Hispanic students were higher than rates of African American students. *(MMWR 51:6–7, 2002)*

42. **(A)** This clinical scenario is classic for a toddler's fracture, which is seen most often in toddlers aged 9–36 months. History of injury may not be elicited, and physical findings often are subtle. Care and time must be taken in the physical examination. Approximately one-fourth of the time, these fractures are not evident radiographically and must be diagnosed by physical examination or bone scan, with confirmatory x-ray revealing subperiosteal new bone 2–3 weeks later. *(Rudolph CD:2451; Fleisher: 1470–1471)*

43. **(G)**, 44. **(H)**, 45. **(F)**, 46. **(B)**, 47. **(D)**, 48. **(C)**, 49. **(I)**, 50. **(A)**, 51. **(D)**, 52. **(E)** There are specific antidotes for a number of toxic ingestions. These antidotes should be readily available in

emergency room settings, and administered as early as possible in the appropriate dose. Antidote administration should be used in conjunction with meticulous ongoing evaluation, management, and supportive care. *(Tobias:420; Fleisher:895)*

BIBLIOGRAPHY

AAP Committee on Injury and Poison Prevention, 2001–2002. Bicycle helmets. *Pediatrics* 2001;108: 1030–1032.

AAP Committee on Injury and Poison Prevention. Drowning in infants, children, and adolescents (RE9319). *Pediatrics* 1993;92:292–294.

AAP Committee on Injury and Poison Prevention. Firearm-related injuries affecting the pediatric population (RE9926). *Pediatrics* 2000;105:888–895.

AAP Committee on Injury, Violence and Poison Prevention. Poison treatment in the home. *Pediatrics* 2003;112:1182–1185.

AAP Committee on Sports Medicine and Fitness. Adolescents and anabolic steroids: a subject review (RE9720). *Pediatrics* 1997;99:6.

Behrman RE, Kliegman RM, Arvin AM. *Nelson Textbook of Pediatrics*, 16th ed. Philadelphia, PA: W.B. Saunders, 1999.

Caffey J. The whiplash shaken infant syndrome. *Pediatrics* 1974;54:396–403.

CDC. Youth risk behavior surveillance—United States, 2001. *MMWR* 2002;51:6–7.

Fleisher GR, Ludwig S. *Textbook of Pediatric Emergency Medicine*, 4th ed. Philadelphia, PA: JB Lippincott, Williams & Wilkins, 2000.

Gaudreault P, Temple AR, Lovejoy FH. The relative severity of acute versus chronic salicylate poisoning in children. *Pediatrics* 1982;70:566–572.

Gunn VL, Nechyba C. *The Harriet Lane Handbook*, 16th ed. Philadelphia, PA: Mosby, 2002.

Hay WH, Hayward AR, Levin MJ, et al. *Current Pediatric Diagnosis & Treatment*, 16th ed. New York, NY, McGraw-Hill, 2003.

Hughes JM, Merson MH. Fish and shellfish poisoning. *N Engl J Med* 1976;295:1117–1120.

Knight ME, Roberts RJ. Phenothiazine and butyrophenone intoxication in children. *Pediatr Clin North Am* 1986;33:299–309.

Koch JJ. Performance-enhancing substances and their use among adolescent athletes. *Pediatr Rev* 2002;23:310–317.

Levine M, Carey WB, Crocker AC, et al. *Developmental-Behaviorial Pediatrics*, 3rd ed. Philadelphia, PA: W.B. Saunders, 1999.

MacDorman MF, Arialdi MM, Strobino DM, Guyer, B. Annual summary of vital statistics—2001. *Pediatrics* 2002;110:1037–1052.

McHugh MJ. The abuse of volatile substances. *Pediatr Clin North Am* 1987;34:333–339.

McMillan JA, DeAngelis CD, Feigin RD, Warshaw JB. *Oski's Pediatrics Principles and Practice*, 3rd ed. Philadelphia, PA: JB Lippincott, 1999.

Poirier MP. Care of the female adolescent rape victim. *Pediatr Emerg Care* 2002;18:53–59.

Reece RM, Grodin MA. Recognition of nonaccidental injury. *Pediatr Clin North Am* 1985;32:41–60.

Rudolph AM, Kamei RK, Overby KJ. *Rudolph's Fundamentals of Pediatrics*, 3rd ed. New York, NY: McGraw-Hill, 2001.

Rudolph CD, Rudolph AM, Hostetter MK, et al. *Rudolph's Pediatrics*, 21st ed. New York, NY: McGraw-Hill, 2003.

Singer HS, Freeman JM. Head trauma for the pediatrician. *Pediatrics* 1978;62:819–825.

Tobias JD. *Pediatric Critical Care: The Essentials*. Armonk, NY: Futura Publishing Co., 1999.

Tong T, Boyer EW. Club drugs, smart drugs, raves and circuit parties: an overview of the club scene. *Pediatr Emerg Care* 2002;18:216–218.

www.rapecrisiscenter.com
www.usdoj.gov/ndic

CHAPTER 4

Feeding and Nutrition

Sara S. Viessman, MD

Historically, as well as currently, the topic of feeding and nutrition has special importance in pediatrics because of the rapid growth and development of the pediatric patient, especially the infant. This rapid growth and development results in both quantitatively and qualitatively different nutritional needs than exist for the adult. Quantitatively, for example, newborns and young infants require more calories and more protein relative to body size than do older individuals. In a qualitative sense, for example, certain amino acids are essential for low-birth-weight and preterm infants but not for children or adults or even for normal term infants. Certain fats are essential for brain growth during the first few years of life but not thereafter.

Breast feeding clearly is the healthiest choice for most babies. We currently are aware of many nutritional, psychologic, and immunologic advantages of breastfeeding. Further advantages likely will be uncovered in years to come. Yet, not all young mothers have the necessary support and encouragement to even give breastfeeding a try! This is a current sociological and financial challenge in our country. It is estimated that if all babies were breastfed for the first 12 weeks of life, the savings recognized by the United States would be about $3 billion per year. If all mothers in the WIC program breastfed their babies for only 4 weeks, an estimated $30 million would be saved.

Malnutrition secondary to medical or socioeconomic conditions remains an important problem in infants and children in the United States. Self-inflicted malnutrition seen with eating disorders (or disordered eating) is increasingly prevalent. Obesity now is a common condition among children in the United States. At both ends of this spectrum, children are at risk for serious long-term medical and psychologic problems.

Although specific nutritional deficiencies, except for iron deficiency, are uncommon in developed countries, deficiencies of vitamins or protein remain a major problem among children in developing countries.

Questions

DIRECTIONS: Each of the numbered items or incomplete statements in this section is followed by answers or by completions of the statement. Select the ONE lettered answer or completion that is BEST in each case.

1. The recommended daily dietary allowance of vitamin A for an infant is

   (A) 50 µg (160 IU)
   (B) 100 µg (320 IU)
   (C) 200 µg (650 IU)
   (D) 400 µg (1300 IU)
   (E) 1000 µg (3300 IU)

2. Parents appear in your office to discuss their considerations for adopting their 11-month-old foster son. They state he has a history of failure to thrive at 6 months of age and they are concerned about the possibility of long-term problems. You inform them undernutrition in the first year of life

   (A) has no permanent effect on physical growth or development of intelligence
   (B) can have permanent effects on physical growth but not on development of intelligence
   (C) can have permanent effects on development of intelligence but not on physical growth
   (D) can have permanent effects on both physical growth and development of intelligence
   (E) can have permanent effects on both physical growth and development of intelligence, but only if coupled with psychosocial deprivation

3. It generally is recommended that *beikost* (infant foods other than milk) be introduced into the infant's diet at about

   (A) 3 weeks
   (B) 6 weeks
   (C) 3 months
   (D) 6 months
   (E) 1 year

4. The administration of parenteral vitamin K is indicated for

   (A) all newborn infants
   (B) infants below 2500 g
   (C) infants of less than 36 weeks' gestation
   (D) jaundiced infants
   (E) infants born outside of hospital

5. A 10-week-old child weighing 5 kg is being fed commercial infant formula. The mother is concerned she is underfeeding her baby. You tell her that, to satisfy both his fluid and caloric requirements, the daily intake ought to be at least

   (A) 12 oz
   (B) 18 oz
   (C) 28 oz
   (D) 36 oz
   (E) 48 oz

6. Which of the following statements concerning vitamin K is most accurate?

(A) The vitamin K content of breast milk is about a third that of cow milk.

(B) The vitamin K content of cow milk is about a third that of breast milk.

(C) The amounts of vitamin K in cow milk and in breast milk are about the same and are adequate for most infants who have received parenteral vitamin K as newborns.

(D) Neither cow milk nor breast milk contains adequate amounts of vitamin K even for infants who received parenteral vitamin K as newborns.

(E) There is no vitamin K in either breast milk or cow milk.

7. The recommended daily dietary allowance of vitamin D for an infant is

(A) 2.5 µg (100 IU)
(B) 10 µg (400 IU)
(C) 20 µg (800 IU)
(D) 40 µg (1600 IU)
(E) 100 µg (4000 IU)

8. A pregnant woman plans to breast-feed her baby. She has read of the nutritional, psychologic, and immunologic advantages but recalled breast-fed babies might still require vitamin supplementation. You recommend she supplement the baby's nutrition with

(A) vitamin A
(B) vitamin E
(C) vitamin C
(D) vitamin B_1
(E) vitamin D

9. The recommended daily intake of protein for optimal growth during the first 6 months of life is about

(A) 0.2 g/kg
(B) 1.0 g/kg
(C) 2.0 g/kg
(D) 5.0 g/kg
(E) 10.0 g/kg

10. The recommended daily intake of dietary protein for optimal growth at the age of 10 years is about

(A) 0.2 g/kg
(B) 0.5 g/kg
(C) 1.0 g/kg
(D) 2.0 g/kg
(E) 3.0 g/kg

11. An 8-month-old female is hospitalized for failure to thrive. She has a 1-day history of fever and cough. On physical examination, you observe a very thin, well-hydrated alert infant in no acute distress. You perform limited laboratory work and order a chest x-ray for further evaluation of a 1-day history of fever and cough. You note the lung fields to be normal but also note an absence of a thymic shadow. You should

(A) obtain an immunology consult
(B) order genetic karyotyping
(C) repeat the chest x-ray in 24 h
(D) order a cardiac ultrasound
(E) feed the infant as tolerated, following weight and intake closely

12. The calcium requirement for a school-age child is in the order of

(A) 0.1 g per day
(B) 1.0 g per day
(C) 10.0 g per day
(D) 50.0 g per day
(E) 100 g per day

13. Vitamin B_{12} deficiency is most likely to occur in a child with

(A) resection of the jejunum
(B) resection of the ileum
(C) resection of the colon
(D) a colostomy
(E) a gastrojejunostomy

14. Folic acid deficiency is most likely to occur in a child with

    (A) malabsorptive disease of the small intestines
    (B) hemangioma of the ileum
    (C) a rectal polyp
    (D) a gastrostomy
    (E) gastroesophageal reflux

15. A strict vegan diet (a diet excluding all animal products, even eggs, milk, and milk products, as well as meats and fish) for a young child is likely to be deficient in

    (A) vitamin C
    (B) vitamin E
    (C) vitamin B_1
    (D) vitamin B_{12}
    (E) vitamin A

16. At a 2-month well child visit, a mother states her family has a history of milk-protein allergies and wonders if soy-protein formula would be better for her baby. Which of the following statements regarding soy-protein formula is correct?

    (A) Infants fed exclusively with soy-protein formula display growth comparable to infants fed cow milk-protein formula.
    (B) The protein in soy-protein formulas is essentially nonallergenic, and clinically significant soy-protein hypersensitivity is extremely rare.
    (C) Soy-protein formula is most useful in children with well-documented, severe, gastrointestinal allergic reactions to cow milk-protein.
    (D) Soy-protein formula should not be used by patients with a family history of celiac disease.
    (E) Infants fed soy-protein formula should receive supplemental dietary calcium.

17. Recent concerns about the prevention of atherosclerotic heart disease have led to recommendations for reducing the fat content, and particularly the cholesterol content, of the diet early in life. This can include the use of skim

milk. It is recommended that the use of skim milk begin no earlier than age

    (A) 4 months
    (B) 6 months
    (C) 1 year
    (D) 2 years
    (E) 5 years

18. A 12-year-old female presents for her well child visit with no complaints. However, she is concerned about her friend who counts calories and seems to be losing too much weight. During a discussion about this issue, you tell her that the recommended energy intake for a 12-year-old female is

    (A) 1500 kcal per day
    (B) 1800 kcal per day
    (C) 2200 kcal per day
    (D) 2600 kcal per day
    (E) 3000 kcal per day

19. Of the following, the best source of vitamin C is

    (A) peanuts
    (B) potatoes
    (C) whole eggs
    (D) dark green vegetables
    (E) soybeans

20. Breastfeeding of infants in the United States is contraindicated in which of the following situations?

    (A) an infant whose mother is seropositive for HIV antibody
    (B) an infant whose mother is seropositive for hepatitis B surface antigen
    (C) an infant whose mother is seropositive for hepatitis C antibody
    (D) an infant whose mother was recently immunized for rubella
    (E) an infant whose mother was recently immunized for hepatitis B

21. A new mother presents for her baby's 2-week well child visit with concerns that she may not be able to continue breastfeeding her baby. She

states her nipples are very sore and cracked. You inquire about her feeding techniques and discover she nurses her baby about 20–25 min on each breast each feeding. You encourage her and inform her that the optimal time a baby should nurse on each breast is

(A) 40–50 min
(B) 30–40 min
(C) 20–30 min
(D) 10–20 min
(E) 5–10 min

22. A mother is concerned because her 20-month-old son prefers to eat with his fingers rather than use a small spoon. Which of the following statements is correct?

(A) At 18 months of age, most toddlers prefer to feed themselves with a spoon.
(B) Most children learn to feed themselves independently during the second year of life.
(C) Self spoon feeding usually begins at 12 months of age when well-defined wrist rotation develops.
(D) Most children can manage a cup by 10 months of age.
(E) Most children prefer to feed themselves with a spoon by 12 months of age.

23. You are following a child with ADHD. His teacher requests information on diet and ADHD. In particular, she is interested in the role of ingestion of sugar in this condition. Which of the following statements is true regarding controlled studies of the effects of sucrose ingestion in children?

(A) Sucrose ingestion has been linked to problem behavior in children with ADHD.
(B) Sucrose ingestion has been linked to increased motor activity in children with ADHD.
(C) Sucrose ingestion is associated with an increase in both motor activity and problem behavior in children with ADHD.
(D) Sucrose ingestion is not associated with problem behavior or increased motor activity in children.
(E) Sucrose ingestion is associated with decreased motor activity in children.

24. Which of the following represents the greatest percentage of calories in human breast milk?

(A) carbohydrate
(B) protein
(C) fat
(D) cholesterol
(E) whey

25. Which of the following represents the greatest percentage of calories in unmodified cow milk?

(A) carbohydrate
(B) protein
(C) fat
(D) cholesterol
(E) whey

26. Which of the following represents the greatest percentage of calories in skim milk?

(A) carbohydrate
(B) protein
(C) fat
(D) cholesterol
(E) whey

27. Which of the following accounts for the greatest percentage of calories in the normal diet of the school-age child?

(A) carbohydrate
(B) protein
(C) fat
(D) cholesterol
(E) whey

28. A serious dietary concern regarding a 2-year-old who drinks six bottles of apple juice per day is

    (A) an inadequate protein intake
    (B) development of diabetes mellitus
    (C) vitamin C deficiency
    (D) vitamin A toxicity
    (E) development of diarrhea

29. The number of primary teeth that generally erupt in children by 3 years of age is

    (A) 4
    (B) 8
    (C) 12
    (D) 16
    (E) 20

30. A 5-month-old male presents with poor weight gain. His diet consists only of goat milk. On examination, he appears tired and is mildly tachycardic. The lab value most likely to be elevated is

    (A) serum albumin
    (B) red blood cell mean corpuscular volume
    (C) hemoglobin
    (D) serum vitamin B_{12} level
    (E) serum sodium

31. A 7-year-old male presents for a well child visit. You note his height at 75th percentile and weight at >95th percentile for age. His examination is otherwise normal. His father is overweight but his mother is thin. The most appropriate next step for you to take is

    (A) obtain T4 and TSH levels
    (B) order serum chromosomes
    (C) refer to an endocrinologist
    (D) place on a diet of 75% of caloric needs for height
    (E) counsel the family on increasing exercise and eliminating target foods from diet

32. The most accurate method for assessing adiposity in the office setting is

    (A) measurement of weight
    (B) calculation of percent above ideal body weight for height using age/sex norms
    (C) calculation of body mass index (weight/height^2)
    (D) measurement of subcutaneous fat thickness
    (E) use of densitometry

33. An 18-month-old Hispanic male presents for a well child check. His parents report he drinks seven to eight bottles of cow milk each day and doesn't like solid foods. His weight is greater than the 95th percentile while height and head circumference are at the 25th percentile. His heart rate is 180 bpm. On examination, you find a chubby, happy, pale, and otherwise normal baby. Which of the following tests most likely will be abnormal?

    (A) sweat test
    (B) serum sodium
    (C) eosinophil count
    (D) serum bicarbonate
    (E) hemoglobin

34. A 2-year-old White male presents with failure to thrive, chronic diarrhea, and recurrent pneumonia. Though his family history is negative for cystic fibrosis, a sweat test reveals a sodium concentration of 120 mg/dL. You should start

    (A) iron
    (B) vitamin B_{12} and folic acid
    (C) pancreatic enzyme supplementation
    (D) copper and magnesium
    (E) parenteral diuretics

35. A 15-year-old White female presents with the complaint that she is always cold. She has no history of illness, but she has not had a period for 4 months. Her mother states she is worried because although her daughter intermittently eats a large amount of food, she seems to be losing weight. On examination, the patient is extremely thin for her age. Which of the following is most likely?

(A) She feels she is too thin, but likes it that way.

(B) She feels she is too thin, and would like to gain weight.

(C) She feels she is too fat, and wants to lose weight.

(D) She feels she is too fat, but likes it that way.

(E) She feels she is normal.

36. A 3-month-old White female is brought to you for cold symptoms. On examination, you note her head circumference is at the 50th percentile, her length at the 25th percentile, and her weight less than the 5th percentile. She appears alert but very thin. She has skin folds on her arms, thighs, and buttocks. Parents state she drinks four 8 oz bottles of premixed formula each day. You feed the baby and she quickly drinks 7 oz. You decide to admit the infant. How many calories will she likely need for weight gain?

(A) 60 kcal/kg per day

(B) 80 kcal/kg per day

(C) 100 kcal/kg per day

(D) 150 kcal/kg per day

(E) 200 kcal/kg per day

Answers and Explanations

1. **(D)** The recommended daily allowance of retinol (vitamin A) for an infant is 375–400 µg (about 1200–1300 IU). Insufficient amounts of vitamin A can lead to visual problems, poor growth, and impaired resistance to infection. Excessive amounts can be just as dangerous as insufficient amounts. Signs of hypervitaminosis A include anorexia, hepatosplenomegaly, and increased intracranial pressure. *(McMillan: 471–472)*

2. **(D)** Serious undernutrition during the first year of life can have deleterious and permanent effects on both mental and physical growth and development. This appears to be an organic effect independent of psychosocial deprivation, although exogenous undernutrition often is compounded by such deprivation. In follow-up, a high frequency of behavior problems and learning difficulties is found, despite adequate weight gain. The recognition of possible permanent effects of malnutrition during infancy and early childhood has led to increased efforts to avoid such undernutrition both in otherwise healthy children and those with chronic disease. *(NEJM 282:933–939, 1970; McMillan:755)*

3. **(D)** It is recommended that the introduction of nonmilk foods (beikost) be delayed until the age of 4–6 months. One stated reason for this is the low intestinal concentration of pancreatic amylase early in life and the desire to avoid the ingestion of starches. The most compelling reason, however, relates to developmental readiness such as disappearance of tongue thrust, acquisition of head control, and ability to sit with support. Admittedly, it often is difficult to convince parents to refrain from introducing

solids at an earlier age. *(McMillan:477; Pediatrics 63:52–59, 1979)*

4. **(A)** Vitamin K is essential for hepatic synthesis of prothrombin (factor II) as well as factors VII, IX, and X. Plasma prothrombin concentrations are low at birth and fall still lower during the first 3 days of life. The parenteral administration of vitamin K to the newborn prevents the postnatal fall in concentration of these factors and thereby prevents hemorrhagic disease of the newborn. It is indicated prophylactically for all newborn infants. Several oral doses of vitamin K may be equally effective and are a feasible alternative for babies born in developing countries. [*Note*: Although answers (B), (C), (D), and (E) are true, the BEST answer is (A).] *(McMillan:367)*

5. **(C)** Be careful here! An infant's fluid requirements are 120–140 mL/kg per day. Yet, to get sufficient calories, an infant must take in 150–180 mL/kg per day. Therefore, this 10-week-old infant (estimated at 5-kg weight) requires 600–700 mL (20–23 oz) of fluid per day. Her caloric requirement is 500–600 calories per day. Most milks (human and cow) and prepared formulas contain 20 cal/oz. Therefore, it would take 25–30 oz of milk or formula to provide the 500–600 calories required each day. *(McMillan:754)*

6. **(A)** Although the vitamin K content of breast milk is only a third that of cow milk, clinical deficiency is rare in normal infants fed either type of milk provided they received prophylactic vitamin K parenterally at birth. The vitamin K in breast milk can be better absorbed than that in cow milk. So, it evens out. Remember, enteric bacteria are an important additional source of

vitamin K. [*Note:* Beware of answers with two parts. Here, the word "and" is the tip-off. Response (C) is only half-true. Although the amount of vitamin K in each milk is adequate, the amounts are not equal.] *(McMillan:367)*

7. **(B)** The recommended daily allowance of vitamin D for an infant is 10 µg or 400 IU. Unfortunately, some texts and some examinations use micrograms (µg) and others use international units (IU) when referring to vitamins. Most now use the preferred term "recomended daily allowance" rather than the expression "minimal daily requirement," acknowledging that we really do not know the minimal requirement. Too much vitamin D can be toxic and just as dangerous as too little. The major target organ of vitamin D poisoning is the kidney. *(McMillan:471, 474)*

8. **(E)** Formulas are fortified with the necessary vitamins and minerals, at least to the best of our current knowledge. Breast milk contains quantitatively small amounts of vitamin D. However, this is sufficient for most babies. Exclusively breast-fed infants who are at risk for vitamin D deficiency include infants with inadequate maternal intake of vitamin D, infants with inadequate sunlight exposure (e.g., dark skin pigmentation, cold climates, urban environments, clothing practices), and older infants still exclusively breast-fed. Therefore, vitamin D supplementation is recommended for most babies who are exclusively breast-fed. *(McMillan:477; AAP Nutrition Handbook:275)*

9. **(C)** The minimum dietary requirement of high-quality protein in early infancy has been estimated at 1.9 g/kg. The recommended daily allowance is 2.2 g/kg. Insufficient protein intake leads to poor growth, hypoproteinemic edema, and other changes. Excessive intake can result in metabolic acidosis, lethargy, and poor feeding. *(McMillan:472)*

10. **(C)** As the child gets older, growth slows and protein requirement falls. By the age of 10 years, the minimum daily protein requirement has fallen to 1 g/kg of body weight, with a recommended daily allowance of 1.2 g/kg. This amount is easily provided by most ordinary American diets. However, in some strict vegan diets, fad diets, or severe low-calorie diets, even this modest amount of protein requirement is not provided. *(McMillan:472)*

11. **(E)** The thymus dramatically decreases in size during periods of undernutrition. Therefore, it is not uncommon to see loss of thymic shadow on the chest x-ray of infants admitted for failure to thrive. Involution of the thymus during starvation accounts for some of the increased suscepti-bility to infection in these children. The combination of thymic dysplasia and failure to thrive could bring to mind DiGeorge anomaly (or DiGeorge syndrome). These infants, however, typically present with cardiac disease or symptoms related to abnormal calcium metabolism during early infancy. *(McMillan: 2099; Pediatrics 59:490–494, 1977)*

12. **(B)** The multiplicity of factors affecting calcium metabolism, not the least of which is the effect of other dietary factors, makes it difficult to give an exact figure for the daily requirement of calcium. For a school-age child it is estimated to be about 1 g per day. (Contrast this with the amount of protein required which for this age group is about 1 g/kg of body weight per day!). This amount of calcium is easily provided by most ordinary diets, and calcium supplementation usually is not necessary, even for the child who drinks little or no milk. Eggs, molasses, nuts, and many fish and vegetables are good sources of calcium. A variety of products (specific brands of cereal, bread, orange juice, and even ice cream) are fortified with added calcium. *(McMillan:472)*

13. **(B)** Vitamin B_{12} is absorbed primarily in the distal portion of the ileum. Vitamin B_{12} deficiency can occur in children who have undergone surgical removal of this portion of the bowel or in children with inflammatory disease involving the distal portion of the ileum. In the former case, deficiency is severe and permanent; in the latter situation, deficiency is mild and often transient. Children who have had surgical removal of the distal ileum should receive prophylactic vitamin B_{12}. *(Rudolph AM:465–466)*

14. **(A)** Folic acid is absorbed primarily in the small intestine. Deficiency is seen commonly in chronic diarrhea and malabsorptive states involving the small bowel. Hypersegmentation of neutrophil nuclei on a peripheral blood smear is usually the first abnormality and is a useful aid to early diagnosis. Folic acid deficiency is not associated with any of the other conditions listed. *(Rudolph AM:541–542)*

15. **(D)** A vegan or strict vegetarian diet provides almost no vitamin B_{12} as well as marginal levels of calcium, vitamin D, and iron. The relatively low caloric density of vegetables also means that a large bulk of food must be ingested to provide adequate calories. However, the content of vitamins other than B_{12} and D is apt to be adequate. *(Pediatrics 70:582–586, 1982)*

16. **(A)** Soy-protein-based commercial infant formulas presently available provide adequate nutrition (including calcium), and infants fed these formulas exhibit normal growth. Soy formulas often are prescribed for infants with personal or family history of allergy in the hope of avoiding the development of milk-protein allergy. Unfortunately, severe gastrointestinal allergic reactions to soy-protein in infants are well recognized and not rare. For this reason, soy-protein formula is not recommended for infants or children already demonstrating significant gastrointestinal hypersensitivity to cow milk-protein. These patients are best prescribed a protein hydrolysate formula. Soy-based formulas are not recommended for premature infants. *(Pediatrics 72:359–363, 1983; AAP Nutrition Handbook:158, 469)*

17. **(D)** Skim milk is essentially free of all fat. If it is used at a time when the infant receives most or all of his calories from milk, this could lead to essential fatty acid deficiency. Fats, especially saturated fats, are essential for myelinization and brain growth. Additionally, since skim milk contains only 10 cal/oz, the infant would need to consume twice the volume in order to obtain sufficient calories. [*Note*: There is a difference between skim milk and low-fat milks. The former has zero fat, whereas the latter has 1/2–2% fat. Two percent fat milk would be permissible

at an earlier age than skim milk. The question specified skim milk.] *(Pediatrics72: 253–255, 1983; McMillan:607)*

18. **(C)** From 11 to 18 years of age, the recommended calorie intake for females remains 2200 kcal per day. For males, the recommended energy intake at 11 years of age is 2500 kcal per day and increases steadily to 3000 kcal per day by 15–18 years of age. *(McMillan:470, 817–818)*

19. **(B)** Potatoes, tomatoes, and cabbage join citrus fruits as good sources of vitamin C. Additionally, breast milk is an excellent dietary source for vitamin C. *(McMillan:474)*

20. **(A)** The human immunodeficiency virus can be transmitted from mother to baby via breastfeeding. In the United States, where other means of infant nutrition are readily available, HIV infected women should be advised not to feed their breast milk to babies. According to WHO recommendations, in developing countries, the risk of HIV transmission from breastfeeding must be weighed against the risk of the replacement feeding. Although hepatitis B surface antigen has been detected in breast milk, studies indicate this does not significantly increase the risk of transmission of hepatitis among breast-fed infants. Transmission of hepatitis C virus via breastfeeding is theoretically possible but not clinically documented in anti-HCV-positive, antihuman immunodeficiency virus (HIV)-negative women. *(2003 Red Book:119)*

21. **(E)** Normal infants will ingest most of the available milk from a breast within 3–5 min. Additional sucking stimulates future milk production, which is necessary for continued successful breastfeeding. Prolonged nursing, especially during the first few weeks, can result in extremely sore or cracked nipples, which can result in early cessation of breastfeeding. *(McMillan:473)*

22. **(B)** Children do learn to feed themselves independently during the second year of life. However, this will not necessarily include the use of utensils. Holding and manipulating a spoon to scoop food and then bring it to the mouth

requires complex development. Most 2-year-old children are *able* to use a spoon to feed themselves, but many still *prefer* to use their fingers. (*AAP Nutrition Handbook:126*)

23. **(D)** Despite public belief, sucrose alone has not been determined to be a cause of problem behavior or increasing hyperactivity in children. Controlled, double blind studies have not shown a difference in behavior measures, motor activity, or cognitive performance of children receiving sucrose compared to those receiving a control substance. (*NEJM 330:301–307, 1994*)

24. **(C)** Fat yields about 9 cal/g, whereas protein and carbohydrate yield only 4 cal/g. More than 50% of the calories in human breast milk are in the form of fat. Of all mammals known, seals have the richest fat content in their milk, which is the consistency of mayonnaise. The milk of seals contains 12–20 times more fat than human milk. This allows short lactation times and high pup growth rates. While human infants will double their birth weight by 2 months of age, seal pups quadruple their birth weight by 2 weeks of age. (*McMillan:478; Miller:40*)

25. **(C)** Fat also accounts for about half of the calories in unmodified cow milk. However, cow milk contains significantly higher amounts of protein. Protein accounts for 22% of calories in cow milk and only 8% of calories in human breast milk. Of note, the protein nitrogen concentration in the ileocecal contents of 1–5-month-old infants fed cow milk formula is three times higher than that found in infants fed breast milk. (*McMillan:478; AAP Nutrition Handbook:99*)

26. **(A)** Skim milk is essentially free of fat. About 60% of the calories are provided as carbohydrate, and the other 40% as protein. (*Pediatrics 72:253–255, 1983*)

27. **(A)** Carbohydrates are the major source of calories in the normal diet throughout life except in the newborn period, when more than half of ingested calories are derived from fat. Excessive carbohydrate intake usually results in obesity. Inadequate intake results in caloric deprivation

and undernutrition rather than any specific deficiency syndrome. (*McMillan:478*)

28. **(A)** Fruit juice is almost pure carbohydrate, mostly sugar rather than starch. Less than 5% of the calories are derived from protein and fat. Excessive intake of fruit juices by a young infant can result in inadequate protein intake despite adequate total calories. (*AAP Nutrition Handbook: 47:131*)

29. **(E)** Twenty primary teeth usually erupt in children during the first 3 years of life. This process begins at about 4–6 months of age. Eruption usually is symmetric and tends to occur in the mandibular arch just ahead of the maxillary arch. (*McMillan:642*)

30. **(B)** Infants fed primarily goat milk are at risk to develop a megaloblastic anemia from folate deficiency. Therefore, the MCV will be elevated. The metabolism of folic acid and vitamin B$_{12}$ is interrelated. Hematologic problems caused by a deficiency in one can be improved with supplementation of either. The neurologic complications of vitamin B$_{12}$ deficiency, however, will not be improved with treatment with folic acid. Therefore, it is important to carefully sort the child's deficiencies. Large doses of folic acid should not be given until vitamin B$_{12}$ deficiency has been excluded. (*McMillan:1449*)

31. **(E)** Childhood obesity is a growing problem in the United States. It is estimated that 20–25% of children in the US are obese. Obesity places these children at risk for lifelong health problems, psychologic issues, and discrimination. There will be an underlying definable cause in less than 5% of children with obesity. This child's adequate linear growth and family history along with an otherwise normal physical examination suggest no further workup is necessary. It generally is not recommended to severely restrict calories in a child who is overweight. The best outcome for an obese child includes a plan that involves the entire family's eating habits and physical activity. It is important to increase the physical activity of the child. This needs to be tailored to the child's interests and should take into account the activities readily available.

Clearly, this requires commitment on the part of the family, child, and practitioner. *(Rudolph AM:12–16)*

32. (D) Although all of the mentioned methods have roles in the assessment of obesity, the best office-based measurement of adiposity is the use of skin-fold measurements. Measuring weight alone does not allow for various size body frames. Using weight for height or body mass index is efficient but does not take into account the variation in lean body mass. *(Rudolph AM:12)*

33. (E) Milk contains very little iron, only about 1.2 mg/L. The average infant requires 1–1.5 mg/kg of iron daily. A diet almost exclusively of milk is a common cause of iron deficiency anemia in the older infant and the toddler. This is especially true when the milk is unmodified cow milk. The iron in cow milk is less well absorbed than that in breast milk. Also, a large intake of unmodified cow milk often is associated with microscopic gastrointestinal blood loss. Cow milk, of course, contains adequate amounts of protein and is fortified with additional vitamin D, so the child described would not be at risk for either hypoproteinemia or rickets. *(McMillan: 1447–1448)*

34. (C) This child presents with cystic fibrosis—the most common genetically transmitted lethal disease among Whites (1/3300). This multisystem disease leads to pancreatic insufficiency in about 85% of patients. This causes fat malabsorption with resultant malabsorption of the fat-soluble vitamins (ADEK). Therefore, all CF patients should receive pancreatic enzyme supplementation. CF patients also are at risk for iron deficiency anemia. Only when anemia or low serum ferritin levels are documented should they receive iron supplementation. *(McMillan:1253; Rudolph AM:717–719)*

35. (C) Adolescents with anorexia nervosa typically perceive themselves as too fat and hope to lose weight, even in the face of emaciation. The degree of distortion of their body image corresponds to the difficulty encountered in treating the patients. This adolescent with anorexia nervosa seems, by history, to have difficulty with bingeing. Because her weight is low for her age, she is likely purging with self-induced vomiting. Therefore, she would be classified as anorexia nervosa, bulimic type. *(McMillan:814–818)*

36. (D) In healthy infants, the nutritional requirements average 100 kcal/kg per day. However, infants who are failing to thrive most often will need more than 100 kcal/kg per day to gain weight. Their intake requirements typically are as much as 50% higher than normal, or 150 kcal/kg per day. *(McMillan:754–755)*

BIBLIOGRAPHY

American Academy of Pediatrics Committee on Nutrition. Use of whole cow milk in infancy. *Pediatrics* 1983;72:253–255.

American Academy of Pediatrics Committee on Nutrition. Soy-protein formulas: recommendations for use in infant feeding. *Pediatrics* 1983;72:359–363.

American Academy of Pediatrics. *Pediatric Nutrition Handbook*, 4th ed. Elk Grove, IL: American Academy of Pediatrics, 1998.

American Academy of Pediatrics. *2003 Red Book, Report of the Committee on Infectious Diseases*, 26th ed. Elk Grove, IL: American Academy of Pediatrics, 2003.

Chase PH, Martin HP. Undernutrition and child development. *N Engl J Med* 1970;282:933–939.

Fomon SJ, Filer LJ, Anderson TA, et al. Recommendations for feeding normal infants. *Pediatrics* 1979;63:52–59.

Katz M, Stiehm ER. Host defenses in malnutrition. *Pediatrics* 1977;59:490–494.

Miller D. *Seals & Sea Lions*. Stillwater, MN: Voyager Press Inc., 1998.

McMillan JA, DeAngelis CD, Feigin RD, Warshaw JB. *Oski's Pediatrics, Principles & Practice*, 3rd ed. Philadelphia, PA: JB Lippincott, 1999.

Rudolph AM, Kamei RK, Overby KJ. *Rudolph's Fundamentals of Pediatrics*, 3rd ed. New York, NY: McGraw-Hill, 2002.

Shinwell ED, Gorodischer R. Totally vegetarian diets and infant nutrition. *Pediatrics* 1982;70: 582–586.

Wolraich ML, Lindgren SD, Stumbo PJ, et al. Effects of diets high in sucrose or aspartamine on the behavior and cognitive performance of children. *N Engl J Med* 1994;330:301–307.

CHAPTER 5

Fluids, Electrolytes, and Metabolic Disorders

R. Blaine Easley, MD
Jeffrey G. Michael, DO
Z. Leah Harris, MD

Fluid and electrolyte abnormalities are common problems in the pediatric population. These disturbances occur secondary to disease (e.g., pyloric stenosis, diarrhea, vomiting, diabetic ketoacidosis), therapeutic interventions (e.g., diuretics), and environmental factors (e.g., diluting of infant formula, hyperthermia, poisonings). Specific metabolic derangements are more commonly associated with certain age groups. For instance, neonates frequently experience hypoglycemia, hyponatremia and hypocalcemia non-specifically with illnesses. Older infants and young children commonly develop dehydration and/or electrolyte abnormalities from gastroenteritis.

Such acquired metabolic abnormalities are clinically and academically relevant and deserve a careful comprehensive review.

While acquired metabolic problems are common in pediatrics, genetic inborn errors of metabolism are rare. Inborn errors of metabolism are relatively unique to pediatrics in their presentation and management. Because of this, these metabolic abnormalities are well reviewed in many texts and are well tested on examinations. This section will attempt to focus the material and to review the more commonly encountered defects in each area of metabolism (e.g., carbohydrates, amino acids, lipids).

Questions

DIRECTIONS (Questions 1 through 34): Each of the numbered items or incomplete statements in this section is followed by answers or by completions of the statement. Select the ONE lettered answer or completion that is BEST in each case.

1. What is the approximate daily fluid requirement for an infant who weighs 3 kg?

   (A) 900 mL
   (B) 700 mL
   (C) 500 mL
   (D) 300 mL
   (E) 100 mL

2. What is the approximate daily fluid requirement of a 30-kg child?

   (A) 3000 mL
   (B) 2400 mL
   (C) 1700 mL
   (D) 1200 mL
   (E) 1000 mL

3. What is the hourly fluid rate for a 15-kg child requiring twice daily maintenance?

   (A) 125 mL/h
   (B) 105 mL/h
   (C) 95 mL/h
   (D) 70 mL/h
   (E) 60 mL/h

4. What is the approximate hourly fluid rate needed to meet maintenance fluid requirements of a 50-kg child?

   (A) 125 mL/h
   (B) 115 mL/h
   (C) 100 mL/h
   (D) 90 mL/h
   (E) 80 mL/h

5. An infant presents with a weight of 8 kg and a 3-day history of diarrhea and vomiting. He appears severely dehydrated with decreased sensorium, sunken fontanelle, poor skin turgor, and decreased urine output. The fluid deficit of this child is approximately

   (A) 1900–2000 mL
   (B) 1300–1500 mL
   (C) 900–1100 mL
   (D) 400–500 mL
   (E) 200–250 mL

6. Normal serum osmolality is between

   (A) 330 and 350 mOsm/L
   (B) 315 and 325 mOsm/L
   (C) 300 and 310 mOsm/L
   (D) 285 and 295 mOsm/L
   (E) 250 and 260 mOsm/L

7. A child with diabetic ketoacidosis has the following serum values: glucose 500 mg/dL; Na^+ 126 meq/L; K^+ 4 meq/L; Cl^- 80 meq/L; BUN 16 mg/dL; and HCO_3^- 6 meq/L. The patient's serum osmolality is approximately

   (A) 285 mOsm/L
   (B) 295 mOsm/L
   (C) 310 mOsm/L

(D) 270 mOsm/L

(E) 260 mOsm/L

8. An infant with diarrhea is 10% dehydrated. Before the onset of illness, the weight was 5 kg and the surface area 0.3 m². The child's serum sodium concentration is normal. Assuming the child will not be fed and the diarrhea ceases, what is the approximate total amount of fluid you should deliver to meet maintenance needs and restore the child to a state of normal hydration in the first 24 h?

(A) 750 mL

(B) 1000 mL

(C) 1250 mL

(D) 1500 mL

(E) 1750 mL

9. A 6-year-old girl has vomiting, headache, and irritability. She does not appear dehydrated. But when reviewing her vitals you notice her weight is up 3 kg from just 3 weeks ago. Laboratory findings are: Na^+ 112 meq/L; K^+ 4.0 meq/L; Cl^- 75 meq/L; HCO_3^- 19 meq/L; BUN 10 mg/dL; and creatinine 0.4 mg/dL. A spot urine sodium concentration is 100 meq/L. The most likely cause of these findings is

(A) decreased glucocorticoid production

(B) decreased mineralcorticoid production

(C) increased oral intake of water

(D) decreased antidiuretic hormone secretion

(E) increased antidiuretic hormone secretion

10. A 10-month-old male infant had multiple episodes of vomiting and diarrhea over the last 24 h. The infant now has slightly sunken eyes, mildly decreased activity, and dry skin. Vital signs are stable. Which of the following is the generally preferred method for rehydration for this patient?

(A) oral administration of a solution containing 75 meq/L of sodium and 5 g/dL of glucose

(B) oral administration of a solution containing 50 meq/L of sodium and 2 g/dL of glucose

(C) oral administration of a solution containing 35 meq/L of sodium and 10 g/dL of glucose

(D) intravenous administration of a solution containing 154 meq/L of sodium and 5 g/dL of glucose

(E) intravenous administration of a solution containing 35 meq/L of sodium and 10 g/dL of glucose

11. A 16-year-old male is brought to the ER by his friends. They relate they were drinking alcohol and that their friend "passed out" about 2 h ago and is increasingly difficult to arouse. Which of the following is MOST useful in your immediate management of this patient?

(A) serum sodium

(B) serum glucose

(C) blood alcohol level

(D) serum calcium

(E) serum drug screen

12. Individuals with homocystinuria (type I) are at higher risk than the general population for

(A) thromboembolic events

(B) arthritis

(C) hypoglycemia

(D) hyperglycemia

(E) renal tubular acidosis

13. Which of the glycogen storage diseases has the worst prognosis?

(A) type Ia (Von Gierke disease)

(B) type Ib (glucose-6-phosphatase microsomal transport defect)

(C) type II (Pompe disease)

(D) type III (debranching enzyme deficiency)

(E) type IV (branch enzyme deficiency)

14. Tyrosinemia type I is caused by a defect of what enzyme?

(A) tyrosine aminotransferase

(B) phenylalanine hydroxylase

(C) fumarylacetoacetate hydrolase

(D) malylacetoacetate isomerase

(E) carbinolamine dehydratase

15. Alcaptonuria is a metabolic disease caused by a defect in or lack of homogentisic acid oxidase which leads to

    (A) kinky hair
    (B) absent patella
    (C) black urine and darkly pigmented sclera, cornea, and ears
    (D) blue sclera
    (E) absent radii

16. Death from tyrosinemia type I is primarily related to

    (A) renal failure
    (B) hepatic failure
    (C) diabetes
    (D) respiratory failure
    (E) infection

17. Subluxation of the ocular lens (ectopia lentis) generally occurs after 3 years of age in children with

    (A) hawkinsinuria
    (B) tyrosinemia
    (C) phenylketonuria
    (D) isovaleric acidemia
    (E) homocystinuria

18. Daily maintenance fluid for a 16-kg afebrile toddler is approximately

    (A) 1000 mL
    (B) 1200 mL
    (C) 1300 mL
    (D) 1400 mL
    (E) 1500 mL

19. With regard to sodium content, which of the following intravenous fluids would be the maintenance fluid of choice for a 12-kg infant?

    (A) 0.9% NaCl
    (B) 0.2% NaCl
    (C) 0.45% NaCl
    (D) lasmalyte
    (E) Ringer lactate

20. A 15-kg toddler with group A coxsackievirus infection is refusing to drink. His serum potassium is normal. For maintenance intravenous fluids, what concentration of KCl should be added?

    (A) 5 meq KCl/L
    (B) 10 meq KCl/L
    (C) 25 meq KCl/L
    (D) 40 meq KCl/L
    (E) 50 meq KCl/L

21. A 15-month-old male presents with moderate dehydration. Resuscitation proceeds with assessment of airway, breathing, and circulation. An isotonic intravenous fluid bolus of 20 cc/kg is administered. Laboratory studies reveal a serum sodium of 165 meq/L and a normal serum potassium. The most appropriate plan for rehydration is

    (A) correct the hypernatremia over 8 h with 0.45% NS without maintenance potassium
    (B) correct the hypernatremia over 8 h with D_5W with maintenance potassium
    (C) correct the hypernatremia over 24–48 h with D_5 0.45% NS with maintenance potassium
    (D) correct the hypernatremia over 12 h with D_5 0.45% NS with maintenance potassium
    (E) correct the hypernatremia over 24–48 h with $D_{10}W$ without maintenance potassium

22. Pyruvate kinase deficiency is the most common glycolytic enzyme deficiency. Which of the following is a common clinical sign in neonatal presentation of this disorder?

    (A) sepsis
    (B) jaundice
    (C) hepatomegaly
    (D) hypertonia
    (E) seizures

23. The major clinical manifestation of Wilson disease in children 8–16 years of age is

(A) hepatic dysfunction

(B) cardiac failure

(C) thromboembolic event

(D) inflammatory bowel disease

(E) blindness

24. Galactokinase deficiency leads to the development of cataracts of the eye by early infancy. Dietary adjustments necessary for treatment and prevention include

(A) eliminating gluten

(B) providing low iron formula

(C) eliminating milk and milk products

(D) providing increased amounts of milk and milk products

(E) providing increased amounts of folate

25. Hurler disease is the most severe of which of the following groups of inherited diseases?

(A) glycogen storage diseases

(B) glycoproteinoses

(C) mucopolysaccharidoses

(D) sphingolipidoses

(E) mucolipidoses

26. Adrenoleukodystrophy (ALD) is an X-linked disorder leading to progressive neurologic deterioration and death. Which of the following substances is found in high plasma levels in this disorder?

(A) lead

(B) iron

(C) short chain fatty acids

(D) long chain fatty acids

(E) very long chain fatty acids

27. Pyruvate dehydrogenase complex deficiency is an autosomal recessive disease and leads to

(A) beta-hydroxybutyric acidosis

(B) acetoacetic acidosis

(C) lactic acidosis

(D) hydrochloric acidosis

(E) hypochloremic alkalosis

28. You are evaluating a 10-month-old infant for recurrent fractures following relatively minor trauma. You note deep blue sclera and bowing of the lower extremities. X-ray examination reveals generalized osteopenia. The child probably has

(A) achondroplasia

(B) histiocytosis X

(C) osteogenesis imperfecta

(D) osteopetrosis

(E) rickets

29. A 2-week-old infant has a 12-h history of recurrent episodes of bilious vomiting. A firm, tender abdomen is noted on physical examination. Flat plate of the abdomen demonstrates a large dilated loop of distended bowel consistent with midgut volvulus. Which of the following best corresponds with this patient's condition?

serum pH		serum electrolytes					
		$[Na^+]$ (meq/L)	$[K^+]$ (meq/L)	$[Cl^-]$ (meq/L)	$[HCO_3^-]$ (meq/L)	[BUN] (mg/dL)	[Cr] (mg/dL)
(A)	7.28	128	5.8	88	16	25	0.2
(B)	7.35	130	2.8	90	21	18	0.1
(C)	7.50	130	3.6	88	34	18	0.1
(D)	7.45	140	4.0	100	22	9	0.1
(E)	7.32	140	3.0	112	18	13	0.2

30. A 4-month-old male with failure to thrive ingests >175 cal/kg per day during 72 h of hospitalization, but does not gain weight. Laboratory values are serum Na^+ 138 meq/L, K^+ 3.5 meq/L, Cl^- 111 meq/L, HCO_3^- 12 meq/L, BUN 2 mg/dL, Cr 0.2 mg/dL, glucose 112 mg/dL; serum pH 7.30 and urine pH 8.0 (under oil). The serum phosphate level is 2.4 meq/L. The most likely condition of this infant is

(A) nonorganic failure to thrive

(B) congenital adrenal hyperplasia

(C) cystic fibrosis

(D) renal tubular acidosis

(E) diabetes insipidus

31. A 5-week-old male presents with poor feeding, poor growth, a peculiar odor, hypertonia, and hyperactive reflexes. He is afebrile. History reveals no problems with labor and delivery and early hospital discharge at 24 h of age. He has not seen a physician since that time. The most likely etiology of this infant's condition is

    (A) sepsis
    (B) pyloric stenosis
    (C) over feeding
    (D) phenylketonuria (PKU)
    (E) hypothyroidism

32. The most important part of management of the infant described above is to restrict consumption of

    (A) iron
    (B) complex carbohydrates
    (C) short chain fatty acids
    (D) phenylalanine
    (E) all proteins

33. In galactosemia, the enzyme most commonly deficient is

    (A) galactokinase
    (B) galactose-1-phosphate uridyl transferase
    (C) pyruvate dehydrogenase
    (D) galactose-1-phosphate dehydrogenase
    (E) uridyl diphosphogalactose-4-epimerase

34. A 6-week-old presents with a history of frequent, nonbilious vomiting, which the parents state "shoots clear across the room." Examination reveals a thin, alert baby. Gastric peristaltic waves are present as well as a small epigastric mass. Which of the following sets of electrolytes, with values in meq/L, is most consistent with this infant's probable condition?

    (A) Na^+ 142, K^+ 4.0, Cl^- 110, HCO_3^- 22
    (B) Na^+ 140, K^+ 3.8, Cl^- 96, HCO_3^- 22
    (C) Na^+ 138, K^+ 3.5, Cl^- 88, HCO_3^- 38
    (D) Na^+ 145, K^+ 2.5, Cl^- 110, HCO_3^- 30
    (E) Na^+ 128, K^+ 6.0, Cl^- 110, HCO_3^- 18

DIRECTIONS (Questions 35 through 46): Each case scenario has one to four associated questions. Read each question carefully and select the ONE lettered answer or completion that BEST fulfills the statement or question. To enhance your learning experience, answer all the questions regarding one case before looking at any of the answers and explanations.

Questions 35 through 37
A 5-month-old male infant, previously well, is admitted to the hospital following 2 days of severe diarrhea. There is no history of fever or vomiting. The infant has been fed unmodified cow milk, orange juice, tea, rice water, and plain water. The child is lethargic and dehydrated with sunken eyes, depressed fontanelle, dry mucous membranes, and poor skin turgor. Pulses are "thready," and capillary refill time is 4 s. BP is 70/30 mmHg, heart rate is 190 bpm, T is 102°F, weight is 6.3 kg. The remainder of the examination is within normal limits.

35. The child should immediately be given a rapid intravenous infusion (bolus) of what amount of normal saline?

    (A) 1 mL/kg
    (B) 5 mL/kg
    (C) 20 mL/kg
    (D) 50 mL/kg
    (E) 100 mL/kg

36. The initial intravenous fluid bolus given to this child should contain

    (A) 140 meq/L of sodium
    (B) 100 meq/L of sodium
    (C) 75 meq/L of sodium, D_5
    (D) 35 meq/L of sodium, D_5
    (E) no sodium, $D_{25}W$

37. This initial intravenous bolus should also contain

    (A) 60 meq/L of potassium
    (B) 40 meq/L of potassium
    (C) 20 meq/L of potassium
    (D) 10 meq/L of potassium
    (E) no potassium

Questions 38 through 41

A 1-week-old female infant was admitted because of vomiting, weight loss, and poor feeding. The infant weighed 2.8 kg at birth. Vomiting and poor feeding started the fourth day of life and loose stools were a problem since birth. The infant was fed a standard prepared cow milk formula. On examination, the child was found to be poorly nourished and mildly dehydrated. Weight was 2.1 kg. The clitoris was large and the posterior aspects of the labia majora were fused. The remainder of the physical examination was normal. Serum electrolytes were Na^+ 110 meq/L; Cl^- 82 meq/L; K^+ 7.2 meq/L; BUN 31 mg/dL; and glucose 56 mg/dL.

38. The most likely cause of this clinical picture is

    (A) viral gastroenteritis
    (B) obstructive uropathy
    (C) adrenal insufficiency
    (D) inappropriate feeding
    (E) inappropriate secretion of ADH

39. This patient's chromosomal analysis would most likely be

    (A) XX
    (B) XY
    (C) XO
    (D) XXY
    (E) XYY

40. Therapy for this child should include

    (A) peritoneal dialysis
    (B) low protein diet
    (C) fluid restriction
    (D) low salt diet
    (E) glucocorticoid and mineralcorticoid replacement

41. Correction of this patient's electrolyte abnormalities is best achieved with intravenous administration of

    (A) an initial bolus with 0.9% NS and rehydration therapy with D_5W
    (B) an initial bolus with 0.9% NS and rehydration therapy with 0.25% NS
    (C) an initial bolus with 0.9% NS and rehydration therapy with 0.9% NS
    (D) an initial bolus with 0.9% NS and rehydration therapy with D_5 0.9% NS
    (E) maintenance with 0.25% NS

Questions 42 through 44

An 8-day-old male infant is brought to clinic for a routine postdelivery evaluation. On examination, the child weighs 6 kg. Multiple pits are present on the posterior helix of the ears. The neonate is excessively jittery. Pregnancy history, labor, and vaginal delivery were unremarkable. The mother states the baby is feeding well.

42. Evaluation of which of the following would be most beneficial in an infant with these physical findings and history?

    (A) calcium
    (B) thyroid
    (C) magnesium
    (D) glucose
    (E) sodium

43. Additional family history is obtained and the siblings examined. There is a history of mental retardation in the family. Some of the siblings are large for their age and have the same lines or pits seen on the posterior helix of their ears. Which of the following genetic disorders does this family most likely have?

    (A) Prader-Willi syndrome
    (B) neurofibromatosis
    (C) DiGeorge sequence
    (D) Sotos syndrome
    (E) Beckwith-Wiedemann syndrome

44. Based on your diagnosis, the most likely etiology of this child's jitteriness and abnormal laboratory study is

    (A) hyperinsulinism
    (B) thyrotoxicosis
    (C) SIADH
    (D) adrenal insufficiency
    (E) excess growth hormone

Questions 45 and 46

A 3-year-old formerly healthy male toddler is seen in clinic with an acute onset of vomiting. On physical examination the child is tachypneic (respirations of 60/min), febrile (temperature of 102°F), sleepy and difficult to arouse. The parents explain they are visiting the child's grandparents. Serum laboratory results are Na^+ 150 meq/L, K^+ 2.9, Cl^- 99, HCO_3^- 18 meq/L, glucose 45 mg/dL, anion gap 26, BUN 16 mg/dL, creatinine 0.3 mg/dL. Blood gas pH 7.25, PCO_2 15, PO_2 88, BE –18.0.

45. This child most likely ingested

    (A) ethanol

    (B) ibuprofen

    (C) acetaminophen

    (D) organophosphate

    (E) oil of wintergreen

46. Treatment beyond acute supportive care should focus on

    (A) alkalization of the urine

    (B) administration of a cathartic

    (C) administration of *N*-acetylcystiene

    (D) peritoneal dialysis

    (E) antibiotic administration

DIRECTIONS (Questions 47 through 58): Each set of matching questions in this section consists of a list of lettered options followed by several numbered items. For each numbered item select the ONE lettered option with which it is most closely associated. Each lettered option may be selected once, more than once, or not at all.

Questions 47 through 50

    (A) hypercalcemia

    (B) porphyria

    (C) abetalipoproteinemia

    (D) familial hypercholesterolemia

    (E) hypertrophic pyloric stenosis

    (F) Gaucher disease (MPS II)

    (G) Wilson disease

    (H) citrullinemia

47. An 11-month-old male infant presents with abdominal distention and vomiting. His oral intake is three times his daily maintenance requirement of formula and his urine output is 10 mL/kg/h. The child is small for age and has abnormal "elfin" facies. Physical examination is remarkable for a loud grade IV/VI systolic ejection murmur at the left sternal border. Echocardiography reveals supravalvular aortic stenosis.

48. A 3-year-old presents to your office for evaluation of recurrent rash with sun exposure. This sun sensitivity seems to be worsening with age. Examination of his skin reveals areas of resolving damage and new areas of exposure which are red, swollen, and excoriated. Additional physical findings are splenomegaly and brownish teeth.

49. A 4-month-old child presents with diarrhea and poor growth since birth. The child has adequate oral intake but recurrent large malodorous stools. He has been evaluated for cystic fibrosis but tests were negative. Stool studies reveal an increased amount of fecal fat. Celiac sprue is considered and the child undergoes colonoscopy. Intestinal biopsy, however, demonstrates normal appearing villi.

50. A 16-year-old male comes to clinic for a routine sports physical examination. His physical examination is unremarkable except for the skin findings of multiple pale masses which appear to be xanthomas. Additional family history is remarkable for the sudden early deaths of two paternal uncles with myocardial infarction.

Questions 51 through 54

    (A) familial hypercholesterolemia

    (B) Tay-Sachs disease

    (C) Wilson disease

    (D) Menkes syndrome

51. Kayser-Fleisher rings

52. Cherry red macular spots

53. Kinky hair

54. Arcus juvenilis

Questions 55 through 58

   (A) PKU

   (B) tyrosinemia

   (C) isovaleric aciduria

   (D) maple syrup urine disease

55. Urine odor of sweaty feet

56. Urine odor of cabbage

57. Urine odor of musty smell

58. Urine odor of syrup

Answers and Explanations

1. **(D)** Infants weighing less than 10 kg expend an average of 100 cal/kg of body weight. A 3-kg infant has a basal caloric requirement of 300 calories. The infant needs approximately 100 mL of water per 100 calories metabolized. This translates to a fluid requirement of 1 mL/cal. This concept is an important one to remember since fluid and caloric calculations for adults are different from those for children. *(McMillan:67; Behrman:138, 141)*

2. **(C)** There is a simple method for calculating the fluid (and caloric) requirements for an infant or child: 100 mL/kg for the first 10 kg of body weight, 50 mL/kg for the second 10 kg of body weight (between 11 and 20 kg), and 20 mL/kg for each kilogram of body weight greater than 20 kg. Using this method, the fluid requirements for this child are calculated as follows:

   For the first 10 kg

   $$100 \text{ mL/kg} \times 10 \text{ kg} = 1000 \text{ mL}$$

   For the second 10 kg

   $$50 \text{ mL/kg} \times 10 \text{ kg} = 500 \text{ mL}$$

   For the remaining 10 kg

   $$20 \text{ mL/kg} \times 10 \text{ kg} = 200 \text{ mL}$$

   This gives the child a total fluid requirement of 1000 mL + 500 mL + 200 mL = 1700 mL. Notice that this child does not require 10 times as much fluid as the 3-kg child or twice as much fluid as a 15-kg child. *(McMillan: 67–68; Behrman:138, 141)*

3. **(B)** First calculate the daily fluid requirements for a 15-kg child as follows: 10 kg × 100 mL/kg = 1,000 mL and 5 kg × 50 mL/kg = 250 mL; then 1000 mL + 250 mL = 1250 mL daily maintenance. Twice daily maintenance is 2500 mL (1250 mL × 2). The intravenous fluid hourly rate is established by dividing the daily total fluid requirement by 24 h as follows: 2500 mL/24 h = approximately 105 mL/h. *(McMillan:67; Behrman:138, 141)*

4. **(D)** Calculate the daily fluid requirements of the patient.

   For the first 10 kg

   $$10 \text{ kg} \times 100 \text{ mL/kg} = 1000 \text{ mL}$$

   For the next 10 kg

   $$10 \text{ kg} \times 50 \text{ mL/kg} = 500 \text{ mL}$$

   For the remainder of the body weight

   $$30 \text{ kg} \times 20 \text{ mL/kg} = 600 \text{ mL}$$

   Adding these together (1000 mL + 500 mL + 600 mL) gives a daily total of 2100 mL. This daily maintenance requirement divided over 24 h (2100 mL/24 h) gives you 88 mL/h, or approximately 90 mL/h. *(McMillan:67; Behrman: 138, 141)*

5. **(B)** The infant described is probably about 15% (severely) dehydrated. In classifying infants and young children, dehydration is divided into mild (5%), moderate (10%), and severe (15%) based on clinical examination. (For an older child and adult, comparable figures

would be 3, 6, and 9%.) An infant that is mildly (5%) dehydrated has a normal to slightly increased heart rate, slightly dry mucous membranes, poor tear production, and slightly decreased urine output. An infant moderately (10%) dehydrated demonstrates worsening of the previous signs along with decreased skin turgor and sunken anterior fontanelle. An infant with severe (15%) dehydration presents with symptoms of hypovolemic shock with decreased blood pressure, delayed cap refill, Kussmaul's respiration, and depressed sensorium.

Many students and physicians would calculate a rough estimate of total body fluid deficit as 8 kg × 15% = 1200 mL deficit. However, this calculation is not entirely correct, or accurate, as dehydration and percent dehydration are related to a premorbid weight (wt_{pre})—in this case, the infant's weight before he became dehydrated. Current weight = wt_{pre} × (1 – percent dehydrated/100). Therefore,

$$wt_{pre} = \frac{\text{current wt}}{1.0 - (\text{percent dehydrated}/100)}$$

and

$$wt_{Pre} = \frac{8\text{kg}}{1.0 - 0.15} = 9.4\text{kg}$$

The deficit, therefore, is 15% of 9.4 kg, or 1400 mL. [*Note:* Total fluid deficit is not the same as total fluid requirement. Daily total fluid requirements in a dehydrated child includes deficit fluid replacement *in addition* to routine daily fluid requirements and any abnormal ongoing losses such as continued diarrhea.] *(Behrman:213–219)*

6. **(D)** Serum osmolality normally is between 285 and 295 mOsm/L, with a range of 275–300 mOsm/L. Serum osmolality is approximately equal to twice the serum sodium concentration. However, serum osmolality can be calculated more accurately by the use of the formula: serum osmolality equals 2(Na) + BUN/2.8 + glucose/18. If a calculated serum osmolality and measured serum osmolality are unequal then there exists some large extracellular fluid

molecule (e.g., when mannitol is used in treating patients at risk for cerebral edema). Abnormalities of consciousness are seen when osmolality is <260 or >330 mOsm/L. *(Behrman:192–193)*

7. **(A)** Total serum osmolality in this patient is normal. The elevated serum glucose increases osmolality, but this is compensated by the lowered sodium concentration which decreases osmolality. By using the calculation 2(Na) + BUN/2.8 + glucose/18, the estimated osmolality is figured as 2(126) + 16/2.8 + 500/18, or 285 mOsm/L. The actual measured osmolality might be a little lower than this calculated figure because some of the ionic material is protein bound and therefore does not actually contribute to osmolality. When managing a patient in diabetic ketoacidosis the abnormalities in osmolarity are important, and warrant slow correction of serum glucose and careful monitoring of serum electrolytes and mental status changes. [*Note:* It is important to recognize that a patient is not necessarily hyperosmolar with a blood glucose of 500 mg/dL or hypoosmolar with a low serum sodium.] *(Behrman:192–193)*

8. **(B)** A child's maintenance requirements might be calculated either on a caloric (weight) basis (5 kg × 100 mL (calories)/kg = 500 mL) or on a surface area basis (0.30 m^2 × 1600 mL/m^2 = 480 mL). For children weighing <10 kg, the preferred method is the use of the caloric basis, or the Holliday-Segar method. The deficit, however, must be calculated on the basis of weight (not surface area): 5 kg × 100 mL/kg = 500 mL. Adding deficit and maintenance: 500 mL + 500 mL = 1000 mL. *(Gunn:233–234; Behrman:212– 217).*

9. **(E)** The diagnosis of the syndrome of inappropriate antidiuretic hormone secretion (SIADH) is made in this patient with a low serum sodium, normal renal function, and inappropriately elevated urine sodium concentration. This increase in the extracellular fluid volume occurs from the action of antidiuretic hormone or vasopressin on the renal collecting tubule, resulting in retention of water and loss of sodium into the urine. Management involves fluid restriction and treating the underlying

cause of the SIADH which includes, among others, central nervous system lesions, pulmonary diseases, and medications.

All of the listed answers are possible causes of hyponatremia, defined as a serum sodium less than 130 meq/L. Symptomatic hyponatremia (e.g., weight gain, nausea, confusion) is not seen until serum sodium concentration ≤120 meq/L. Seizures and coma occur when the serum sodium value drops quickly or becomes less than 110 meq/L. Adrenal insufficiency, with deficiency of glucocorticoid/mineralcorticoid, as a cause of hyponatremia often will be accompanied by acidosis and hyperkalemia. Psychogenic polydypsia can cause a dramatically low serum sodium, but urine is dilute with a low sodium level. Depending on the laboratory method used, hypertriglyceridemia can result in a fictitiously low sodium; it is a rare cause of hyponatremia in children. SIADH is the most likely etiology of this child's hyponatremia. *(Behrman:196, 221–222: 1684)*

10. **(A)** Infants that present with these physical findings are mildly to moderately dehydrated and are candidates for oral rehydration therapy. Consistent administration of small volumes is effective in correcting dehydration even with continued diarrhea. Composition of the oral replacement fluid should be designed to optimize repletion of the ECF space and provide some carbohydrate to give minimal calories in order to avoid catabolism. The relationship of sodium concentration to carbohydrate concentration is important for appropriate absorption of sodium without worsening the fluid losses from an osmotic diarrhea caused by over administered and/or inappropriate carbohydrate solutions. Most household liquids (tea and koolaid) are inappropriate because of their hypotonic (low sodium) content. However, commercially available rehydration formulas (i.e., Pedialyte) are useful. Intravenous therapy is necessary only when the child refuses fluids orally or has severe dehydration with impending circulatory collapse. *(Behrman:854)*

11. **(B)** In an obtunded or comatose patient, regardless of suspected etiology, a serum glucose measurement is useful in directing acute management efforts. The change in sensorium can be a result of the direct effects of alcohol or a result of hypoglycemia which occurs secondary to the effect of alcohol on gluconeogenesis. Gluconeogenesis is impaired in two ways. First, ethanol is an acid in the blood stream and creates a metabolic acidosis which directly reduces the activity of the metabolic pathway responsible for glucose mobilization. Second, the depletion of NADH in the system by the metabolism of alcohol to acetaldehyde (via reduction of NAD by alcohol dehydrogenase) indirectly stops glucose production, as NADH depletion halts gluconeogenesis. The other pathway of alcohol metabolism, which utilizes the microsomal system, results in the abnormal clearance of other drugs metabolized by this same pathway in the body. The preferential metabolism of ethanol by this system often causes the clearance of other drugs to be slowed and their blood levels to rise, resulting in their additive toxic effects to ethanol toxicity. *(Behrman:446, 567; Tobias:423)*

12. **(A)** People with homocystinuria type I are at increased risk for thromboembolic events due to changes in their vascular walls from increased homocystine levels leading to increased platelet adherence and thrombus formation. *(McMillan: 1833; Jones:478–479)*

13. **(C)** Pompe disease is an abnormality of carbohydrate metabolism with autosomal recessive inheritance. Clinically normal at birth, the infants have a deficiency of acid maltase that leads to a build-up of glycogen products in cells. This in turn leads to marked muscle weakness, hypotonia, and severe cardiomegaly. Children with Pompe disease often die within the first 2 years of life from cardiac or respiratory failure. *(Behrman:407–409, 411–412)*

14. **(C)** A deficiency in the enzyme fumarylacetoacetate hydrolase results in moderate elevations of tyrosine. This is thought to lead to accumulation of intermediate metabolites, primarily succinylacetone, leading to damage of

the liver, kidney, and central nervous system. *(Behrman:347–349)*

15. **(C)** The defect seen in alcaptonuria leads to increased amounts of homogentisic acid which is excreted in the urine. Alkaline urine appears black secondary to oxidation and polymerization of the homogentisic acid. This unusually colored urine helps establish the diagnosis. Additionally, the sclera, cornea, and ear cartilage of patients with alcaptonuria become darkly pigmented (ochronosis) secondary to the black polymer of homogentisic acid. Later in life they develop arthritis, which is the only disabling aspect of the illness. *(Behrman: 347–349)*

16. **(B)** Tyrosinemia primarily affects the liver, peripheral nerves, and kidneys. Early death most often is a result of hepatic failure. Affected infants may become symptomatic as early as 2 weeks of age, or may appear normal during the first year of life. Commonly, affected infants will first present with an acute hepatic crisis precipitated by an intercurrent illness and resultant catabolic state. *(Behrman:347–349)*

17. **(E)** Subluxation of the ocular lens known as ectopia lentis occurs generally after 3 years of age in homocystinuria, leading to severe myopia and iridodonesis (quivering of the iris). These patients lack the enzyme cystathionine synthase and have multiple problems including severe mental retardation, increased thromboembolic events, psychiatric disorders, skeletal abnormalities resembling Marfan disease, generalized osteoporosis and seizures. *(McMillan:1833–1834)*

18. **(C)** Using the Holliday-Segar method (i.e., 100 mL/kg for the first 10 kg, then 50 mL/kg for the next 10 kg, then 20 mL/kg for each additional kg > 20 kg), this child should receive 1300 mL per day. A short cut method is the "4-2-1" method: 4 cc/h/kg for the first 10 kg, 2 cc/h/kg for the next 10 kg, plus 1 cc/h/k > 20 kg. In this child, that would be 52 cc/h which is close to 1300 cc per day. This short cut method is useful for double checking accurate fluid calculations. *(Gunn:233–234)*

19. **(B)** Sodium and chloride requirements are approximately 3 meq/kg per day, or 36 meq NaCl in a 12 kg infant. Requirements for fluids in a 12-kg infant are approximately 1100 mL per day. Therefore, 36 meq of NaCl must be provided in 1100 mL of fluid each day to meet requirements ($36/1100 \times 1000 = 32$ meq NaCl/L IVF). Of the choices listed, 0.9% NaCl contains 155 meq NaCl/L, 0.45% NaCl contains 77 meq NaCl/L, 0.2% NaCl contains 35 meq NaCl/L, LR contains 130 meq NaCl/L and plasmalyte contains 140 meq NaCl/L. Thus, the best choice for intravenous fluids in this child is 0.2% NS. *(McMillan:68; Gunn:250)*

20. **(C)** Potassium requirement generally is calculated at 2–2.5 meq KCl/kg/day. For this 15 kg child that would be 30–37 meq KCl per day. Using the Holliday-Segar method, the child's maintenance fluid requirement is 1250 cc per day; 30 meq KCl/1.250 L = 24 meq KCl/L, or approximately 25 meq KCl/L. *(McMillan:68; Gunn:250)*

21. **(C)** Evaluation of dehydration must always include the "ABCs" to evaluate for hypovolemic shock. Following initial fluid resuscitation the serum sodium should be corrected over 24–48 h. The duration of the hypernatremic state determines the body's level of compensation of osmolality. The brain has been found to make "idiogenic osmoles" in order to preserve cerebral oncotic pressure and to prevent neuronal shrinkage. Administering too much free water too quickly can lead to cerebral edema and seizures, thus the hypernatremic dehydration must be corrected slowly. *(Rudolph CD:1651–1652)*

22. **(B)** Pyruvate kinase deficiency causes a congenital nonspherocytic hemolytic anemia with resultant hyperbilirubinemia. The breakdown may be so severe as to put the neonate at risk for bilirubin encephalopathy and require exchange transfusion. Blood transfusion may be indicated for the anemia. Splenectomy improves the anemia but does not cure the underlying defect. *(Rudolph CD:1542; McMillan: 1455)*

23. **(A)** Wilson disease is an autosomal recessive disorder associated with progressive

accumulation of intracellular copper in the liver, brain, kidneys, and eyes. This accumulation of copper results from impaired incorporation of copper into ceruloplasmin and decreased biliary copper excretion. The gene for Wilson disease is located on the long arm of chromosome 13 and is designated ATP7B. Typically the first organ to demonstrate signs of dysfunction from copper deposition is the liver. *(McMillan: 1721–1722; Rudolph CD:1491–1493)*

24. **(C)** Strict elimination of mammalian milk, which is the natural source of lactose (and therefore galactose) is the treatment for galactokinase deficiency. Avoidance of milk products and other products, such as some medications or candy that contain lactose, is important. If started early in the neonatal period, this diet can prevent the formation of nuclear cataracts, usually the sole manifestation of this disease. Once formed, the cataracts are not reversible. The disease is autosomal recessive with gene coding located on chromosome 17q24. *(Rudolph CD:641)*

25. **(C)** The mucopolysaccharidoses (MPS) form a group of diseases associated with lysosomal accumulation of partially degraded acid mucopolysaccharides. Hurler disease, the most severe of the MPS disorders, is autosomal recessive and occurs in about 1:100,000 births. It is associated with coarse facial features, clouding of the corneas, deafness, airway obstruction, thickening of the cardiac valve leaflets, cardiomyopathy, congestive heart failure, poor growth and development, mental retardation, and early death often secondary to cardiopulmonary problems. *(McMillan: 1870–1871; Rudolph CD:2329)*

26. **(E)** ALD is an X-linked disease characterized by progressive neurologic degeneration and adrenal insufficiency. Patients with ALD have elevated plasma levels of very long chain fatty acids (VLCFAs), which accumulate in cerebral white matter and adrenal cortex. Treatment includes hormone replacement for adrenal insufficiency, restriction of dietary VLCFAs, provision of C18:1 and C22:1 fatty acids, and bone marrow transplant. The dietary supplements and bone marrow therapy seem to be more successful when instituted prior to onset of neurologic symptoms. Death generally occurs 3–5 years after onset of symptoms. *(Rudolph CD:2324)*

27. **(C)** Pyruvate is converted to acetyl-CoA during glycolysis via the pyruvate dehydrogenase complex. The complex is made up of three enzymes, pyruvate dehydrogenase (E1), dihydrolipoyltransacetylase (E2), and dihydrolipoyldehydrogenase (E3). Babies with this defect may have a severe lactic acidosis with resultant tachypnea, hypotonia, lethargy, and coma in the first few days of life, or the disease may not manifest itself for months to years until the child is stressed by infection, prolonged fasting, or other conditions requiring increased gluconeogenesis. Treatment centers on reducing gluconeogenesis (the major pathway is through pyruvate) by providing a high-fat, low carbohydrate diet, normalizing blood sugars, and administering sodium bicarbonate and carnitine. *(McMillan:1982)*

28. **(C)** The child described probably has osteogenesis imperfecta, a disorder characterized by osteoporotic bones that fracture easily. Blue sclera, present in infancy, is a common feature. Some patients also have opalescent dentin (dentinogenesis imperfecta), and many develop conductive hearing loss in adolescence. At least four types have been described, with differing modes of inheritance and varying degrees of severity. *(Rudolph CD:2161)*

29. **(B)** Bilious vomitus consists of gastric and duodenal (pancreatic secretions and bile) contents. Pancreatic secretions contain sodium at 140 meq/L, potassium at 5 meq/L, chloride at 50–100 meq/L, bicarbonate at 100 meq/L; bile contains sodium at 130 meq/L, potassium at 5 meq/L, chloride at 100 meq/L, and bicarbonate at 40 meq/L. Knowledge of body fluid composition is useful in understanding the metabolic derangement seen. Typically, bilious vomiting results in isotonic dehydration and either a neutral pH or acidic pH. This contrasts with pure gastric losses, such as those seen in pyloric stenosis, where the dehydration typically results in a hypochloremic, metabolic alkalosis. *(Randolph CD:1376–1379, 1401; Gunn:240)*

30. **(D)** This patient most likely has renal tubular acidosis (RTA), described as Fanconi or a Fanconi-like syndrome. This is a proximal RTA heralded by urinary losses of bicarbonate and phosphate. Classic findings are aminoaciduria, phosphaturia, and glycosuria with resultant hyperchloremic metabolic acidosis with normal anion gap. There are multiple causes of this disorder including inborn errors of metabolism (cystinosis, galactosemia, tyrosinemia, and Wilson disease), and acquired forms from heavy metal toxicity and drug toxicity (i.e., gentamicin, valproic acid, cisplatin). The metabolic acidosis and phosphate loss seen in this disorder lead to growth failure and vitamin D-resistant rickets. *(Rudolph CD:1708–1709; Finberg 114, 228)*

31. **(D)** Classic phenylketonuria results from the lack of, or near complete lack of, phenylalanine hydroxylase. Impaired metabolism of the common essential amino acid phenylalanine to tyrosine leads to build-up of phenylpyruvic acid and phenylethylamine. These products as well as excess phenylalanine lead to central nervous system damage. As of December 1995, all states mandate newborn screening for at least phenylketonuria (PKU) and hypothyroidism, and in most states, newborns are secreened for galactosemia. The introduction of tandem mass spectrometry is driving reconsideration of expanding newborn screening. The screening is performed by collecting blood spots on filter paper at the time of discharge from the hospital to home and before 7 days of life. Infants discharged at less than 24 h of age should have the screening test repeated prior to 14 days of life. Unfortunately, this baby did not have adequate newborn screening. For PKU, presymptomatic diagnosis allows control of the disease through control of the diet of the infant. Though further CNS damage can be prevented in this case with dietary control, the signs and symptoms this baby displays are, for the most part, irreversible. *(Rudolph CD:579, 609–610; Pediatrics: 473–475, 1996)*

32. **(D)** Treatment of PKU consists of a very strict diet low in phenylalanine. Reducing phenylalanine in the diet will then reduce the serum levels and help reduce the consequences of the disease, which include brain damage, mental retardation, seizures, athetosis, hyperactivity, and behavioral problems. The diet is difficult to adhere to, and creates increased stress on the child and the family, which adds to the complexity of the disease. *(Behrman:344–346)*

33. **(B)** Classic galactosemia occurs in 1 in 60,000 newborns. Defective or total lack of galactose-1-phosphate uridyl transferase causes an inability to convert galactose into glucose. Normally galactose converts to galactose-1-phosphate by galactokinase. Galactose-1-phosphate is then converted to glucose-1-phosphate by the enzyme in question. Without the enzyme, galactose-1-phosphate accumulates causing parenchymal damage to the kidneys, liver, and brain. Indirect hyperbilirubinemia, acidosis, and urosepsis frequently are seen at presentation. *(Rudolph CD:1486–1487)*

34. **(C)** Pyloric stenosis with persistent vomiting leads to loss of hydrochloric acid. The resultant hypochloremic metabolic alkalosis can be profound, and must be corrected prior to surgery. The incidence is approximately 1/150 male infants and 1/750 female infants and the risks are greatly increased in male infants born to mothers who had pyloric stenosis. *(Rudolph CD:722:1402)*

35. **(C)** In this child immediate treatment indicated is a 20 mL/kg rapid infusion of fluid to quickly expand the extracellular fluid volume. Such aggressive fluid resuscitation is the mainstay of preventing and treating shock. *Only isotonic fluids should be used.* Use of hypotonic fluids results in loss of fluid intracellularly, cell lysis, and potentially life-threatening cerebral edema. Other fluids such as albumin and blood can be used for volume expansion, but usually are not as readily available as crystalloid solutions in emergent rehydration situations. Depending on the degree, severity, and nature of the volume loss, two to three isotonic fluid boluses of normal saline (154 meq/L of sodium and chloride) may be required. *(Rudolph CD: 1644–1646; Tobias:289–290)*

36. **(A)** The initial hydrating solution should contain 135–154 meq/L of sodium for two reasons. One reason is that sodium will effectively stay in the intravascular space and help to expand the intravascular volume because it does not readily cross intracellularly. The second reason is the record of safety in administering isotonic fluid as opposed to hypertonic or hypotonic fluid. Even in cases of severe hypernatremic or hyponatremic dehydration the additional sodium and free water provided with even two to three boluses of the isotonic fluid is negligible in its impact on the serum sodium level, especially when repleting the intravascular space of a patient in shock or near-shock. *(Tobias:288–291; Rudolph CD:650–653)*

37. **(E)** Because of the concern about renal impairment/damage from the dehydration and hypoperfusion of the kidneys, potassium should be withheld from the rehydration solutions until the patient has voided or the serum potassium level is known. In addition, potassium chloride should be administered as a bolus *only* in specific situations and in a carefully controlled manner because of the possibility of precipitating EKG abnormalities, arrythmias, and muscle weakness. *(Rudolph CD:1645–1647)*

38. **(C)** The history of vomiting and diarrhea, the weight loss >10% of birth weight, low serum sodium and elevated serum potassium are highly suggestive of adrenal insufficiency. The findings on physical examination of a prominent clitoris and labial fusion are suggestive of virilization, and further support the diagnosis of adrenal insufficiency. Adrenogenital disorder, or congenital adrenal hyperplasia (CAH), could explain all of these findings. CAH is a condition resulting from an inherited defect in cortisol synthesis. Ninety to ninety-five percent of cases are caused by 21-hydroxylase deficiency. Most forms of this disorder are associated with virilization and/or salt wasting. Although a viral gastroenteritis could explain the dehydration in an older infant or child, it would be less likely in a neonate this age. Those affected by inappropriate secretion of ADH also have low sodium, but often experience abnormal increases in weight secondary to fluid retention. *(Rudolph CD:2038–2041)*

39. **(A)** Congenital adrenal hyperplasia is an autosomal recessive genetic disorder associated with either XX or XY genotype. However, because of the virilization associated with CAH, many affected XX females are evaluated for ambiguous genitalia in the newborn period. CAH occurs from a spontaneous mutation. Some ethnic bias is seen with 1 of 20,000 Japanese births affected, 1 of 10,000–16,000 North American births affected, and 1 of 300 Yupik Eskimos in Alaska affected. Males and females are affected equally, though diagnosis in males is often delayed outside the newborn period until they experience a "salt-losing" crisis or show evidence of increased masculinization. Prenatal diagnosis is available for at risk families. Screening methods include HLA typing, DNA probe hybridization and measurements of 17-hydroxyprogesterone in the amniotic fluid. *(Behrman:1732–1736)*

40. **(E)** Therapy for the salt-losing form of adrenal hyperplasia requires replacement of both mineralcorticoids and glucocorticoids. In stressed children (i.e., those experiencing illness or salt-losing crisis) a "stress" dosage should be administered of the glucocorticoid that is two to three times the daily calculated replacement. A high salt intake is also useful depending on the degree of salt wasting. For infants, NaCl is added to the formula (1 g NaCl/10 kg of weight). *(Behrman:1735)*

41. **(D)** Many authors point out that adrenal crisis is similar to diabetic ketoacidosis in that the patients are often more dehydrated than they appear clinically. Replacement of 25% of the total fluid deficit in the first 2 h is advocated with early addition of glucose to the fluids. D_5 NS (same as D_5 0.9% NS) should be used the first 24 h for replacement and maintenance. Potassium should be withheld until serum electrolyte values have normalized. The presence of hypoglycemia should be evaluated and treated immediately. Stress doses of steroids should be administered. *(Behrman:1735; Finberg: 211–212)*

42. **(D)** Although jitteriness in neonates can result from abnormalities of each of the possible answers, this infant has qualities that make hypoglycemia the most likely cause. The size of the infant is well above the 90th percentile for newborn males. Many causes of macrosomia (e.g., previous large for gestational age infants and maternal diabetes) are associated with abnormal glucose metabolism. The additional findings of ear anomalies could implicate a calcium abnormality (e.g., DiGeorge anomaly/sequence) but the child has no heart murmur and is not failing to thrive at this point, making this a less likely diagnosis. *(McMillan: 346–347)*

43. **(E)** There is a well-known association of Beckwith-Wiedemann syndrome (BWS) with hypoglycemia affecting up to 50% of children with the disorder. Physical findings are characterized by macrosomia, microcephaly, visceromegaly, and macroglossia. Other associated anomalies are an increased incidence of hemihypertrophy, omphaloceles, cryptorchidism, and renal tumors. The ear pits or creases are not always present in affected patients but are highly characteristic of BWS. Transmission is often from a sporadic mutation on chromosome 11, although familial cases have been reported. The frequency of occurrence is 1:15,000, with variable expression. Mild to moderate mental deficiency has been reported in this disorder and is thought to be related to neonatal hypoglycemia. *(McMillan: 346)*

44. **(A)** The exact etiology of hypoglycemia in a neonate can be difficult to determine and involves a differential that is very different from that seen in an older infant, child, or adult. Small for gestational age infants and premature infants both have increased incidence of symptomatic hypoglycemia. A majority of their glucose problems are related to deficient glycogen stores, muscle protein, and body fat needed for metabolization to meet energy requirements. Infants born to diabetic mothers also experience an increased incidence of hypoglycemia. However, hypoglycemia in infants of diabetic mothers is not due to insufficient stores, but is due to hyperinsulinemia and low glucagon levels. Beckwith-Wiedemann syndrome infants also experience hyperinsulinemia which causes hypoglycemia. Their increased insulin secretion is caused by pancreatic islet cell hypertrophy. Treatment for these infants is the same as for other causes of hyperinsulinism; supportive administration of intravenous glucose at a rate of 6–8 mg/kg/min. At times, more aggressive treatments are warranted (e.g., increased rates of glucose administration and supplementation of regulatory hormones by injections of steroids and growth hormone). *(McMillan: 346–347)*

45. **(E)** Oil of wintergreen is a solution containing methylsalicylate, a form of salicylic acid. When ingested, a small quantity can cause a rather toxic ingestion because one teaspoon (5 cc) of this liquid contains 5 g of methylsalicylate. Salicylate ingestions are impressive in the unique metabolic derangements comprised of a mixed respiratory alkalosis with metabolic acidosis. Initially, the salicylate is absorbed rapidly and directly stimulates the respiratory center causing tachypnea and a respiratory alkalosis. Unfortunately, this tachypnea is short lived in infants before more severe symptoms are seen. Potassium and sodium are lost in the urine from the alkalosis and a compensatory acidosis begins. Lactic acid levels, along with other metabolic acid levels, begin to rise in the serum resulting in a severe acidosis. In addition, the patient is probably 5–10% dehydrated from urinary losses. Oxidative phosphorylation is uncoupled by the salicylate and the patient's acidosis worsens. Symptoms of hyperpnea, tachycardia, lethargy, vomiting, dehydration, and coma can occur. Treatment is directed at primarily supportive care until the toxicity has been corrected. *(Behrman: 2016–2018; McMillan 837–838)*

46. **(A)** The mainstay of management with any ingestion is (1) preventing further absorption of the toxic material, (2) facilitating removal of the toxin from the system, and (3) administering an antidote to the toxin/poison if one is available. These management steps along with good supportive care will minimize the duration of toxicity and facilitate rapid recovery of the patient with the least amount of adverse effects.

Patients with salicylate toxicity typically are approximately 5–10% dehydrated and have experienced losses of potassium and hydrogen via the urine. Therapy includes both aggressive rehydration and alkalinization of the urine with administration of sodium bicarbonate. Unfortunately, no antidote is available for salicylate poisoning. In severe ingestions, hemodialysis may be necessary if the quantity of ingestion, level of salicylates, and observed toxicity are not responding to conventional measures. (Behrman:2016–2018; McMillan 837–838)

47. **(A)** This patient shows symptoms of hypercalcemia (increased drinking and voiding) commonly associated with Williams syndrome. Williams syndrome is a genetic disorder that commonly results from sporadic mutations on chromosome 7 (a microdeletion of the elastin gene). The syndrome is characterized by its unique facial features of prominent lips and thin philtrum as well as cardiac anomalies (e.g., supravalvular aortic stenosis). Infantile hypercalcemia often is noted and can lead to problems of nephrocalcinosis, constipation, and mental status changes. (Rudolph CD:163, 859, 1805; Jones:118–121)

48. **(B)** This child is suffering from one of the porphyrias, a group of relatively rare inherited disorders that result in defects in heme biosynthesis and a build-up of heme precursors. These precursors exist in elevated amounts in the skin creating the reactions to ultraviolet light. Some forms cause repetitive attacks of abdominal pain (neurovisceral attacks). (McMillan:1999–2003)

49. **(C)** This patient's history is most suggestive of abetalipoproteinemia, or Bassen-Kornsweig disease. This disease is an autosomal recessive disorder resulting in absence of the betalipoproteins in the plasma. The resultant features are fat malabsorption, failure to thrive, cerebellar ataxia, retinitis pigmentosa, and changes in red blood cell morphology (acanthocytosis). Management includes supplementation of fat soluble vitamins (ADEK) and maintenance of a low fat diet. (McMillan: 1700–1701)

50. **(D)** This patient's history is most suggestive of familial hypercholesterolemia, an autosomal dominant disorder with a prevalence of 1/500 individuals. Additional evaluation of a fasting serum cholesterol level (with HDL and LDL levels), triglyceride levels, and 12-lead ECG is indicated. Dietary reduction of cholesterol can be effective treatment; however, cholesterol lowering agents such as cholysteramine (ion exchange resin) or lovastatin (HMG-CoA reductase inhibitor) are usually necessary. (McMillan: 1865–1866)

51. **(C)** Wilson disease is an autosomal recessive disorder associated with increased deposition of copper into tissues, primarily the liver initially, then other parts of the body. The basic defect appears to be an inability to excrete hepatic copper into bile and an inability to incorporate copper into apoceruloplasmin. Storage of copper in the cornea may result in brownish green granular copper deposits in Descemet's membrane, given the name Kayser-Fleisher rings. The presence of these often correlates with neurologic involvement. (McMillan: 1721–1722)

52. **(B)** Tay-Sachs disease is one of the sphingolipidoses and produces disease secondary to abnormal lysosomal accumulation of glycosphingolipids, gangliosides, and sphingomyelin. Faulty degradation due to absent or deficient lysosomal acid hydrolases is the defect. Tay-Sachs is associated with storage of G_{M2} ganglioside in the nervous system. Cherry red spots represent a normal red macular area of the eye surrounded by a white area of storage material. Later the spots will turn darker as macular degeneration progresses. The disease is associated with progressive CNS degeneration, seizures, blindness, respiratory problems, and death, usually by 3 or 4 years of age. (McMillan:1875)

53. **(D)** Menkes syndrome is an X-linked recessive disease associated with faulty copper transport. In part, the basic defect includes an impaired ability to incorporate copper into certain enzymes that need it as a cofactor. Children with the disease develop progressive neurologic

deterioration, seizures, and eventual death (primarily from infection) by 3 years of age. The most characteristic aspect of the disease is the "kinky hair" which is brittle, depigmented, dull, short, and brush-like. *(Jones: 198–199)*

54. **(A)** Arcus juvenilis is the appearance of an opaque ring close to the periphery of the cornea associated with hypercholesterolemia and hyperlipidemia. Other ocular findings are xanthomas of the eyelids and pale deposits in the retina (lipemia retinalis). Familial hypercholesterolemia results in accelerated cholesterol synthesis leading to increased risk of atherogenesis leading to peripheral vascular disease, heart attack, or stroke. The disease is also associated with the more commonly known xanthomas of the skin. *(McMillan:1865–1866; Campbell: 1674)*

55. **(C)** Isovaleric aciduria results from defective catabolism of leucine and may produce severe metabolic abnormalities in the first days of life. The odor of isovaleric acid resembles the odor of "sweaty feet." It is an autosomal recessive disorder and results in early death in severe cases and mental retardation in milder cases. *(Rudolph CD:623–624)*

56. **(B)** Tyrosinemia type 1 is associated with a deficiency of fumarylacetoacetase leading to elevated levels of toxic metabolites succinylacetone and succinylacetoacetone. Clinical findings at infancy include vomiting, diarrhea, the odor of rotten cabbage in the body fluids, jaundice, hepatomegaly, and liver damage. *(McMillan:1830–1831)*

57. **(A)** Phenylketonuria is a disorder of phenylalanine metabolism due to lack of phenylalanine hydroxylase which leads to accumulation of its metabolites (phenylpyruvic acid and phenylethylamine). The disorder results in mental retardation, seizures, movement disorders, and behavioral problems. The symptoms can be prevented with timely dietary restriction of phenylalanine. For this reason, newborn screening is essential. *(McMillan:1829–1830)*

58. **(D)** Maple syrup urine disease is named after the sweet syrupy smell of the urine in affected infants. The classic form is the most severe and often, at presentation, is confused with sepsis. Affected infants may require dialysis in the acute phase to eliminate the high levels of leucine, valine, and isoleucine in the blood. Lifelong treatment consists of limiting amounts of branched chain amino acids in the diet. *(McMillan:1841–1842)*

BIBLIOGRAPHY

Behrman RE, Kliegman RM, Arvin AM. *Nelson Textbook of Pediatrics*, 16th ed. Philadelphia, PA: W.B. Saunders, 1999.

Campbell AGM, McIntosh N. *Forfar's and Arneil's Textbook of Pediatrics*, 5th ed. New York, NY: Churchill-Livingstone, 1998.

Committee on Genetics. Newborn screening fact sheets. *Pediatrics* 1996;98(3):473–501.

Finberg L, Kravath RE, Hellerstein S. *Water and Electrolytes in Pediatrics.* 2nd ed. Philadelphia, PA: W.B. Saunders, 1993.

Gunn VL, Nechyba C. *The Harriet Lane Handbook*, 16th ed. Philadelphia, PA: Mosby, 2002.

Jones KL. *Smith's Recognizable Patterns of Human Malformations*, 5th ed. Philadelphia, PA: W.B. Saunders, 1997.

McMillan JA, DeAngelis CD, Feigin RD, Warshaw JB. *Oski's Pediatrics: Principles and Practice*, 3rd ed. Philadelphia, PA: JB Lippincott, 1999.

Rudolph CD, Rudolph AM, Hostetter MK, et al. *Rudolph's Pediatrics*, 21st ed. New York, NY: McGraw-Hill, 2003.

Tobias JD. *Pediatric Critical Care, The Essentials.* Armonk, NY: Futura Publishing Co., 1999.

CHAPTER 6

Growth and Development

Shiv Someshwar, MD

The area of growth and development occupies an important and unique position in the field of pediatrics. Both national general medical examinations and pediatric specialty examinations devote a significant percentage of questions to growth and development. Although this is a topic rich in concepts, it is also an area where memorization is important. The age at which a specific function or ability appears, or at which a child normally masters a certain skill, is called a developmental landmark. Unfortunately, a number of these landmarks must be committed to memory, either by study or by examining a sufficient number of children at different ages. Observing the behavior and abilities of normal children in nonmedical settings can be a helpful and enjoyable way to learn about landmarks and other aspects of child development, and the student should make the most of every opportunity to do so. The student also must commit to memory a number of normal values relating growth, as well as physiologic parameters such as weight, head circumference, and blood pressure, to age. Finally, although some national examinations provide a list of normal laboratory values with the examination booklet, they usually provide adult norms only rather than age-related norms. Many laboratory values (e.g., hemoglobin and serum alkaline phosphatase) are very age dependent, and the examinee will need to know these norms. Don't be discouraged by the amount of such numerical information asked for in this chapter. There also is a great deal of conceptual material about growth and development.

Questions

1. Weight gain in an infant is a good parameter of overall well-being. After 2 weeks of age, a term neonate will gain an average of

    (A) 15 g per day or 1/2 oz per day
    (B) 30 g per day or 1 oz per day
    (C) 45 g per day or 1 1/2 oz per day
    (D) 60 g per day or 2 oz per day
    (E) 120 g per day or 4 oz per day

2. Object permanence, the understanding that objects continue to exist even when not seen, is a major milestone in the cognitive development of a young infant. This occurs closest to

    (A) 2 months
    (B) 4 months
    (C) 6 months
    (D) 9 months
    (E) 15 months

3. All 20 primary teeth typically have erupted by age

    (A) 9–12 months
    (B) 15–18 months
    (C) 30–33 months
    (D) 4 years
    (E) 5–6 years

4. Handedness is established by age

    (A) 12 months
    (B) 24 months
    (C) 3–5 years
    (D) 7 years
    (E) 9 years

5. Visual acuity reaches 20/20 at age

    (A) 1 week
    (B) 6 months
    (C) 1 year
    (D) 4–5 years
    (E) 7–9 years

6. Frontal sinuses can be visualized radiologically by age

    (A) 1 week
    (B) 1 year
    (C) 3 years
    (D) 4 years
    (E) 6 years

7. Denver developmental screening exam

    (A) tests all five domains of development
    (B) can be used in children 0–6 years
    (C) can be administered in 5–10 min
    (D) requires extensive training to administer
    (E) is useful only in infants

8. The embryonic period ends and the fetal period begins at gestational age

    (A) 5 weeks
    (B) 9 weeks

(C) 12 weeks

(D) 16 weeks

(E) 20 weeks

9. Gender of the external genitalia becomes clearly distinguishable by gestational age

   (A) 4 weeks

   (B) 8 weeks

   (C) 12 weeks

   (D) 16 weeks

   (E) 20 weeks

10. Vocabulary of 100–200 words is characteristic of age

   (A) 12 months

   (B) 15 months

   (C) 18 months

   (D) 24 months

   (E) 36 months

11. A child attains 50% of adult height by about age

   (A) 6 months

   (B) 12 months

   (C) 24 months

   (D) 36 months

   (E) 60 months

12. The first visible sign of puberty in girls is

   (A) development of breast buds

   (B) appearance of early public hair

   (C) menarche

   (D) enlargement of the clitoris

   (E) appearance of axillary hair

13. Median age for entering puberty in boys is

   (A) 8 years

   (B) 10 years

   (C) 12 years

   (D) 13 years

   (E) 15 years

14. Maximal height gain velocity in girls occurs during sexual maturity rating (SMR)

   (A) I

   (B) II

   (C) III

   (D) IV

   (E) V

15. Prepubertal annual increase in height in children is closest to

   (A) 1–2 cm

   (B) 3–4 cm

   (C) 5–7 cm

   (D) 8–10 cm

   (E) 12–14 cm

16. Obesity is defined as weight for height exceeding what percentage of the median?

   (A) 50%

   (B) 75%

   (C) 95%

   (D) 120%

   (E) 150%

17. The upper segment/lower segment body ratio which is 1.7:1 at birth reaches 1:1 at about age

   (A) 1 year

   (B) 3 years

   (C) 7 years

   (D) 10 years

   (E) 18 years

18. In constitutional growth delay, the child

   (A) has a history of being short at birth

   (B) is short during early adolescence

   (C) will have stunted height as an adult

   (D) has a normal bone age

   (E) frequently has growing pains

19. Delayed dental eruption is considered when the child has no teeth by age

   (A) 6 months

   (B) 8 months

   (C) 11 months

   (D) 13 months

   (E) 18 months

20. In the Freudian theory of psychosexual development, the Oedipal phase

    (A) precedes the oral phase
    (B) directly follows the oral phase
    (C) precedes latency
    (D) occurs during adolescence
    (E) is a sign of abnormal development

21. A mother is concerned that her 30-month-old son occasionally repeats words spoken to him. Physical and neurologic examinations are entirely normal, and the child's developmental landmarks are within normal limits. This child probably

    (A) is displaying precocious verbal behavior
    (B) has a subtle neurologic abnormality
    (C) has poor language development
    (D) has infantile autism
    (E) is normal

22. The neonate

    (A) has a visual preference for geometric shapes over faces
    (B) needs 4–6 h after birth to suck well at the breast
    (C) is farsighted
    (D) is unable to hear well
    (E) learns to differentiate the voice of her mother from that of other women by 4 weeks of age

23. Correct sequence for attainment of gross motor milestones is

    (A) head control, rolling over, hands together in midline, sits without support
    (B) head control, hands together in midline, rolling over, pulls to stand
    (C) rolls over, sits without support, hands together in midline, pulls to stand
    (D) sits without support, hands together in midline, pulls to stand, walks along
    (E) pulls to stand, walks along table, sits without support, hands together at midline

24. Correct sequence of fine motor development is

    (A) thumb–finger grasp, grasps rattle, transfers objects from hand to hand
    (B) grasps rattle, thumb–finger grasp, reaches for objects, transfers objects from hand to hand
    (C) grasps rattle, transfers objects from hand to hand, builds tower of two cubes, thumb–finger grasp
    (D) reaches for objects, transfers objects from hand to hand, turns pages of book, builds tower of two cubes
    (E) grasps rattle, transfers objects from hand to hand, thumb–finger grasp, builds tower of two cubes

25. Correct sequence for eruption of permanent teeth is

    (A) central incisors, first premolars, canines, second molars
    (B) central incisors, first molars, canines, first premolars
    (C) central incisors, lateral incisors, canines, first molars
    (D) first molars, lateral incisors, canines, first premolars
    (E) lateral incisors, first molars, canines, first premolars

26. Correct sequence for eruption of primary teeth includes

    (A) central incisors, first molars, second molars, canines
    (B) central incisors, lateral incisors, canines, first molars
    (C) central incisors, canines, first molars, second molars
    (D) central incisors, lateral incisors, first molars, canines
    (E) canines, central incisors, lateral incisors, first molars

27. Ossification centers present at birth usually include the

    (A) patella
    (B) lunate (carpal)

(C) proximal tibia

(D) head of the femur

(E) distal tibia

28. Which of the following sequence best demonstrates the correct attainment of motor milestones?

(A) runs, rides tricycle, skips, hops

(B) runs, hops, skips, rides tricycle

(C) runs, goes upstairs alternating feet, rides tricycle, skips

(D) hops, skips, rides tricycle, goes upstairs alternating feet

(E) goes upstairs alternating feet, rides tricycle, runs, skips

29. Which of the following sequences does social development of toddlers follow?

(A) feeds self, helps to undress, washes hands, domestic role-playing

(B) handles spoon well, plays in parallel, dresses and undresses, washes hands

(C) feeds self, dresses and undresses, washes hands, plays in parallel

(D) plays in parallel, dresses and undresses, washes hands, feeds self

(E) washes hands, dresses herself, plays in parallel, handles spoon well

30. Language is a critical barometer of both cognitive and emotional development. With which of the following is speech delay most closely associated?

(A) DiGeorge syndrome

(B) Williams syndrome

(C) diabetes

(D) child abuse

(E) asthma

31. Which of the following statements regarding temper tantrums is correct?

(A) most often indicate a serious psychosocial problem

(B) usually appear at the end of the first year

(C) peak prevalence is between 4 and 6 years

(D) routinely occur 8–10 times per day

(E) usually last between 30 and 45 min

32. Typically, infants and children stay within one or two growth chart channels. A normal exception to this rule exists

(A) for female infants

(B) during preschool years (3–6 years)

(C) up to age 2 years

(D) for male infants

(E) during adolescence

33. As part of a routine 18-month check-up, your nurse administers the Denver Developmental Screening Test (DDST) to the child. She reports to you that the child appeared to function at about a 15–18-month level, but he was noncompliant and difficult to test. You tell her that the child probably is developmentally

(A) advanced and was stressed by the test

(B) delayed and psychologically disturbed

(C) delayed and was stressed by the test

(D) normal and noncompliance is common at this age

(E) normal but psychologically disturbed

34. Evaluation of academic failure at school typically includes

(A) hearing and visual evaluation

(B) personality testing

(C) magnetic resonance imaging (MRI) of head

(D) home visit

(E) computed tomography (CT) scan of head

35. Fixation and tracking through the visual field are well developed

(A) at 7 months gestation

(B) at birth

(C) at 2 months

(D) at 6 months

(E) at 1 year

36. At the 2-month well child visit, the mother states that her baby boy is crying a lot. She states he is feeding and sleeping well but cries for a total of 3 h each day. The baby's examination is normal. Which of the following statements about crying is correct?

    (A) Crying increases through the entire first year of life.
    (B) Crying usually is a result of hunger.
    (C) Any baby crying 3 h per day, even in light of a normal examination, warrants a medical workup.
    (D) This amount of crying is normal for this age.
    (E) This degree of crying warrants an immediate skeletal survey.

37. Separation anxiety usually first manifests at age

    (A) 1 week
    (B) 3–4 months
    (C) 8–9 months
    (D) 2–3 years
    (E) 5–6 years

38. At birth the head is what percentage of adult size?

    (A) 25%
    (B) 43%
    (C) 62%
    (D) 75%
    (E) 100%

39. Persistence of neonatal reflexes is an indicator of developmental delay. The Moro reflex should disappear by age

    (A) 3 months
    (B) 4 months
    (C) 6–8 months
    (D) 12–16 months
    (E) 17–20 months

40. The Tonic neck reflex should disappear by age

    (A) 3 months
    (B) 4 months
    (C) 6–8 months
    (D) 12–16 months
    (E) 17–20 months

41. The Babinski (upgoing plantar) reflex should disappear by age

    (A) 3 months
    (B) 4 months
    (C) 6–8 months
    (D) 15–18 months
    (E) 20–24 months

42. The Palmar grasp reflex should disappear by age

    (A) 3 months
    (B) 4 months
    (C) 6–8 months
    (D) 12–16 months
    (E) 17–20 months

43. The pubertal growth spurt in females on average begins at age

    (A) 8 years
    (B) 10 years
    (C) 12 years
    (D) 14 years
    (E) 16 years

44. The pubertal growth spurt in males

    (A) precedes the growth spurt in females by 2 years
    (B) has its onset at the same age as in females but lasts longer
    (C) follows the growth spurt in females by 2 years
    (D) coincides with attainment of the ability to ejaculate
    (E) begins at Tanner IV stage of sexual maturity

45. Peak velocity of growth during adolescence averages

    (A) 1–2 cm per year
    (B) 3–4 cm per year

(C) 5–6 cm per year

(D) 7–8 cm per year

(E) 9–10 cm per year

46. Gynecomastia in males during adolescence

(A) is distinctly uncommon

(B) usually occurs at age 14–15 years

(C) is synonymous with lipomastia

(D) is often a continuing problem in adulthood

(E) necessitates basic laboratory testing

47. The average growth in head circumference during the first year of life is about

(A) 4 cm

(B) 12 cm

(C) 25 cm

(D) 37 cm

(E) 50 cm

48. Which of the following statements is true regarding parental depression?

(A) Postpartum depression is seen in over half of all new mothers.

(B) Children who are seen frequently by their pediatrician are less likely to have a depressed parent.

(C) Teenage mothers do not have a high rate of depression.

(D) After the depressed parent is treated successfully, their children's functioning returns to normal.

(E) In the majority of cases of postpartum depression, intervention is necessary for resolution of symptoms.

49. Major depressive disorder in children

(A) is not diagnosed before 6 years of age

(B) is seen in less than 1% of pediatric inpatients

(C) can be associated with rumination, enuresis, and encopresis

(D) should not be screened for by the primary care pediatrician

(E) is seen in 5–10% of child psychiatry inpatients

50. Colic is a particularly frustrating problem for parents. Which of the following statements regarding colic is correct?

(A) Colic usually is associated with infants who are bottle-fed.

(B) Colic typically begins at 41–42 weeks gestational age regardless of gestational age at birth.

(C) Colic is most prevalent among White neonates.

(D) Colic occurs more commonly among females than males.

(E) There are very predictable long-term temperamental outcomes that emerge from a colicky infancy.

51. Disruptive behavioral disorders (DBD) constitute a group of behavioral problems that are symptomatic of diverse underlying problems. Which of the following is correct regarding these disorders?

(A) They are equally common in boys and girls.

(B) They are more prevalent in African American children.

(C) Significant stealing occurs in approximately 5% of children.

(D) They do not include attention-deficit hyperactivity disorder.

(E) They are strongly associated with childhood asthma.

52. Failure to thrive is

(A) more common among Hispanic children

(B) extremely rare in the United States

(C) most often caused by an organic problem

(D) more common among female infants than male infants

(E) a major risk factor for later developmental and behavioral difficulties

53. Some behavior patterns are considered appropriate at certain developmental stages but are obviously pathologic if present later on in life. Other behavior patterns are considered pathologic at all ages. Which of the following is an example of the latter?

    (A) temper tantrums
    (B) lying
    (C) oppositional behavior
    (D) truancy
    (E) rebellion

54. Childhood aggression is more common among

    (A) girls compared to boys
    (B) children small for their age compared to children large for their age
    (C) children from smaller families compared to children from larger families
    (D) children diagnosed with attention-deficit hyperactivity disorder
    (E) children with borderline personality disorder

55. Pica is the ingestion of nonnutrient substances like dirt and chalk. Which of the following statements regarding pica is true?

    (A) The median age of onset is 6 years.
    (B) It is often a symptom of family disorganization, poor supervision, and affectional neglect.
    (C) It is caused by iron poisoning and parasitic infestations.
    (D) It usually persists into adolescence.
    (E) It is caused by viral infections.

56. Which of the following statements regarding enuresis is true?
    (A) Prevalence at age 10 years ranges from 7 to 10%.
    (B) A marked familial pattern is often noted.
    (C) Workup routinely recommended in the management includes renal ultrasound and micturating cystourethrogram to rule out kidney disease and vesicoureteric reflux.

    (D) Bed wetting alarms are rarely useful in the management of some children with enuresis.
    (E) Among 5-year-old children, enuresis is more common in females.

57. In the normal infant and child, neuromotor development progresses in a

    (A) cephalocaudal and proximodistal manner
    (B) cephalocaudal and distoproximal manner
    (C) caudocephalal and proximodistal manner
    (D) caudocephalal and distoproximal manner
    (E) random manner

58. Which of the following is a criterion for the diagnosis of learning disorder?

    (A) above average intelligence
    (B) reversal of letter in writing
    (C) absence of emotional, behavioral, or motivational problems
    (D) discrepancy between intelligence and achievement in one or more areas
    (E) evidence of visual or auditory perceptual defects

59. A newborn infant is noted to have the physical characteristics of Down syndrome. In regard to telling the parents the presumed diagnosis, which of the following would be most appropriate?

    (A) delay any discussion with either parent until the diagnosis is confirmed by chromosomal analysis
    (B) permit the mother to bond to the infant (1–3 days) before discussing the diagnosis
    (C) explain the diagnosis to the father and have him tell the mother, either privately or with a physician present as he prefers

(D) inform both parents of the presumed diagnosis as soon as possible

(E) explain the diagnosis to the father at once, but delay discussion with the mother for 48–72 h

60. Which of the following laboratory values is normally higher in childhood than in adulthood?

(A) hemoglobin concentration

(B) serum alkaline phosphatase

(C) serum bicarbonate

(D) serum cholesterol

(E) serum sodium

61. The developmental thrust of the toddler is best expressed by the phrase

(A) "me do it"

(B) "show me how"

(C) "that can't be right"

(D) "why"

(E) "you do it"

62. Which of the following statements regarding total body water (TBW) expressed as a percentage of body weight is most correct?

(A) The percentage of TBW is less in the infant than in the older child.

(B) The percentage of TBW is greater in the infant than in the older child.

(C) The percentage of TBW is the same in the infant as in the older child.

(D) The percentage of TBW is less in the male infant than in the older male, but the same in the female infant as in the older female.

(E) The percentage of TBW is more in the female infant than in the older female, but the same in the male infant as in the older male.

63. In the male, body fat expressed as a percentage of total body weight peaks at about the age

(A) 1 week

(B) 1 year

(C) 5 years

(D) 10–12 years

(E) 13–17 years

64. A child who can walk downstairs alternating his or her feet, do a broad jump, and throw a ball overhand, also would be expected to

(A) add five and five

(B) identify three or four coins

(C) name two or three colors

(D) multiply three times three

(E) write his or her name

65. A toddler who resists going to bed at the appropriate time probably is

(A) emotionally deprived and eager for human contact

(B) being intentionally negative to get attention

(C) preoccupied with current activities

(D) physically ill

(E) depressed

66. The ability to copy forms develops in a regular order. Which of the following is the correct sequence?

(A) copy a square, a cross, a circle

(B) copy a square, a circle, a cross

(C) copy a cross, a circle, a square

(D) copy a circle, a square, a cross

(E) copy a circle, a cross, a square

67. In the term newborn, which of the following statements regarding fetal hemoglobin is correct?

(A) Essentially all the hemoglobin is fetal hemoglobin.

(B) Fetal hemoglobin binds oxygen less tightly than adult hemoglobin.

(C) Oxygenated fetal hemoglobin is blue rather than red.

(D) Fetal hemoglobin prevents sickling of sickle cells.

(E) Fetal hemoglobin hemolyzes easily and is a major cause of neonatal jaundice.

68. The normal respiratory rate of a 1-year-old child is

    (A) over 80/min
    (B) between 60 and 80/min
    (C) between 35 and 50/min
    (D) between 20 and 30/min
    (E) between 10 and 12/min

69. As compared to older children and adults, the electrocardiogram (ECG) of an infant normally shows

    (A) a shorter RR and shorter PR interval
    (B) a shorter RR and longer PR interval
    (C) a longer RR and shorter PR interval
    (D) a longer RR and shorter PR interval
    (E) an equal RR and PR interval

70. The average blood pressure at 2 years of age is

    (A) 50/30 mmHg
    (B) 60/30 mmHg
    (C) 75/50 mmHg
    (D) 95/60 mmHg
    (E) 120/80 mmHg

71. The concentration of protein in the cerebrospinal fluid of infants during the first few weeks of life normally may be as high as

    (A) 20 mg/dL
    (B) 45 mg/dL
    (C) 125 mg/dL
    (D) 500 mg/dL
    (E) 1000 mg/dL

72. By 4 years of age one would expect a child's conversation to be

    (A) fully understandable, although mispronunciations and grammatical errors are common
    (B) fully understandable, with few if any mispronunciations and grammatical errors
    (C) fully understandable to the parent but not necessarily to others
    (D) somewhat understandable although garbled and indistinct
    (E) somewhat understandable, with mostly correct use of nouns and mostly incorrect use of verbs

73. A child with an intelligence quotient (IQ) of 65 would be classified as

    (A) at the lower limits of normal
    (B) mildly retarded and educable
    (C) moderately retarded and trainable
    (D) moderately retarded and untrainable
    (E) severely retarded and untrainable

74. Development of the skeleton is by progression from connective tissue to cartilage to bone. At birth, the anterior fontanel is

    (A) bone
    (B) cartilage
    (C) connective tissue
    (D) a combination of cartilage and bone
    (E) a combination of connective tissue and cartilage

75. The anterior fontanel usually feels closed on physical examination (palpation)

    (A) by 3 months
    (B) between 3 and 9 months
    (C) between 9 and 18 months
    (D) between 18 and 24 months
    (E) between 24 and 36 months

76. In regard to puberty, maximal growth in muscle mass

    (A) occurs just before the onset of puberty
    (B) precedes the maximal growth in height
    (C) parallels the maximal growth in height
    (D) follows the maximal growth in height
    (E) is sporadic and unpredictable

77. The growth curve shown below is most compatible with a diagnosis of

(A) androgen excess
(B) constitutional growth delay
(C) craniopharyngioma
(D) normal variant
(E) thyroid dysgenesis

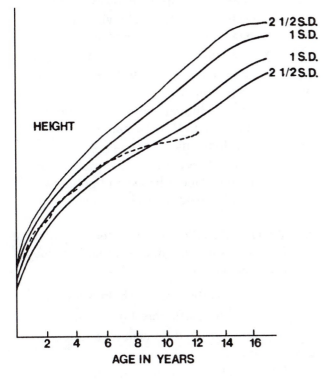

78. Children with isolated growth hormone (GH) deficiency usually

(A) have a normal bone age
(B) have associated mild hypothyroidism
(C) grow parallel to, but below, the normal growth curve
(D) have an associated (*compensating*) hyperthyroidism
(E) show deceleration of growth velocity and fall away from the growth normal curve

79. Children with delayed puberty (without endocrine abnormality) generally can expect to be ultimately

(A) very short and obese
(B) short but of proportionate weight
(C) of normal height and weight

(D) very tall but of proportionate weight
(E) very tall and obese

80. It is estimated that the average school-age American child watches television for about

(A) 1–2 h a week
(B) 3–4 h a week
(C) 5–10 h a week
(D) 30–40 h a week
(E) 70–100 h a week

81. A mild lumbar lordosis and a protuberant abdomen are most characteristic of the

(A) infant
(B) toddler
(C) preschooler
(D) school-age child
(E) adolescent

82. Adolescence is best defined as the period

(A) immediately before, during, and after puberty
(B) of maximal physical growth
(C) of maximal sexual development
(D) of physiologic adjustment to maturity
(E) of psychosocial transition from childhood to adulthood

83. Declining scholastic grades, refusal to participate in family activities, and unwillingness to communicate with either parent in an adolescent usually indicates

(A) a normal stage of development
(B) a normal response to peer pressure
(C) a normal reaction to overprotective parents
(D) a transient phase of ambivalence
(E) an emotional or psychiatric problem

84. Ovulation usually

(A) precedes menarche by 12–24 months
(B) precedes menarche by 1–2 months
(C) occurs at the same time as menarche
(D) follows menarche by 1–2 months
(E) follows menarche by 12–24 months

85. The normal (average) hemoglobin concentration at 1 year of age is about

    (A) 17 g/dL
    (B) 15 g/dL
    (C) 12 g/dL
    (D) 10 g/dL
    (E) 8 g/dL

86. The number of alveoli present in the term infant lung is

    (A) equal to that of the adult
    (B) twice that of the adult
    (C) 5–10 times that of the adult
    (D) one-half that of the adult
    (E) 1/10–1/5 that of the adult

87. The number of glomeruli in the kidney of a term infant is

    (A) equal to that of the adult
    (B) twice that of the adult
    (C) five times that of the adult
    (D) one-half that of the adult
    (E) one-fifth that of the adult

88. During the first year of life, an infant who weighs 7.5 lb (3.4 kg) at birth ordinarily would gain about

    (A) 5 lb (2.3 kg)
    (B) 10 lb (4.5 kg)
    (C) 15 lb (6.8 kg)
    (D) 20 lb (9 kg)
    (E) 25 lb (11.4 kg)

89. During the second year of life, the average child grows about

    (A) 12–15 cm
    (B) 20–25 cm
    (C) 30–40 cm
    (D) 40–50 cm
    (E) over 50 cm

90. During the first month of life, head circumference grows about

    (A) 0.5 cm
    (B) 1.25 cm
    (C) 2.5 cm
    (D) 5 cm
    (E) 7.5 cm

91. Menarche in the adolescent girl

    (A) precedes the spurt in linear growth
    (B) occurs simultaneously with Tanner stage II breast development
    (C) generally occurs when Tanner stage III breast and pubic hair development have been achieved
    (D) occurs simultaneously with Tanner stages IV to V pubic hair and breast development
    (E) generally occurs a year or more after Tanner stage V breast and pubic hair development have been achieved

92. Which of the following statements about renal function of the infant, as compared to that of the adult, is true?

    (A) The bicarbonate threshold is lower.
    (B) The phosphate threshold is lower.
    (C) The threshold for acid excretion is lower.
    (D) The ability to concentrate the urine is greater.
    (E) The GFR is lower because there are 50% fewer glomeruli.

DIRECTIONS (Questions 93 through 100): This section consists of a list of five lettered answers followed by several numbered statements. For each numbered statement select the ONE lettered option with which it is most closely associated. Each lettered option may be selected once, more than once, or not at all.

Questions 93 through 96

    (A) Clinical neruologic examination
    (B) Electroencephalogram
    (C) Gesell schedules
    (D) Thematic apperception test (TAT)
    (E) Wechsler Intelligence Scale (WISC) test

93. Measure development of a 1-year-old

94. Measure intelligence of a 10-year-old

95. Detection of hemiparesis in a 3-month-old

96. Detection of blindness or deafness in a 2-month-old

Questions 97 through 100

   (A) 0–2 years

   (B) 3–6 years

   (C) 6–12 years

   (D) 12–14 years

   (E) 14–19 years

97. Suicidal behavior

98. Gender identity

99. Oedipal years

100. Latency

Answers and Explanations

1. **(B)** Newborns may lose up to 10% of their birth weight in the first few days of life, but with normal nutrition birth weight is regained in approximately 10 days. The infant subsequently gains approximately 30 g per day for the first several months. *(Behrman:35)*

2. **(D)** At 9–12 months, infants gradually develop the concept of object permanence, or the understanding that objects exist even when they are not seen. Around the time this milestone is achieved, infants develop frontal activity on the electroencephalogram. Infants first apply this concept of object permanence to the image of their mother because of her emotional importance; this realization is a critical part of attachment behavior. *(Hay:76)*

3. **(C)** Primary or milk teeth are the initial dentition of children. The first teeth to erupt are the central incisors, at 6–10 months of age. Typically, the mandibular central incisors erupt before the maxillary. The lateral incisors (typically maxillary, followed by mandibular) come in next at 9–13 months of age. The first molars follow at 13–19 months. The canines erupt at around 16–23 months. The second molars are the last to come in at 23–33 months of age. *(Rudolph AM:2167)*

4. **(C)** Handedness frequently is established by the third year. Frustration may result from attempts to change children's hand preference once handedness is established. Unusually early appearance of handedness, such as before the second year, should raise suspicion of motor weakness of an upper extremity. *(Rudolph CD:2167)*

5. **(D)** At birth, the retina is well developed, but the lens is rather immobile. Fixation and tracking through the visual field are well developed by 2 months of age. Infants prefer to gaze at a human face rather than geometrical designs and they also prefer curved lines, bright colors, and high contrast. Strabismus is common after birth but usually resolves by 3 months of age. Although visual acuity is poor at birth, approximately 20/400, it improves rapidly in the first 6 months of life to 20/40. However, it does not reach 20/20 until about 4 years of age. *(Hay:79, 444–447)*

6. **(E)** Development of the paranasal sinuses continues throughout childhood. The ethmoid and maxillary sinuses are present from birth; the frontal and sphenoid sinuses usually appear radiologically around 6 years of age, and frequently develop asymmetrically. Frontal sinuses are absent in 1–5% of adults. *(Rudolph CD:1258)*

7. **(B)** The Denver developmental exam is one of the most widely used developmental screening tools. It tests four domains of development: personal-social, fine motor-adaptive, language, and gross motor. It can be used from birth to 6 years of age and can be administered in 20–30 min. There is no extensive training or expensive equipment required to complete the screening. It is said to have limited predictive validity to foresee cognitive delays at a later age. The new expanded form (DDST-II) includes expanded language testing and is reported to have greater sensitivity, particularly for language delays. *(Hay:81)*

8. **(B)** The fetal period begins at the ninth week of gestation and ends at birth. It is preceded by the embryonic period, during which the rudiments of all major organ systems develop. *(Behrman:29)*

9. **(C)** By 10 weeks gestation the face is recognizably human, and by 12 weeks gestation the gender of the external genitalia is clearly distinguishable. *(Behrman:28)*

10. **(D)** Following the realization that words can stand for things, the child's vocabulary balloons from about 10–15 words at 18 months to 100 or more at 2 years. After 18 months, there is a dramatic increase in expressive and receptive vocabulary and by the end of the second year, a quantum leap occurs in language development. *(Behrman:34; Hay:80–81)*

11. **(C)** Average length at birth is around 20 in or 50 cm. The newborn averages a gain in length of 3.5 cm per month through the first 3 months of life. From 3–6 months of life, the infant grows by about 2 cm per month. The growth velocity tapers off gradually. By 9–12 months of life the child grows 1.2 cm per month. Between 1 and 3 years of life the child grows 1 cm per month. By age 2 the child is about 35 in or 87 cm which is about 50% of adult height. *(Rudolph CD:5; Behrman:32–33)*

12. **(A)** Teenagers have been entering puberty at increasingly earlier ages during the last century, presumably because of better nutrition and improved socioeconomic conditions. The age of menarche decreased by about 4 months per decade during the last century. In the United States, the average age at menarche is 12 years, the average weight is 48 kg and the average height is 158.5 cm. Although the first measurable sign of puberty in girls is the beginning of the height spurt, the first conspicuous sign usually is development of breast buds between the ages of 8 and 11 years. *(Behrman: 53–55)*

13. **(B)** The first sign of puberty in boys, testicular enlargement, begins as early as 9.5 years. The appearance of pubic hair is an early event in puberty but can occur any time between ages 10 and 15 years. The penis begins to grow significantly a year or so after the onset of testicular and pubic hair development, usually between the ages of 10 and 13.5 years. The median age for entering SMR 2 or puberty in boys is 10.5 years. However, great variability exists in the timing and onset of puberty and growth, and psychosocial development does not necessarily parallel physical changes. *(Behrman:52–55)*

14. **(C)** Growth acceleration begins in early adolescence, although peak growth velocity is not reached until SMR 3 in girls and SMR 4 in boys. Girls reach their peak height velocity between 11.5 and 12 years of age. The height spurt usually ends by age 14. Girls who mature early will reach their peak height velocity sooner and attain their final height earlier. Girls who mature late will attain a greater ultimate height because of the longer period of growth before the growth spurt. Final height is related to skeletal age at onset of puberty as well as genetic factors. *(Behrman:55)*

15. **(C)** Growth is rapid in the first 2 years of life. Infants increase their length by 50% the first year and 25% the next. They triple their birth weight in the first year. After 2 years of age, the growth velocity curve stabilizes into the rate for mid childhood, which is a weight gain of 2–3 kg or 4.5–6.5 lbs per year and a height gain of 5–7 cm or 2–3 in per year. *(Rudolph CD:5)*

16. **(D)** Growth charts can confirm an impression of obesity if the weight for height exceeds 120% of the standard (median) weight for height. Obesity is the most common form of malnutrition in the United States. Other parameters used to detect and quantify obesity include body mass index (BMI) and measurement of skinfold thickness in triceps and subscapular regions. BMI is calculated as (weight in kilograms)/(height in meters)^2. BMI varies with age and BMI curves are available. *(Rudolph CD:478–480, 2140)*

17. **(C)** Body proportions follow a sequence of regular changes with development. The head and

trunk are relatively large at birth, with progressive lengthening of the limbs during puberty. Proportionality can be assessed by measuring the lower body segment, defined as the length from the symphysis pubis to the floor, and the upper body segment, defined as the height minus the lower body segment. The ratio of upper body segment divided by lower body segment equals approximately 1.7 at birth, 1.3 at 3 years, and 1.0 after age 7. Higher U/L ratios are characteristic of short-limbed dwarfism or bone disorders such as rickets. *(Behrman:59)*

18. **(B)** Constitutional growth delay has a characteristic pattern of having a late growth spurt during adolescence, therefore in early adolescence the child will be short as compared to his or her peers. However, he or she will continue to grow later in adolescence and reach a normal adult height. Children with constitutional growth delay will be of normal size at birth. Bone age is delayed and is comparable to the height age. Children with constitutional growth delay must be differentiated from those with undernutrition and endocrinologic short stature who also have delayed bone age. *(Behrman:1679)*

19. **(D)** The first teeth to erupt are the central incisors, at 5–7 months of age. These are followed by the lateral incisors, the first molars, the canines, and the second molars. Delayed eruption is usually considered when there are no teeth at approximately 13 months of age (mean + 3 standard deviations). Delayed eruption of all teeth may indicate systemic or nutritional disturbances such as hypopituitarism, hypothyroidism, cleidocranial dysostosis, trisomy 21, progeria, Albright osteodystrophy, incontinentia pigmenti, rickets, and multiple syndromes (Hunter, Dubowitz, Goltz, de Lange, Gardner, Maroteaux-Lamy). Failure of eruption of single or small groups of teeth may arise from local causes such as supernumerary teeth, cysts, or retained primary teeth. Premature loss of primary predecessors is the most common cause of premature eruption of teeth. If the entire dentition is advanced for age and sex, precocious puberty should be considered. *(Behrman:1108–1109)*

20. **(C)** Freud describes the first year of life as the oral stage because so many of the infant's needs are fulfilled by oral means. The next period from 18 months to 3 years is termed the anal stage because the developmental issue of bowel control is the major task requiring mastery. It basically represents a more generalized theme of socialized behavior and overall body cleanliness which is begun to be taught to or imposed on the child at this age. Freud describes the Oedipal phase between the ages of 3 and 6 years when there is a strong attachment to the parent of the opposite sex. The child's fantasies may focus on play acting the adult role with that parent. By 6 years of age, Oedipal issues are usually resolved and attachment is redirected toward the parent of the same sex. The next phase (6–12 years) is described as the latency phase, since children are not bothered by significant aggressive or sexual drive but instead devote most of their energies to school and peer group interactions. *(Behrman:25–26)*

21. **(E)** Some echolalia (echoing spoken words) during toddlerhood is common and usually of no concern. When severe or persistent beyond toddlerhood, echolalia may be a sign of disturbed language development, mental retardation, or neurologic disease. Although echolalia is common in infantile autism, most toddlers who display word repetition are not autistic. [*Note*: The question did not ask whether autism should be considered (it should) but whether the child probably has autism (he probably does not).] *(Behrman:87)*

22. **(E)** Normal newborns are endowed with a set of reflexes to facilitate survival, including rooting and sucking reflexes, and remarkable sensory abilities. The newborn is no longer considered a blank slate. Instead, the newborn is seen as having genetic strengths and weaknesses in neurocognitive organization that are reflected in temperament, adaptability, responsiveness, and general interaction with the environment. Hearing is well developed at birth, and speech sounds are preferred. The infant learns to recognize his mother's voice and differentiate it from other female voices within

the first 3 weeks of life. At birth infants prefer to gaze at a human face rather than geometric designs, and they also prefer curved lines, bright colors, and high contrast. Infants are myopic at birth. They are able to suckle at the breast immediately after birth. *(Behrman:32–34)*

23. **(B)** The attainment of gross motor milestones begins at approximately 2 months of age with steady head control. This allows better visual interaction between infants and parents. The child is then able to be pulled to sit without head lag at around 3 months of age. Putting hands together in the midline at around 3 months of age allows the infant to examine objects in the midline and manipulate them with both hands. Once the asymmetric Tonic neck reflex is gone, at around 4 months of age, infants are able to begin to roll over, first from stomach to back and finally around 6 months of age from back to stomach. Infants will sit without support at approximately 6 months of age and will pull to stand and cruise around furniture by 9 months of age. The average age of beginning to walk alone is 12 months. *(Behrman: 34–36)*

24. **(E)** Around the same time as the infant is able to put hands together in the midline he is able to grasp objects and examine them. This occurs at an average of 3.5 months of age. He can transfer objects from hand to hand at approximately 5.5 months of age, allowing him to compare objects. He attains thumb–finger grasp at approximately 8 months of age, at which time he begins to feed himself finger foods. At around 1 year of age he is able to turn pages in a book, and by 13 months of age he has attained sufficient visual-motor coordination to scribble. By 15 months of age he can build a tower of two cubes, using objects in combination, and by 22 months of age he can build his tower up to six cubes, which requires visual, gross, and fine motor coordination. *(Behrman:34–35)*

25. **(B)** Growth of the midface and lower face in children occurs gradually. Loss of the deciduous (baby) teeth is a more dramatic sign of maturation, beginning at around 6 years of age, after eruption of the first molars. Replacement with adult teeth occurs at a rate of about 4 per

year. The central incisors are replaced at the same time as the first molars erupt, around 6–7 years of age; after this, the lateral incisors erupt, at around 7–8 years of age. The adult canines replace the baby teeth at around 9–11 years of age, and next to erupt are the first premolars and then the second premolars. The second molars erupt at around 12 years of age but the third molars (wisdom teeth) do not erupt until 17–22 years of age. *(Behrman:1109)*

26. **(D)** The primary teeth form in dental crypts that arise from a band of epithelial cells incorporated into each developing jaw. Organization of adjacent mesenchyme takes place in each area of epithelial growth, and the two elements together comprise the beginning of a tooth. The first primary or deciduous teeth to erupt are the central incisors at 5–7 months of age, followed by the lateral incisors at around 7–10 months of age and the first molars at around 10–16 months of age. The canines do not erupt until 16–20 months of age. *(Behrman:1108–1109)*

27. **(C)** Ossification centers usually present at birth include the distal femur and the proximal tibia. Reference standards for bone maturation facilitate estimation of bone age. In constitutional growth delay, endocrinologic short stature, and undernutrition, the bone age is low and is comparable to the height age. In familial short stature, the bone age is normal (compared to chronological age). The most commonly used standards are those of Gruelich and Pyle, which require radiographs of the left hand and wrist; knee films are sometimes added for younger children. *(Rudolph CD:2420)*

28. **(C)** Most children begin to walk independently around the time of their first birthday; some do not walk until 15 months. At 18 months of age, the infant shows improvements in balance and agility, and the ability to run and climb stairs while holding a parent's hand emerges. By 30 months of age, the child is able to go upstairs by himself, alternating feet. By 3 years of age, the child has attained the motor coordination to ride a tricycle. A child is usually hopping by 4 years of age and skipping by 6 years of age. *(Behrman:34)*

29. (A) At approximately 18 months, several cognitive changes come together to mark the conclusion of the sensorimotor period. At this time, the infant can feed himself, seek help when in trouble, and complain when wet or soiled. From this age forward, the child is increasingly independent. By 24 months of age, he helps to undress himself and is able to handle a spoon well. As a 3-year-old, he helps in dressing and undressing, washes his own hands, and engages in "parallel play." By age 5, he is able to fully dress and undress himself. At this time he is likely to engage in domestic role-playing. *(Behrman:33–35)*

30. (D) Child abuse and neglect are correlated with delayed language, particularly the ability to convey emotional states. Such delays may contribute to problems of behavior, socialization, and learning. Mental retardation may first become apparent with delayed speech at approximately 2 years, although earlier signs may have been overlooked. Hearing loss is a common cause of speech delay. Consequently, hearing evaluation should be an integral part of the management of delayed speech. The other choices listed do not have a proclivity for speech delay. *(Behrman:49)*

31. (B) As children mature, they learn what behaviors are acceptable and how much power they are able to wield by testing limits. Control is a central issue. Inability to control some aspect of the external world, such as how to make a certain toy work or when to leave, often results in a loss of internal control, that is, a temper tantrum. Fear, overtiredness, or physical discomfort can also evoke tantrums. When they are reinforced by intermittent rewards, as when the parent occasionally gives in to the child's demands, tantrums can also become an entrenched strategy for exerting control by the toddler. Tantrums lasting more than 15 min or happening regularly more than three times daily can reflect underlying medical, emotional, or social problems. Tantrums normally appear at the end of the first year of life and peak at 2–4 years. Frequent tantrums after 5 years of age usually persist throughout childhood. Clearly, this is an undesirable outcome which, in nearly all children, is avoidable. *(Levine:28–29)*.

32. (C) A newborn's birth weight correlates with the size, nutritional state, and general health of the mother and represents the influence of uterine constraints on ultimate size. After the first 6 months of life, genetic factors influencing ultimate height begin to exert their effect. The growth percentile, therefore, may shift significantly in the first 4–18 months of life. This shift can be either up or down. An infant who is small for gestational age and has a genetic predisposition to larger stature usually experiences accelerated growth in the first 6 months, and by 18 months a stable growth percentile is established. A downward shift is seen in large infants who have a genetic predisposition to short stature. A stable growth percentile should be established by 18 months of age. *(Behrman:32, 58–59)*

33. (D) About half of normal children during the second year of life are noncompliant when faced with a task such as the DDST. This is itself a developmental phenomenon, reflecting the child's movement toward independence and his newfound ability to resist control and do things himself. The range of normal on-screening tests such as the DDST is broad, and a score in the 15–18-month range for an 18-month-old child is not bothersome. Usually, more formal and complete evaluation is indicated for the child who is functioning more than one-third below his chronologic age. *(Hay:80–82)*

34. (A) In evaluation of academic failure at school, neuropsychological and educational testing is completed, as well as audiometry and visual testing by the school or the pediatrician. Evaluation for attention-deficit hyperactivity disorder (ADHD) may form part of the evaluation for academic failure. Neuroimaging typically is not part of this evaluation process. Although a home visit may be particularly helpful, it is not commonly carried out by the school personnel. *(Rudolph AM:123–124)*

35. (C) At birth, the retina is well developed but the lens is rather immobile. Fixation and tracking through the visual field are well developed by 2 months of age. The length of time that an infant fixates on a paired visual stimulus has been interpreted as visual preference, and has also been correlated with later cognitive development. Visual fixation tasks are the basis of infant IQ testing marketed recently. *(Hay:79, 444–447)*

36. **(D)** Crying gradually increases during the first 6–12 weeks of age because it is the main modality by which infants express responses to stimuli, both aversive and nonaversive. Crying can be a response to a variety of stimuli, including hunger, a wet diaper, fear, fatigue, and overstimulation. Crying gradually decreases after 12 weeks of age as the infant develops other responses, such as smiling or reaching, or becomes more adept at self-soothing, such as sucking the fingers or the thumb. In the first weeks of life, however, crying can become a distressing problem for the parents, and crying associated with irritability is often labeled as colic. *(Behrman:32)*

37. **(C)** The advent of object constancy corresponds with qualitative changes in social and communicative development. The infant looks back and forth between an approaching stranger and a parent, as if to contrast known from unknown, and may cling or cry anxiously. This occurs around 8–9 months of age. Separations often become more difficult, and infants who have been sleeping through the night for months begin to awaken regularly and cry, as though remembering that parents are in the next room. This is a normal developmental milestone not to be confused with *separation anxiety disorder* which occurs in school-age children. *(Behrman:34; Rudolph CD:451)*

38. **(D)** At birth, the head is 75% of its adult size and makes up 25% of the baby's length. This changes dramatically in time, so that at 25 years of age the head measures only one-eighth of the body length. After birth, the brain continues to grow rapidly, completing half of its lifetime growth in the first year. Postnatal brain growth is the result of an increase in white matter and a proliferation of synaptic connections. After 2 years of age, the head circumference increases only 2 cm per year in middle childhood. By

7 years of age, 90% of brain growth is completed. *(Behrman:33)*

39. **(C), 40. (C), 41. (D), 42. (C)**
Reflex movement begins in fetal development as early as 9 weeks gestation. However, most of the reflexes associated with the newborn develop between 20 and 38 weeks gestation. The Moro reflex disappears by 7 months of age. Palmar grasp usually disappears by 6 months of age, facilitating release of objects. The Tonic neck reflex, which is elicited by turning the infant's head, resulting in extension of the arm and leg on the side toward which the head is turned and flexion of the opposite side, disappears by 8 months of age, unless myelinization or brain development is pathologic. The Babinski (upgoing toes) sign, which develops in an infant just prior to term, does not disappear until 16 months of age, when adequate myelinization has occurred. *(Rudolph AM:799)*

43. **(B)** Growth acceleration begins in early adolescence, although peak growth velocities are not reached until SMR 3 or SMR 4. The pubertal growth spurt begins at about 10 years in females and about 12.5 years in males. Different areas of the skeleton attain their peak growth at different times. This is seen most dramatically in the feet, which first develop a growth spurt. This is followed by a rapid increase in leg length, and subsequently in truncal growth. Facial growth occurs after peak height velocity. This asymmetric growth gives the young adolescent a gawky look. *(Behrman:54–55)*

44. **(C)** The first sign of puberty in the male, usually between the ages of 10 and 12, is scrotal and testicular growth. The first ejaculation is a notable event and usually begins 1 year after the beginning of testicular growth, but its timing is highly variable. Ninety percent of boys have this experience between the ages of 11 and 15 years. The pubertal growth spurt begins at about 10 years in females and about 2 years later in males. Boys have just over 2 more years of preadolescent growth than girls do; during this time, leg growth increases more dramatically than trunk growth. Girls have a

greater spurt in hip width related to stature than boys do, although boys exceed girls in most other areas of bone growth. The growth spurt begins at SMR 2 and peaks at SMR 4. *(Behrman:54–57)*

45. **(E)** The peak velocity of growth among adolescent girls corresponds with SMR 3, and among boys with SMR 4. This growth averages 9–10 cm per year, although this growth is somewhat lower in girls than in boys. However, the period of pubertal development lasts much longer in boys and may not be completed until the age of 18 years. Thelarche (breast development) in girls occurs much earlier than the period of peak growth velocity; it is the first visible sign of puberty and may begin as early as age 8 years. *(Behrman:54–56)*

46. **(B)** Gynecomastia significant enough to be embarrassing for adolescent males occurs in less than 10% of boys, although some degree of breast tissue enlargement is seen in 40–65% of adolescent boys in the ages of 14–15. This resolves within 2 years on its own in the majority of cases, and rarely is pathologic. Lipomastia refers to soft subcutaneous fat often seen in obese boys and sometimes confused with gynecomastia. *(Rudolph AM:101)*

47. **(B)** During the first year of life, the average total increase in head circumference is about 12 cm (5 in): 6 cm (2.5 in) during the first 3 months; 3 cm (1.25 in) from 3 to 6 months; and another 3 cm from 6 to 12 months. A convenient rule to remember is that growth in head circumference averages 2 cm per month during the first 3 months (equals 6 cm), 1 cm per month during the next 3 months (equals 3 cm), and 1/2 cm per month for the last 6 months of the year (equals 3 cm). This totals (6 + 3 + 3) 12 cm for the year. *(Rudolph CD:5)*

48. **(A)** Postpartum depression is a common occurrence among new mothers, affecting up to 80%. This usually resolves itself with hormonal changes back to normal homeostasis, but in 10% a major depression occurs. Depressed parents tend to bring their children to the pediatrician more often. Teenage mothers are particularly

vulnerable to depression, especially if there is poor social structure. Even after treatment of a parent with major depression, the children tend to have ongoing problems of functioning. The adjustment of children is related not only to their exposure to psychiatric symptomatology but also to longer-term patterns of dysfunctional parenting behaviors and aberrant social interactions. *(NEJM 347(3):194–199, 2002; JAMA 287(6):762–765, 2002)*

49. **(C)** Major depressive disorder (MDD) can be diagnosed in infants and preschoolers (1%) and is seen in greatest numbers in adolescents (5%). In infants, MDD is seen as failure to thrive, in preschoolers it is seen as behavioral problems and separation anxiety. It may be associated with rumination, enuresis, and encopresis. MDD is common in the hospitalized child. As high as 7% of general inpatients and 28% of child psychiatry inpatients have MDD. Physicians should screen patients for this disorder by taking a thorough history on behavior and mood of the child. *(Levine:633–635)*

50. **(B)** Colic typically begins at 41–42 weeks gestational age in both term and preterm infants. There are two patterns of colic, the most common being associated with fussiness beginning in the early evening hours and occurring in paroxysms of crying. The second pattern is characterized by paroxysms of crying throughout the day in a hyperirritable infant. There are no differences in prevalence of colic among race, gender, or method of feeding (breast vs. bottle). The presence of colic during infancy gives no predictive value for long-term behavioral, temperamental, or psychologic outcomes. *(Levine:365–369)*

51. **(C)** Disruptive behavioral disorders, a group of behavioral syndromes symptomatic of diverse underlying problems, include conduct disorder, oppositional defiant disorder, attention-deficit hyperactivity disorder, adjustment disorder, and posttraumatic stress disorder. These disorders are three to four times more common in boys than in girls but there are no differences in ethnicity or race. These disorders frequently are associated with familial psychosocial dysfunction and poverty. Significant stealing occurs in

approximately 5% of children; other significant manifestations of conduct disorder include fire setting, assault on people and animals, and truancy. Psychologic testing may be helpful to assess cognitive functioning. Differential diagnosis includes CNS abnormalities, lead poisoning, and substance abuse. *(Behrman:82–84)*

52. **(E)** Failure to thrive is a major risk factor for later behavioral and developmental problems. It is diagnosed by persistent and significant deviation from the growth curves along time. Poverty-stricken children are likely to be affected, at 8–12% prevalence. Although this could represent an organic disorder, by far the most common cause of failure to thrive is psychosocial: the so called non-organic failure to thrive. *(Rudolph CD:5–9)*

53. **(D)** In children less than 6 years of age, oppositional behavior, rebellion, and lying are common as children are just learning to follow societal rules. Temper tantrums may persist from preschoolers up until 5 years of age, usually without pathologic origin. Truancy, or intentional school avoidance, is pathologic at any age. *(Behrman:82–84)*

54. **(D)** Several factors contribute to childhood aggression. Boys almost universally are reported to be more aggressive than girls. Larger children often are more aggressive than smaller ones. Children from larger families often are more aggressive than those from smaller families. Conduct-disordered behavior often is associated with psychopathologic conditions. Both attention-deficit hyperactivity disorder and borderline personality disorder (BPD) correlate with aggression. However, ADHD is much more common than BPD, so (D) is the best answer. Of interest is the correlation in boys between severe reading retardation and the development of aggressive conduct disorder. *(Behrman:83)*

55. **(B)** Pica is a chronic eating disorder which involves the eating of nonnutritive substances such as dirt, clay, and peeling paint. The age of onset usually is 1–2 years but may be earlier. This disorder usually remits by middle childhood.

Lack of parental nurturing and mental retardation are predisposing factors. Children with pica are at an increased risk for lead poisoning and parasitic infections. Differential diagnoses for this behavior include autism, schizophrenia, and certain physical disorders such as Kleine-Levin syndrome. *(Behrman:72)*

56. **(B)** Enuresis, the repeated involuntary or voluntary discharge of the bladder after the age at which bladder control should be maintained, is among the most common problems brought to the pediatrician. Among 5 year olds, enuresis occurs in 7% of males and 3% of females. Twin studies reveal a marked familial pattern. Enuresis is associated with immigration, socioeconomic disadvantage, and family psychopathology. Organic pathology can be found in only a very small number of cases; physical examination and urinalysis are the only routinely indicated tests in enuresis. *(Behrman:72–73)*

57. **(A)** Normal neuromotor development progresses in a cephalocaudal and proximodistal order. Control of the eyes and head precedes control of the arms and legs. Control of the arms precedes control of the hands, which precedes control of the fingers. Although the rate of development varies considerably, even among normal infants, the pattern and sequence of acquisition of neuromotor control is relatively constant. *(Hay:64, 74, 81)*

58. **(D)** The key criterion to the diagnosis of learning disorder is a significant discrepancy between the child's estimated intelligence and his or her achievement in one or more learning areas. Although reversal of letters is common in these children, it is not present in all patients and is not a criterion for diagnosis. Furthermore, some reversal of letters may occur in normal children as they begin to learn to write. Children with learning disorders are usually of average or above average intelligence, but above average intelligence is not a criterion for diagnosis. Similarly, visual or auditory perceptual defects are frequently seen in these patients but are not criteria for diagnosis. Many of these patients do have emotional,

behavioral, or motivational problems in addition to, or in reaction to, their learning disorder. *(Rudolph CD:435–437)*

59. (D) Studies have shown that the majority of parents prefer to be informed of Down syndrome and other causes of impairment or mental retardation in their baby as soon as possible. Delay only makes the shock greater. The diagnosis should be presented to both parents together, gently and compassionately, preferably by a physician with whom they are familiar. It is not necessary to delay informing the parents while awaiting the results of chromosomal analysis or other tests. Most parents will accept the fact that the diagnosis is less than 100% certain while confirmation is pending. Often, the small ray of hope that this permits eases the acceptance of reality. *(Rudolph CD:726; Pediatr Clin North Am 22:561, 1975)*

60. (B) Serum concentration of alkaline phosphatase is consistently higher throughout childhood than in adulthood. It is very high at birth. Although it falls during childhood, it still remains considerably above adult values and then peaks again during adolescence. Hemoglobin concentration at birth is higher than normal adult values, falls to a physiologic nadir of 10–12 g/dL at 2–4 months, and then rises, remaining at or below adult values for the rest of childhood. Serum bicarbonate and cholesterol concentrations are slightly low in infancy but then reach levels that are about equal to adult values. Serum sodium concentration is not different in children than in adults. [*Note*: The question specifies that the value normally be higher in childhood. Hemoglobin values are normally higher than adult values in early infancy only. It is especially important in reading pediatric questions to pay careful attention to any indication of age or stage of childhood.] *(Hay:1311)*

61. (A) Toddlerhood is the period of developing autonomy, when the child normally is seeking to establish his or her own identity and to prove his or her own ability. Toddlers want to control and do everything by themselves. They are too impatient and immature to seek or accept explanations. The toddler's slogan is "me do it." *(Rudolph CD:403–405)*

62. (B) Total body water, as a percent of total body weight, is greater in the infant than in the child or adult. The percentage of TBW is highest at birth and decreases steadily from infancy to late childhood, averaging almost 70% of body weight in early infancy and only 60% in late childhood. Age-related changes in body composition and water content have clinical significance. Daily fluid needs in relation to body weight are greatest in the young infant. The infant who is moderately to severely dehydrated will have lost 10–15% of his body weight as water, whereas the corresponding figure for the older child or adult is only 6–9%. *(Rudolph CD:1315; Hay:1281)*

63. (B) Body fat comprises about 16% of body weight at birth, increases to about 22% at about a year of age, and then gradually declines. At adolescence there is a second marked increase in body fat in females but not in males. In the normal male, percentage of body fat is at its relative highest at about 1 year of age. *(Rudolph CD:223; Behrman:58–59)*

64. (C) The gross motor tasks described (walking downstairs with alternate feet, throwing overhand, broad jump) are accomplished at 3–4 years of age. A child of this age also should be able to identify two or three colors. The other abilities listed generally come at, or after, 5 years of age. [*Note*: This format is common in pediatric examination questions about development. The student should recognize that often, as is the case in this question, the correct answer can be surmised even if the reader cannot identify the age of the child described in the body of the question. Logically, in this case, the correct choice must be the one corresponding to the youngest age. The ability to name colors precedes all the other items listed and therefore must be the correct answer. Knowing the sequence of development without knowing the corresponding ages would be sufficient to answer this question.] *(Hay:74–75, 81)*

65. **(C)** Resistance to going to bed is a common pattern of normal maturation in the young child. The toddler is preoccupied with current activities and unaware of tomorrow and the need for sleep. Consequently, she frequently is unwilling to suspend her present activity. At this age, resistance to going to bed (unless extreme) is unlikely to represent an emotional problem, although it may present a management problem for the parents. *(Pediatrics 50:312–324, 1972; Rudolph CD:418–420).*

66. **(E)** The ability to copy certain printed forms is considered a fine motor-adaptive characteristic and develops in a regular order. The ability to copy a vertical line appears first, at about 2–3 years. The following abilities then appear in sequence: a circle at $2^{1/2}$ to $3^{1/2}$ years, a cross at $3^{1/2}$ to $4^{1/2}$ years and finally, a square at 5–6 years. *(J Pediatr 71:181, 1967;Hay:81)*

67. **(D)** At term birth (40 weeks gestation), the percentage of fetal hemoglobin varies greatly from infant to infant but usually is between 60 and 90%. Fetal hemoglobin binds more tightly to oxygen than does adult hemoglobin, giving the newborn infant a relative advantage in picking up oxygen in the lung but a disadvantage in releasing oxygen to the tissues. The presence of significant amounts of fetal hemoglobin (which protects the sickle erythrocyte against sickling) is the major reason that young infants with sickle cell disease rarely are symptomatic. Oxygenated fetal hemoglobin is red, just like adult hemoglobin. Fetal hemoglobin does not predispose the red cell to hemolysis. *(McMillan:358–359:1450)*

68. **(D)** Both heart rate and respiratory rate are greater in infants and young children than in adults, reflecting the relatively larger surface area and higher metabolic rate of the youngsters. The respiratory rate of most normal 1-year-old children is between 20 and 30 times per minute. This is slower than a neonate and faster than an older child or adult. *(McMillan: 1429)*

69. **(A)** For the reasons explained in answer 68 above, the infant normally has a more rapid heart rate than an adult. Rates of up to 180 bpm can be normal in the first year of life. This increased rate is associated with both a shorter RR and a shorter PR interval on the electrocardiogram. *(Rudolph CD:1757–1760)*

70. **(D)** The blood pressure of a normal 2-year-old child averages about 95/60 mmHg. There is almost no change in normal blood pressure values between 2 and 6 years, but after 6 years there is a gradual increase to an average of 120/75 mmHg at 16 years. It is generally recommended that routine measurement of blood pressure in children commence at 2–3 years of age; however, blood pressure should be measured in younger children, including neonates, whenever clinically indicated. *(Hay:708)*

71. **(C)** The cerebrospinal fluid concentration of protein in the immediate newborn period normally may be as high as 125 mg/dL; some series have suggested normal values up to 200 mg/dL. The concentration gradually falls to "normal values" of less than 45 mg/dL by 6–8 weeks. *(Hay:49, 719)*

72. **(A)** The physician needs to distinguish speech (pronunciation, articulation, and fluency) from language (content, meaning, vocabulary, and grammar) and to evaluate each separately. Normally, both speech and language are sufficiently developed by 4 years so that the child's verbal communications are fully understandable, even by strangers. Mispronunciations and grammatical errors, however, remain common until about $4^{1/2}$ years or even 5 years. *(Hay:77, 80–82; Pediatrics 82:447, 1988; Rudolph CD:18)*

73. **(B)** An IQ between 50 and 70 or 75 (depending on the test employed) usually indicates mild mental retardation. Such children generally are educable if given appropriate support and opportunity. An IQ between 30 and 50 is considered moderate retardation; less than 30 is considered severe and profound retardation. *(Rudolph CD:438)*

74. **(C)** At birth, the anterior fontanel, which is the junction of the coronal and sagittal sutures in the region between the frontal and parietal

bones, is composed of connective tissue, which is why it feels like a hole or soft spot. It will be replaced gradually by bone. Examination of the anterior fontanel during infancy can provide information about intracranial pressure. A full or bulging fontanel may indicate meningitis or intracranial hemorrhage. A sunken fontanel can be seen in dehydrated infants. (Rudolph CD:87)

75. **(C)** Despite wide variations in size and rate of closure, it is generally accepted that the anterior fontanel closes some time between 9 and 18 months. That is, by this time, it is composed of cartilage and bone and no longer is palpable as a soft spot. Early closure may be indicative of a disorder such as premature cranial synostosis. Late closure may be seen in conditions such as hypothyroidism, rickets, hypophosphatasia, hydrocephalus, or trisomy 18 syndrome. (Rudolph CD:11)

76. **(D)** Growth in muscle mass is a relatively late event of puberty. Maximal growth of muscle follows maximal growth in height. First the adolescent grows taller; then he or she fills out. Knowledge of this normal pattern can help the adolescent, and his or her parent, deal with aspirations and expectations regarding physical appearance and performance. (Rudolph CD:223)

77. **(C)** Craniopharyngioma often is associated with hypothalamic and pituitary destruction, which may present as growth failure any time during later childhood or adolescence. A rather sudden arrest of previously normal linear growth should make one consider this diagnosis. Thyroid dysgenesis would cause growth failure from early infancy. The growth impairment shown is too severe to be considered either a normal variation or constitutional growth delay. Although androgen excess can lead to ultimate short stature because it stimulates closure of the skeletal growth centers, it also stimulates linear growth, so the child initially is tall for his age. (Behrman:1675–1680)

78. **(E)** About 50% of patients with isolated GH deficiency grow normally during the first year of life. Growth then decelerates, and both height and weight fall further and further away from the normal curves. Bone age generally is delayed. By definition, in isolated growth hormone deficiency other endocrine functions are normal; there is no associated disturbance of thyroid function. Before concluding that a child has isolated growth hormone deficiency, however, it is necessary to rule out physical destruction of the pituitary gland (e.g., by a craniopharyngioma), or an associated pituitary abnormality such as ACTH deficiency. Isolated growth hormone deficiency can be sporadic or genetic. [Note: The astute student will realize that it is very unlikely that statements (C) and (E) are both correct and will concentrate on these, even if uncertain about the remaining choices.] (Behrman:58)

79. **(C)** Children with delayed puberty not associated with an endocrine abnormality are initially short but have a longer than normal period of growth and a later than normal adolescent growth spurt. Ultimate height, therefore, generally is normal, and ultimate weight is normal and proportionate to height. (Rudolph CD:2103; Behrman:58)

80. **(D)** Remarkable as it seems, American children spend an average of 30–40 h a week in front of the television set, whereas, in general, they spend only 25–30 h a week in school. Television has a major influence on children's knowledge, attitude, and behavior. The nature and quality of the program material is, of course, as much a problem as the volume. There are considerable concerns and some data that such excessive viewing adversely affects children's attitudes toward violence, gender roles, concepts of racial stereotypes, and commercialism. (Am J Dis Child 140:78–79, 1986; Pediatrics 75:233, 1985; Rudolph CD:528)

81. **(B)** A relatively large abdomen is common throughout infancy and early childhood, reflecting a relatively large liver and considerable gas in the small bowel. This is most noticeable during toddlerhood, from 1 to 3 years. It is also during this period of early ambulation that a lumbar lordosis is common. The lordosis exaggerates

the large and protuberant abdomen, resulting in the typical "pot-bellied" appearance of the toddler. This normal pot-bellied appearance may be one reason that abdominal tumors (Wilms tumor or neuroblastoma) at this age are often diagnosed late. *(Behrman:1101)*

82. **(E)** Adolescence is the period of psychosocial transition from childhood to adulthood. Puberty is a physiologic event. Adolescence is a psychosocial phenomenon, albeit strongly influenced by the child's reaction to the physical and physiologic changes of puberty. Adolescence cannot be defined by a fixed temporal relation to puberty. Often, adolescence appears to occur some time after the onset of puberty. *(Rudolph CD:223)*

83. **(E)** Although adolescence is characteristically a difficult period of psychosocial and emotional growth, change, and adjustment, current understanding of this period indicates that emotional turmoil, disruptive behavior, and family crises are not the norm and, when present, represent significant pathology. Declining scholastic grades are always worrisome. Such behavior warrants investigation and intervention rather than acceptance and reassurance. The differential diagnosis includes emotional problems, maladjustment, psychosis, drug abuse, and, rarely, organic disease. *(Rudolph CD:2166; Hay:111–113)*

84. **(E)** The first menstrual cycles following menarche generally are anovulatory. Most, but not all, girls do not begin to ovulate for 12–24 months following menarche. Anovulatory cycles tend to be irregular. The onset of ovulation a year or more after menarche can be associated with surprise pregnancy in the girl who had been sexually active while using no method of contraception. *(McMillan:540)*

85. **(C)** The average hemoglobin value at birth is about 17 g/dL. It then falls rapidly over the next 2–3 months to a low of about 11 g/dL in the term infant. Hemoglobin values then gradually rise, although remaining below adult values until the early teen years. The mean value at 1 year of age is about 12 g/dL. *(McMillan:2224)*

86. **(E)** The number of alveoli present at birth is only about 1/10–1/30 that of the adult. As the child grows, new terminal bronchioles and alveoli will form from the distal airways. Clinically, this is an important factor that permits the infant eventually to recover from pulmonary diseases such as bronchopulmonary dysplasia, a protracted postinflammatory state following respiratory distress syndrome (hyaline membrane disease). *(Rudolph CD:1905)*

87. **(A)** At term, the formation of nephrons in the kidney is complete, and generally no new units are formed after birth. Recovery from destroyed glomeruli, therefore, is minimal. Each kidney, in newborns and adults, contains approximately 1 million nephrons. In cases of premature infants, however, it is believed that some new nephrons are formed postnatally. *(Behrman:1573)*

88. **(C)** Although there is great variation within the normal range, the average infant roughly triples his or her birth weight by the first birthday. This means an increase from an average of 7.5 lb (3.4 kg) at birth to 22 lb (10 kg) at 1 year. Thus, the weight gain during the first year of life is about 15 lb (6 kg). [*Note:* The tables and figures on this reference page are worth studying!] *(Rudolph CD:5)*

89. **(A)** As with weight gain, gain in height during the second year of life is considerably less than during the first year. During the first year, the child grows about 25 cm (10 in). Between the first and second birthdays, the youngster grows an average of only 13 cm (about 5 in), about half that of the first year. *(Rudolph CD:5)*

90. **(C)** Head circumference increases relatively rapidly after birth, growing about 2.5 cm (1 in) the first month. Of course, this is related to the rapid growth of the brain that occurs during infancy. A greater than normal increase in head circumference may indicate subdural effusions or hydrocephalus. Less than normal head growth may reflect brain injury, for example, from intrauterine infection, or it may represent primary microcephaly. *(Behrman:33–35)*

91. **(D)** Menarche usually occurs as, or shortly after, breast and pubic hair development reach SMR 4. Menarche generally follows rather than precedes the adolescent growth spurt. In fact, for most girls, menarche heralds the end of the adolescent growth spurt, and there is little further increase in height following menarche. *(McMillan:531)*

92. **(A)** Infants have a lower bicarbonate threshold than do older children or adults. This is why they normally have a lower serum bicarbonate (17–22 meq/L) than older individuals. They also have impairment of phosphate excretion (higher threshold) and a relative inability to increase acid excretion in response to an acid load. This adds to their risk for metabolic acidosis at times of stress. Infants also have an impaired ability to excrete a sodium load and a relative inability to concentrate the urine maximally. *(J Pediatr 86:485, 1975)*

93. **(C)** The Gesell schedules are designed to evaluate the developmental achievements of infants and children less than 5 years of age. *(Levine:8; Pediatr Clin North Am 29:359, 1982)*

94. **(E)** The Wechsler Intelligence Scale is designed to measure the intelligence of children from 5 to 15 years of age. The WISC and the Gesell are different in what they measure as well as in the age groups for which they are designed. The thematic apperception test assesses the personality and adjustment patterns of the subject (4 years to adult). *(Levine:729; Pediatr Clin North Am 29:359, 1982)*

95. **(A)** Neurologic defects such as a hemiparesis are best detected by a thorough neurologic examination. Neither the Gesell nor the WISC is designed to detect visual, auditory, or focal motor impairment, although, of course, such impairment could result in a diminished performance. *(Pediatr Clin North Am 29:359, 1982)*

96. **(A)** Blindness or deafness is best detected by the routine neurologic examination. Confirmation may require specific testing such as measurement of visual or auditory evoked brain potentials. *(Pediatr Clin North Am 29:359, 1982)*

97. **(E)** Suicide is the third leading cause of death during adolescence. Although suicide is seen during childhood and preadolescence (12–14 years), it is decidedly uncommon before adolescence. *(McMillan:9)*

98. **(A)** Current studies indicate that gender identity is well established by 2 years of age. The major determinant of gender identity appears to be the parents' attitudes, behavior, and expectations rather than genetic or biologic factors. *(Pediatr Clin North Am 22:643, 1975)*

99. **(B)** According to classic psychodevelopmental theory, some time around 3 years children become aware of the anatomic differences between the sexes. The child develops erotic feelings toward the parent of the opposite sex and feelings of rivalry toward the parent of the same sex. This stage in psychosocial development has been labeled the Oedipal period and is characterized by a great deal of curiosity about the genitalia (self and others) and a strengthening or reaffirmation of gender identity. *(Pediatr Clin North Am 22:643, 1975)*

100. **(C)** The term latency, which may be a misnomer, refers to the period between the Oedipal stage and adolescence (i.e., from 6 to 12 years). During this period, genital and sexual curiosities are less overt than before or after but, nevertheless, are present. During latency, sexual feelings and curiosity can be recognized in sexual references in games and in the well-recognized propensity of young children to repeat "bad words." *(Pediatr Clin North Am 22:643, 1975)*

BIBLIOGRAPHY

Anders TF, Weinstein P. Sleep and its disorders in infants and children: a review. *Pediatrics* 1972;50:312–324.

Behrman RE, Kliegman RM, Arvin AM. *Nelson Textbook of Pediatrics*, 16th ed. Philadelphia, PA: W.B. Saunders, 1999.

Coplan J, Gleason JR. Unclear speech: recognition and significance of unintelligible speech in preschool children. *Pediatrics* 1988;82:447–452.

Frankenburg WK, Dodds JB. The Denver Developmental Screening Test. *J Pediatr* 1967;71:181–191.

Gayton WF. Management problems of mentally retarded children and their families. *Pediatr Clin North Am* 1975;22:561–570.

Hay WW, Hayward AR, Levin MJ, Sondheimer JM. *Current Pediatric Diagnosis & Treatment*, 16th ed. New York, NY: McGraw-Hill, 2003.

Horowitz FD. Child development for the pediatrician. *Pediatr Clin North Am* 1982;29:359–375.

Levine M, Carey WB, Crocker AC, et al. *Developmental-Behavioral Pediatrics*, 3rd ed. Philadelphia, PA: W.B. Saunders, 1999.

Loggie JHM, Kleiman LI, Van-Maanen EF. Renal function and diuretic therapy in infants and children. *J Pediatr* 1975;86:485–496.

McMillan JA, DeAngelis CD, Feigin RD, Warshaw JB. *Oski's Pediatrics: Principles & Practice*, 3rd ed. Philadelphia, PA: JB Lippincott, 1999.

Miller LJ. Postpartum depression. *JAMA* 2002; 287(6): 762–765.

Rudolph AM, Kamei RK, Overby KJ. *Rudolph's Fundamentals of Pediatrics*, 3rd ed. New York, NY: McGraw-Hill, 2002.

Rudolph CD, Rudolph AM, Hostetter MK, et al. *Rudolph's Pediatrics*, 21st ed. New York, NY: McGraw-Hill, 2003.

Satterfield S. Common sexual problems of children and adolescents. *Pediatr Clin North Am* 1975;22: 643–652.

Smith RD, Fosarelli PD, Palumbo F, et al. The impact of television on children. *Am J Dis Child* 1986;140: 78–79.

Wisner KL, Parry BL, Piontek CM. Postpartum depression. *N Engl J Med* 2002;347(3):194–199.

Zuckerman DM, Zuckerman BS. Television's impact on children. *Pediatrics* 1985;75:233–240.

CHAPTER 7

Infectious Disease

Mary Anne Jackson, MD
Emily A. Thorell, MD

An estimated 80% of child health visits relate to infectious disease. Public health programs directed toward improvements in water, nutrition, and immunization against communicable diseases resulted in significant declines in infant mortality of up to 200-fold between the mid-1800s and late-1990s. Still, half of all postneonatal deaths in the United States result from infections and injuries, both potentially preventable. The advent of *Haemophilus influenzae* type b vaccine in the late 1980s virtually eradicated the most important pathogen of sepsis and meningitis in the infant population. However, the persistence of such pathogens as tuberculosis, HIV, and malaria, and the emergence of new infectious agents offset the gains of the last century and continue to underscore the importance of the study of infectious diseases, particularly for those involved in the care of children. The following questions address appropriate knowledge of pediatric infections with focus on specific etiologic agents, epidemiology of disease, clinical manifestations, diagnostic tests, treatment, and control measures.

Questions

1. Frequent features of staphylococcal toxic shock syndrome include

   (A) pneumonia and pleural effusion
   (B) erythroderma and conjunctival hyperemia
   (C) exudative tonsillitis and cervical adenitis
   (D) arthritis and myositis
   (E) intraabdominal abscess and ascites

2. Histoplasmosis in the young child is acquired when spores are

   (A) ingested
   (B) spread person to person
   (C) inhaled
   (D) inoculated onto skin
   (E) transmitted by contaminated fomites

3. Passively transferred maternal IgG antibody reaches a nadir at

   (A) 1–2 months
   (B) 3–6 months
   (C) 12–18 months
   (D) 18–24 months
   (E) 24 months

4. Which of the following parasites gains entry by direct larval penetration of the skin?

   (A) *Enterobius vermicularis*
   (B) *Trypanosoma brucei gambiense*
   (C) *Trichinella spiralis*
   (D) *Strongyloides stercoralis*
   (E) *Taenia solium*

5. Infants with congenital rubella infection

   (A) are virus-free by the time of birth
   (B) have virus in their blood but not in their nasopharyngeal secretions
   (C) excrete virus in urine and nasopharyngeal secretions for a few days after birth
   (D) excrete virus but are not infectious
   (E) excrete virus and may be infectious for up to 1 year after birth

6. Patients with smallpox are contagious for

   (A) the duration of the febrile prodrome
   (B) the duration of the first week of rash
   (C) the duration of the prodrome and the first week of rash
   (D) 7–8 days until lesions crust
   (E) 3–4 weeks after rash onset

7. A 6-year-old unimmunized child has fever of 38°C and cropped vesicles on the trunk with scattered scabbed lesions. Which of the following infections is the likely diagnosis?

   (A) measles
   (B) mumps
   (C) roseola
   (D) herpes simplex virus
   (E) varicella

8. Ordinarily, the first dose of live attenuated measles vaccine (as MMR) should be administered

    (A) at 2 months of age
    (B) at 6–9 months of age
    (C) at 12–15 months of age
    (D) at 24 months of age
    (E) at the time of school entry

9. Combined diphtheria-tetanus-acellular pertussis (DTaP) vaccine for primary immunization of children is contraindicated

    (A) if a prior dose was associated with a protracted focal seizure without recovery in 24 h
    (B) for those with family history of seizures
    (C) for a preterm infant who is 2 months of age
    (D) in the internationally adopted child
    (E) if a prior dose was associated with temperature of ≥39.5°C.

10. The standard method of immunizing normal infants and children against polio in the United States involves the use of

    (A) inactivated vaccine alone
    (B) live oral vaccine alone
    (C) inactivated vaccine followed by live vaccine
    (D) live vaccine followed by inactivated vaccine
    (E) inactivated and live vaccines simultaneously

11. In children, risk factors for drug-resistant tuberculosis disease include contact with an infected individual

    (A) from eastern Europe
    (B) from Scandinavia
    (C) from the Pacific Islands
    (D) with HIV infection
    (E) who has been incarcerated

12. Mosquitoes are recognized vectors in the transmission of encephalitis caused by

    (A) arbovirus
    (B) coxsackievirus
    (C) enterovirus
    (D) influenza virus
    (E) mumps virus

13. A 3-year-old child has a positive tuberculin test. Which of the following would be most concerning for extrapulmonary disease?

    (A) fever
    (B) hilar lymphadenopathy on roentgenograph
    (C) night sweats
    (D) weight loss
    (E) hepatosplenomegaly

14. In addition to pneumonia and rash, infection with *Mycoplasma pneumoniae* has been associated most commonly with

    (A) hepatic complications
    (B) renal complications
    (C) neurologic complications
    (D) aplastic anemia
    (E) immunologic suppression

15. Acute bronchiolitis is

    (A) usually associated with high fever and rash
    (B) commonly associated with lobar infiltrates on chest roentgenogram
    (C) commonly associated with retractions, tachypnea, and wheezing
    (D) characterized by the absence of cough despite respiratory distress
    (E) most common between 2 and 5 years of age

16. On tuberculin skin testing, a well 5-year-old who traveled last year to Mexico is found to have 8 mm of induration to 5 tuberculin units (TU) of purified protein derivative (PPD). There is no history suggestive of contact with tuberculosis. This reaction probably indicates

    (A) sensitivity to the diluent
    (B) subcutaneous rather than intradermal injection of test material
    (C) cross-sensitivity to nontuberculous mycobacteria
    (D) tuberculosis infection
    (E) tuberculosis disease

17. Infants and children with uncomplicated tuberculosis disease can attend school or child care

    (A) as soon as effective therapy has been instituted
    (B) 2 weeks after therapy is initiated
    (C) once negative sputum smears are confirmed
    (D) once therapy is completed
    (E) whether they are receiving therapy or not

18. Children with enteric fever secondary to *Salmonella* infection frequently have

    (A) rectal prolapse
    (B) hepatosplenomegaly and abdominal pain
    (C) intensely pruritic skin rash
    (D) cough and lymphadenopathy
    (E) toxic megacolon and perforation

19. Children with chronic granulomatous disease have a defect in

    (A) leukocyte migration
    (B) synthesis of collagen
    (C) capillary permeability
    (D) tissue repair following injury
    (E) leukocyte killing

20. The rash of scabies in infants

    (A) is maculopapular
    (B) is rarely seen in children

    (C) characteristically spares the face
    (D) usually begins with fever
    (E) is papulovesicular

21. Which of the following is seen most commonly as a complication of shiga toxin-producing *E. coli* (formerly known as enterohemorrhagic *E. coli*) diarrhea?

    (A) meningitis
    (B) hemolytic-uremic syndrome
    (C) chronic diarrhea
    (D) endocarditis
    (E) pneumonia

22. A characteristic of the cutaneous manifestations of congenital syphilis is

    (A) that the lesions are sterile
    (B) that lesions are most numerous on the trunk
    (C) a fleeting pink macular rash
    (D) a papular purpuric eruption on the legs and buttocks
    (E) vesiculobullous lesions of the palms and soles

23. The most likely serious bacterial infection encountered in a febrile 1-month-old infant is

    (A) *E. coli* urinary tract infection
    (B) *Salmonella* enteritis
    (C) group A streptococcal bacteremia
    (D) meningococcemia
    (E) *H. influenzae* type b meningitis

24. Findings at birth in an infant with congenital syphilis may include

    (A) osteochondritis and pseudoparalysis
    (B) a primary chancre of the umbilicus
    (C) a high incidence of cardiovascular involvement
    (D) Clutton's joints
    (E) interstitial keratitis

25. The most common manifestation of infection with *Neisseria gonorrhoeae* in prepubertal girls is

(A) arthritis
(B) conjunctivitis
(C) peritonitis
(D) salpingitis
(E) vaginitis

26. Symptomatic gonococcal disease in the adolescent female is most often characterized by

(A) hematuria
(B) salpingitis
(C) fever and shaking chills
(D) arthritis
(E) painless chancre

27. Staphylococcal food poisoning

(A) usually is associated with a high fever
(B) usually begins within minutes of ingestion of the toxin
(C) often is accompanied by staphylococcal bacteremia
(D) is characterized by vomiting, abdominal cramps, and diarrhea
(E) is frequently accompanied by a rash

28. Group A streptococcal infection in a 1-year-old child is likely to present as

(A) meningitis
(B) scarlet fever
(C) peritonsillar abscess
(D) acute rheumatic fever
(E) fever and serous rhinitis

29. Which of the following CSF findings is most likely in a 12-year-old 48 h into the course of enteroviral meningitis?

(A) 5000 WBC, 90% PMNs
(B) 100 WBC, 90% eosinophils
(C) 500 WBC, 90% lymphs
(D) 50 WBC, 90% PMNs
(E) 50 WBC, 40% monocytes

30. Which of the following children is most likely to have group A streptococcal infection?

(A) exudative pharyngitis in a 1-year-old
(B) tonsillitis, rash, and fever in a 5-year-old
(C) cough and pharyngitis in a 15-year-old
(D) "slapped cheeks" appearance in a 5-year-old
(E) empyema in a 1-year-old

31. Pneumococcal pneumonia

(A) is rare before 2 years of age
(B) is most commonly seen in neonates
(C) is associated with vesicular rash
(D) is usually preceded by, or associated with, a viral respiratory infection
(E) usually presents with fever, retractions, and stridor

32. Which of the following staphylococcal infections is toxin-mediated and caused by circulation of exfoliative toxins A and B?

(A) scalded skin syndrome
(B) food poisoning
(C) empyema
(D) toxic shock syndrome
(E) bullous impetigo

33. The clinical manifestation of rotavirus infection in infants is usually

(A) fever and cough
(B) winter diarrhea
(C) summer febrile convulsions
(D) opisthotonos
(E) difficulty sucking and swallowing

34. The rash of Rocky Mountain spotted fever is characterized by

(A) discrete red papules on the trunk
(B) sparing of the palms and soles
(C) vesicular lesions on the face
(D) petechial rash on the wrists and ankles
(E) urticarial rash on the trunk

35. The usual course of pertussis in an infant is characterized by

    (A) 4 or 5 days of high fever followed by croupy cough
    (B) sudden onset of fever and cough
    (C) gradual onset of cough, followed by abrupt onset of fever and whooping
    (D) rhinitis followed by paroxysmal cough
    (E) protracted fever and paroxysmal cough

36. Which of the following white blood cell counts is most suggestive of pertussis?

    (A) 3000/mm^3 with 75% lymphocytes
    (B) 20,000/mm^3 with 65% lymphocytes
    (C) 7000/mm^3 with 65% polymorpho-nuclear leukocytes
    (D) 25,000/mm^3 with 65% polymorpho-nuclear leukocytes
    (E) 12,000/mm^3 with 20% eosinophils

37. A 12-year-old child developed fever about 1 week after visiting relatives in India. The fever has persisted for about 10 days. Diarrhea, present for a few days, has cleared, and the child is now constipated. The child appears moderately acutely ill. The liver and spleen are enlarged. There are palpable, small (2–4 mm) erythematous spots on the trunk only. This child probably has

    (A) measles
    (B) typhoid fever
    (C) *N. meningitidis* bacteremia
    (D) rat-bite fever
    (E) leptospirosis

38. You are working in a clinic in rural Mexico and examine an 8-year-old boy who has a rectal temperature of 38°C (100°F), bilateral tender parotid swelling, and pain when you flex his neck. He has been complaining of a headache. His immunization history is unknown. Your most likely diagnosis is

    (A) brucellosis
    (B) cysticercosis
    (C) Epstein-Barr virus infection
    (D) mumps
    (E) leukemia

39. A previously well 3-year-old child has fever, headache, photophobia, and stiff neck. Your major concern is that the child may have

    (A) brain tumor
    (B) optic neuritis
    (C) subarachnoid hemorrhage
    (D) meningitis
    (E) bacterial sepsis

40. The combination of fever, hemorrhagic skin lesions, and shock in a 6-year-old child is most suggestive of infection with

    (A) *Neisseria meningitidis*
    (B) *Haemophilus influenzae*
    (C) *Streptococcus pneumoniae*
    (D) *Staphylococcus aureus*
    (E) group B β-hemolytic *Streptococcus*

41. Subdural effusions in association with acute bacterial meningitis are

    (A) the result of inadequate treatment
    (B) indicative of a bleeding disorder
    (C) usually fatal
    (D) caused by incidental trauma rather than the infection itself
    (E) a common occurrence

42. A 3-year-old child presents with fever for 8 days, lymphadenopathy, splenomegaly, and numerous reactive or atypical lymphocytes on peripheral blood smear. The monospot test is negative. A likely cause of this clinical picture is infection with

    (A) adenovirus
    (B) respiratory syncytial virus
    (C) herpesvirus
    (D) Epstein-Barr virus
    (E) rubella virus

43. Which of the following drug regimens is the most appropriate chemoprophylaxis for adult

household contacts of a child with meningo-coccal meningitis?

(A) single dose ciprofloxacin

(B) penicillin for 2 days

(C) rifampin for 4 days

(D) trimethoprim/sulfamethoxazole for 7 days

(E) penicillin and rifampin for 2 days

44. Early-onset group B streptococcal infection in the neonate

(A) is more common in infants born at <37 weeks gestation

(B) usually presents with meningitis

(C) is associated with good prognosis if treated promptly

(D) commonly presents with osteomyelitis

(E) is frequently associated with recurrent disease

45. *Listeria monocytogenes* infection in the pediatric age group is seen primarily in

(A) patients receiving broad-spectrum antibiotics

(B) children with chronic otitis media

(C) newborn infants

(D) children with defect of WBC function

(E) children with ventriculoperitoneal shunts

46. A 3-year-old nonimmunized child has had fever for 4 days and now has a maculopapular rash. She is seen in clinic and diagnosed as having measles. There is a 4-month-old sibling at home. Appropriate management of this sibling would include

(A) immediate immunization with live attenuated measles vaccine

(B) immediate immunization with killed measles vaccine

(C) a single dose of immune globulin (IG)

(D) IG plus live attenuated measles vaccine

(E) no treatment necessary

47. A young child with fever, cough, hepatos-plenomegaly, and eosinophilia has negative examinations of the stool for ova and parasites. The most likely parasite to cause this combination of findings is

(A) *Ascaris lumbricoides*

(B) *Toxocara canis*

(C) *Dracunculus medinensis*

(D) *Enterobius vermicularis*

(E) *Trichuris trichiura*

48. Of the following parasitic infections, which is most likely to present with intestinal obstruction?

(A) *Enterobius vermicularis*

(B) *Necator americanus*

(C) *Ascaris lumbricoides*

(D) *Strongyloides stercoralis*

(E) *Trichuris trichiura*

49. Which of the following sequelae of Kawasaki syndrome is most common?

(A) fulminant hepatitis

(B) coronary artery aneurysm

(C) recurrent pericarditis

(D) cerebral edema

(E) renal failure

50. The rash of parvovirus B-19 infection

(A) is a papulovesicular facial rash

(B) is an urticarial truncal rash

(C) is a red rash on the cheeks with circum-oral pallor

(D) is a pustular rash on the face and trunk

(E) is petechial involving the palms and soles

51. Of the following extragenital complications of gonorrhea in the adolescent female, which is most common?

(A) arthritis

(B) carditis

(C) meningitis

(D) pneumonia

(E) anterior uveitis

52. The most common bacterial causes of meningitis in childhood (excluding the neonatal period) are

(A) *Neisseria meningitidis* and *Streptococcus pneumoniae*

(B) *Streptococcus pneumoniae* and *Escherichia coli*

(C) *Neisseria meningitidis* and group A *Streptococcus*

(D) *Neisseria meningitidis* and *Listeria monocytogenes*

(E) group A *Streptococcus* and *Escherichia coli*

53. Neonatal herpes simplex disease

(A) commonly occurs in infants whose mothers have a history of recurrent genital herpes

(B) may present with pneumonitis, hepatitis, and coagulopathy

(C) usually presents within 24 h of delivery

(D) rarely recurs in infants who have had skin only presentation

(E) rarely is seen in infants whose mothers have primary infection at delivery

54. Hepatitis A virus infection is

(A) usually associated with jaundice in the preschool age child

(B) often associated with fulminant disease

(C) subclinical in infants

(D) commonly associated with vertical (mother to newborn) transmission

(E) highly contagious in those who are jaundiced

55. The preicteric phase of hepatitis B virus infection may be associated with

(A) pneumonia

(B) generalized lymphadenopathy

(C) protracted fever

(D) papular acrodermatitis

(E) encephalopathy

56. Which of the following markers identifies the patient with chronic HBV infection who is most likely to transmit infection?

(A) HBsAg

(B) HBeAg

(C) IgM anti-HBc

(D) antibody to HBc

(E) antibody to HBs

57. A 10-month-old child has a temperature of 40°C (104°F) for 4 days without other signs. On the fourth day, a rose pink maculopapular rash appears and the temperature returns to normal. The most likely diagnosis is infection caused by

(A) echovirus

(B) human herpesvirus 6

(C) measles virus

(D) group A *Streptococcus*

(E) typhus

58. Gonococcal infection

(A) can be prevented by use of a killed vaccine

(B) can be prevented by use of a live vaccine

(C) confers immunity to subsequent infection only if the initial infection involves extragenital sites

(D) confers no immunity against repeated infection

(E) can be prevented by intravenous immune globulin

59. Characteristic oral findings in herpangina include

(A) a confluent exudate on the tonsils and uvula

(B) small vesicles or ulcers on the tonsillar fauces, tonsils, uvula, and pharynx

(C) large ulcers on the tongue and gingiva

(D) inflammation and ulceration of the gingiva and buccal mucosa

(E) white plaques opposite the molars

60. Hand-foot-and-mouth syndrome is usually caused by infection with

    (A) adenovirus
    (B) coronavirus
    (C) *Arcanobacterium haemolyticum*
    (D) coxsackievirus A16
    (E) herpes simplex virus

61. You are taking care of a 26-month-old child with bacterial meningitis. Blood and spinal fluid cultures are positive for *Neisseria meningitidis*. The child's household consists of the parents, one grandparent, a 6-month-old sibling, a 5-year-old sibling, and a 14-year-old exchange student who has been living with the family for about 1 month. You advise chemoprophylaxis for

    (A) everyone in the household
    (B) everyone except the grandparent
    (C) everyone except the grandparent and the visiting student
    (D) the siblings only
    (E) the 6-month-old sibling only

62. Which of the following may be associated with exudative pharyngitis?

    (A) Kawasaki syndrome
    (B) *Yersinia enterocolitica*
    (C) adenovirus
    (D) parainfluenza
    (E) respiratory syncytial virus

63. A previously well 12-year-old presents with fever, splenomegaly, and elevated serum transaminase levels. The organism most likely responsible for these findings is

    (A) *Treponema pallidum*
    (B) hepatitis B virus
    (C) rubella virus
    (D) Epstein-Barr virus
    (E) *Toxoplasma gondii*

64. A 15-year-old presents with pain, photophobia, and blurred vision in one eye. Examination reveals chemosis of the affected eye and small vesicular lesions below the eye and on the nose. Application of fluorescein dye reveals branching, dendritic lesions on the cornea. The most likely cause of this clinical picture is

    (A) staphylococcal impetigo
    (B) adenoviral infection
    (C) retinoblastoma
    (D) herpes simplex infection
    (E) trauma

65. Which of the following is the most commonly encountered opportunistic infection in infants with perinatally acquired HIV infection?

    (A) *Pneumocystis* pneumonia
    (B) disseminated cytomegalovirus infection
    (C) disseminated toxoplasmosis
    (D) cryptococcal meningitis
    (E) isosporiasis

66. A newborn infant has microcephaly, periventricular calcifications, jaundice, and thrombocytopenia. Infection with which of the following is most likely?

    (A) Epstein-Barr virus
    (B) cytomegalovirus
    (C) coxsackievirus B
    (D) human immunodeficiency virus
    (E) human parvovirus B-19

67. Which of the following is suggestive diagnosis of the primary pulmonary tuberculosis in childhood?

    (A) papular acrodermatitis
    (B) hilar lymphadenopathy
    (C) cavitary pneumonia
    (D) exudative pharyngitis
    (E) neutrophilic meningitis

68. A 12-year-old who went camping 2 weeks ago in Oklahoma now presents with fever and headache. Laboratory studies demonstrate leukopenia, thrombocytopenia, and hyponatremia. You suspect infection caused by

    (A) *Rickettsia prowazekii*
    (B) *Rickettsia typhi*
    (C) *Ehrlichia chaffeensis*
    (D) *Coxiella burnetii*
    (E) *Borrelia burgdorferi*

69. Case fatality rates from pneumococcal infection are highest in children

    (A) with underlying liver disease
    (B) with asplenia
    (C) with underlying cardiac disease
    (D) with cystic fibrosis
    (E) who are adolescents

70. Varicella infection is associated with

    (A) an incubation period of 5–7 days
    (B) a confluent centrifugal pustular rash
    (C) Koplik spots
    (D) high risk for shingles
    (E) visceral dissemination in the immunocompromised

71. Maternal infection with rubella virus is most commonly associated with congenital defects if infection occurs

    (A) in the first 4 weeks of gestation
    (B) during the second month
    (C) during the third or fourth month
    (D) during the last trimester
    (E) anytime during pregnancy

72. A 15-year-old has exudative tonsillitis, cervical adenitis, and splenomegaly. Which of the following is the most common complication encountered?

    (A) chronic fatigue lasting >6 months
    (B) hemorrhage
    (C) pneumonia

    (D) encephalitis
    (E) airway obstruction

73. Clinical manifestations of adenovirus infection most commonly involve

    (A) the upper respiratory tract
    (B) the lower respiratory tract
    (C) the urinary tract
    (D) the pericardium
    (E) the musculoskeletal system

74. The rash associated with *Arcanobacterium haemolyticum* infection

    (A) has a rough sandpaper-like texture
    (B) has a tendency to involve the palms and soles
    (C) has a tendency to become vesicular within 24 h
    (D) is pustular
    (E) has a predilection for the face

75. Recognized dermatologic manifestations of staphylococcal toxic shock syndrome include

    (A) petechiae on the wrists and ankles with spread to the trunk
    (B) vesicles of the face and trunk
    (C) localized bullous impetigo
    (D) diffuse macular erythema that desquamates in 1–2 weeks
    (E) morbilliform eruption on the trunk

76. Which of the following is a common manifestation of brucellosis in children?

    (A) hepatosplenomegaly
    (B) glaucoma
    (C) meningitis
    (D) endocarditis
    (E) osteomyelitis

77. Which of the following is the most common clinical manifestation that follows infection with *Campylobacter*?

    (A) Guillain-Barré syndrome
    (B) polyarticular arthritis

(C) encephalitis

(D) inguinal lymphadenitis

(E) anterior uveitis

78. Which of the following clinical features is most commonly found in infants and young children with cat-scratch disease?

(A) aseptic meningitis

(B) autoimmune hemolytic anemia

(C) regional lymphadenopathy

(D) hepatosplenomegaly

(E) pneumonia

79. Which of the following roentgenographic findings is most commonly seen in infants with bronchiolitis caused by respiratory syncytial virus?

(A) hyperinflation

(B) hilar adenopathy

(C) multilobar infiltrate

(D) lower lobe infiltrates

(E) pleural effusion

80. Which of the following would be most commonly seen in a child with *Giardia lamblia* infection?

(A) watery diarrhea

(B) fever

(C) bloody diarrhea

(D) failure to thrive

(E) cough

81. Which of the following is characteristic of the CSF in tuberculous meningitis?

(A) The color is blood tinged.

(B) Protein is normal.

(C) Culture reveals tuberculous organisms within 1 week.

(D) Glucose is low.

(E) Leukocytes predominate.

82. Which of the following is characteristic of summer outbreaks of echovirus infection in young children?

(A) conjunctivitis and generalized lymphadenopathy

(B) postauricular and occipital lymphadenopathy

(C) fever, rash, and aseptic meningitis

(D) a pink-red maculopapular rash and exudative conjunctivitis

(E) mild fever, vesicular truncal rash, and gingival ulcers

83. Which of the following infections is associated with bacteremia in a child with sickle cell disease?

(A) *Candida albicans*

(B) *Coccidioides immitis*

(C) *Cryptococcus neoformans*

(D) *Histoplasma capsulatum*

(E) *Yersinia enterocolitica*

84. A common complication of pelvic inflammatory disease secondary to chlamydia infection of the lower genital tract is

(A) perihepatitis

(B) coagulopathy

(C) arthritis

(D) meningitis

(E) endocarditis

DIRECTIONS (Questions 85 through 95): Each set of matching questions in this section consists of a list of lettered options followed by several numbered items. For each numbered item select the ONE lettered option with which it is most closely associated. Each lettered option may be selected once, more than once, or not at all.

Questions 85 through 88

The following questions refer to exanthematous infections in children:

(A) Rocky Mountain spotted fever
(B) measles
(C) Kawasaki syndrome
(D) herpes simplex virus
(E) parvovirus B-19

85. Polymorphous rash and mucositis

86. Petechiae on palms and soles

87. Cropped vesicles

88. Koplik spots

Questions 89 through 92

(A) *Toxocara canis*
(B) *Ascaris lumbricoides*
(C) *Necator americanus*
(D) *Trichuris trichiura*
(E) *Enterobius vermicularis*

89. Anemia

90. Hepatomegaly

91. Rectal prolapse

92. Rectal itching

Questions 93 through 95

(A) dogs
(B) fish
(C) rats, mice
(D) pigeons, parakeets
(E) cattle, swine

93. *Streptobacillus moniliformis*

94. *Pasteurella multocida*

95. *Chlamydia psittaci*

Questions 96 through 98

(A) respiratory infection with *Chlamydia trachomatis*
(B) respiratory infection with *Bordetella pertussis*
(C) respiratory infection with influenza
(D) respiratory infection with respiratory syncytial virus

96. Most common cause of bronchiolitis in infants

97. High fever and toxic appearance in young infants

98. Mortality highest in infants with cyanotic heart disease

Questions 99 through 103

(A) Gram-stained smear of blood
(B) PCR detection of antigen
(C) culture
(D) IgA antibody

99. Preferred diagnostic test for congenital cytomegalovirus infection

100. Preferred diagnostic test for neonatal herpes simplex virus encephalitis

101. Preferred diagnostic perinatal HIV infection

102. Preferred diagnostic group B streptococcal meningitis

103. Preferred diagnostic congenital toxoplasmosis

Questions 104 through 108

(A) tetanus
(B) rabies
(C) diphtheria
(D) *Streptococcus pneumoniae*

104. Trismus

105. Toxic myocarditis

106. Meningitis

107. Encephalitis

108. Heroin addiction

Questions 109 through 116

(A) measles (rubeola)
(B) German measles (rubella)
(C) mumps
(D) varicella

109. Cough, coryza, and conjunctivitis

110. Necrotizing fasciitis

111. Orchitis

112. Cataracts

113. Aseptic meningitis

114. Reye syndrome

115. Subacute sclerosing panencephalitis

116. Severe disease in vitamin A deficiency

Questions 117 through 121

(A) *Staphylococcus aureus*
(B) group B *Streptococcus*
(C) *Streptococcus pneumoniae*
(D) coagulase-negative *Staphylococcus*

117. Most common cause of meningitis in 4-week-old

118. Most common cause of meningitis in 4-year-old

119. Most common cause of ventriculitis in infants with ventriculoperitoneal shunt

120. Meningitis in basilar skull fracture

121. Most common cause of meningitis in sickle cell anemia patient

Questions 122 through 127

(A) X linked agammaglobulinemia
(B) severe combined immunodeficiency syndrome
(C) chronic granulomatous disease
(D) common variable immunodeficiency

122. *Giardia lamblia* infection

123. Enterovirus encephalitis

124. *Pneumocystis jiroveci* pneumonia (PCP)

125. Adenosine deaminase deficiency

126. Liver abscess

127. Diagnosis may not be made until adulthood

Questions 128 through 133
Regarding the preferred timing for routine immunization of normal children:

(A) age 12–15 months
(B) primary series 2, 4, and 6 months
(C) age 11–12 years
(D) age 24 months or older

128. Diphtheria-tetanus-acellular pertussis vaccine

129. Measles-mumps-rubella vaccine

130. Varicella vaccine

131. Pneumococcal conjugate vaccine

132. Hepatitis A vaccine

133. Tetanus-diphtheria vaccine

Answers and Explanations

1. **(B)** Manifestations of the staphylococcal toxic shock syndrome, which include fever, mental status changes, conjunctivitis, diffuse macular erythroderma, and multiple organ failure, are caused by a toxin elaborated by the staphylococci rather than by tissue invasion by the organism. The organism usually can be cultured from skin or mucous membrane and only rarely from the blood. The organism has been recovered from the vagina and has been associated with the use of tampons, especially those designed to be changed infrequently. *(Long:100; Red Book:625)*

2. **(C)** As in adults, the respiratory tract is the portal of entry for histoplasmosis in essentially all cases in children. Inoculation other than by inhalation is exceedingly rare. *(Long:1233; Red Book:354)*

3. **(B)** Passively transferred maternal IgG decreases commensurate with the half-life, which is approximately 30 days. Therefore, the nadir occurs in infants at the age of 3–6 months. *(Long:625; Rudolph CD:791)*

4. **(D)** Like *Ancylostoma duodenale* (hookworm), *Strongyloides stercoralis* enters the human host by penetration of the skin by larvae in the soil. The larvae migrate to the intestines, where they set up residency and mature. *(Red Book:594)*

5. **(E)** Infants congenitally infected with rubella excrete the virus in urine and pharyngeal secretions and can be infectious for many weeks or months. Such infants pose a definite hazard to nonimmune family members, caretakers, and medical and nursing personnel. Pregnant females who are not certain of their rubella immune status should not handle these infants or their secretions. *(Red Book:537)*

6. **(E)** Routine childhood smallpox immunization was discontinued in 1971 and in 1980, the World Health Organization was able to declare the entire globe as certifiably free of smallpox. Following the terrorist attacks on the World Trade Center, the Pentagon, and the suspected attempt at attack on the U.S. Capitol which led to the airplane crash in Pennsylvania on September 11, 2001, concern arose regarding the possible use of smallpox virus as a bioterroristic weapon. This prompted renewed educational efforts focusing on the epidemiology, typical clinical manifestations, diagnosis, and management of smallpox. Regarding infectivity, patients are most contagious during the first week of rash; however, infected individuals remain contagious until all scabbed lesions have separated, usually 3–4 weeks after rash onset. *(Red Book:554)*

7. **(E)** Of the so-called common childhood diseases listed in this question, primary varicella infection (or chickenpox) is most likely to present with a generalized, pruritic vesicular rash and mild fever. The typical exanthem appears first on the scalp, face, or trunk. New crops of lesions develop over a 1–7-day period. Progression from vesicle to pustule to crusted scab occurs quickly such that lesions of all stages are present after the first 48 h. *(Red Book:672; Long:1042)*

8. **(C)** Ordinarily, the first dose of live attenuated measles vaccine (combined with mumps and

rubella as the MMR vaccine) should be administered between 12 and 15 months of age to maximize the likelihood that transplacentally acquired antibodies have disappeared completely from the child's blood. Otherwise, these antibodies may blunt the infant's immunologic response to the vaccine. On the other hand, administration of the vaccine should not be delayed much beyond 15 months because of the seriousness of measles infection. It is now recommended that a second dose of the vaccine be given when the child enters elementary school. In areas where, or at times when, measles is epidemic, it is recommended that an initial dose of monovalent measles vaccine be given as early as 6 months of age, followed by the two MMRs as noted. (*Red Book:424, 426; Long:1152*)

9. **(A)** The use of a combined DTaP vaccine is routine and is the method of choice for the primary immunization of infants and young children. There are two contraindications to pertussis immunization: an immediate anaphylactic reaction, or encephalopathy within 7 days of a prior dose manifested by major alterations in consciousness or protracted generalized or focal seizures without recovery within 24 h. (*Red Book:24:483*)

10. **(A)** The standard method of immunization against polio for normal infants and children in the United States is with four doses of inactivated (killed) vaccine; the first two are given at 2-month intervals beginning at age 2 months and the third is recommended at 6–18 months, with a supplemental dose at school entry. Oral poliovirus vaccine is no longer distributed in the United States but remains the vaccine of choice for global eradication programs. (*Red Book:507–508; Long:1177–1178*)

11. **(A)** In the United States, isoniazid is recommended for the management of latent tuberculosis infection. The incidence of isoniazid resistance in tuberculosis is estimated to be 9%. For the pediatric patient with tuberculosis infection or disease, contact with an individual born in areas including Russia and the former Soviet Union, Asia, Africa, and Latin America or with anyone treated previously for tuberculosis disease are risk factors for drug resistance and such history would influence the type of therapy recommended for such patients. (*Long:807; Red Book:654*)

12. **(A)** Mumps virus, enterovirus, coxsackievirus, and influenza virus are spread primarily by direct contact (e.g., respiratory droplets, hands) and not through an arthropod vector. A number of viruses, notably the arboviruses, are spread by mosquito vectors. Examples in North America include eastern and western equine encephalitis, St. Louis encephalitis, LaCrosse encephalitis, and West Nile encephalitis. (*Long: 1110*)

13. **(E)** Fever, cough, hilar lymphadenopathy, and elevated sedimentation rate are seen commonly in uncomplicated primary pulmonary tuberculosis. Hepatosplenomegaly is generally not seen in uncomplicated primary pulmonary tuberculosis but does occur in more than 50% of children with disseminated disease. (*Long:795*)

14. **(C)** *Mycoplasma pneumoniae* has long been known to cause pneumonia, bronchitis, otitis media, myringitis bullosa, and nonspecific upper respiratory infection. More recently, this organism also has been recognized as a cause of various nonrespiratory manifestations such as polymorphous mucocutaneous eruptions including Stevens-Johnson syndrome, encephalitis, and meningitis. Other neurologic manifestations reported with *M. pneumoniae* infection include transverse myelitis, psychosis, poliomyelitis-like syndrome, and Guillain-Barré syndrome. (*Long: 1008; Red Book:443*)

15. **(C)** In infants with bronchiolitis, fever is usually mild, and a rash is not noted. Cough is characteristic and frequently severe, as are retraction, tachypnea, and wheezing. The disease is most frequent, as well as most severe, in the first 2 years of life. The chest roentgenogram usually reveals hyperaeration only, although pneumonia is an occasional complication. (*Long:1142; Red Book:523*)

16. **(C)** In healthy children over age 4 years, reactions of less than 5-mm induration to 5 TU are considered negative. Reactions between 5 and 15 mm are considered doubtful and usually represent infection with nontuberculous mycobacteria. Reactions of 15 mm or more induration generally are considered positive and indicative of infection with *Mycobacterium tuberculosis* but do not necessarily mean clinically evident disease. The point to remember is that the threshold for interpreting a tuberculin skin test as positive is lower for children with signs or symptoms suggestive of tuberculosis or with a history of contact with tuberculosis. *(Long:798; Red Book:643)*

17. **(A)** In general, children with uncomplicated primary pulmonary tuberculosis are noninfectious and do not require isolation. This is believed to relate to the scanty sputum production, lack of expectoration, and the small number of organisms that can be recovered from sputum or gastric culture. In contrast, children with laryngeal involvement, with cavitary pulmonary tuberculosis, extensive pulmonary infection, positive sputum AFB smears, or suspected congenital tuberculosis should be considered contagious and appropriate precautions should be taken. Children with tuberculosis disease can attend school or child care if they are receiving therapy. *(Feigin:1200; Red Book:658)*

18. **(B)** In enteric *Salmonella* infections, fever is characteristic; diarrhea may or may not be present. Some features highly suggestive of *Salmonella* infection include leukopenia and a relative bradycardia; that is, the heart rate is slower than would be anticipated for the degree of fever present, though this is seen more commonly in adults than in children. Clinical manifestations such as fever, abdominal pain, hepatomegaly, splenomegaly, rose spots, and changes in mental status are reported. *(Long:833; Red Book:542)*

19. **(E)** The defect in chronic granulomatous disease (CGD) is the inability of polymorphonuclear leukocytes to effect intracellular killing of certain phagocytosed bacteria. The neutrophils can ingest bacteria normally but cannot produce the intracellular hydrogen peroxide needed to kill certain organisms. CGD is inherited primarily as a sex-linked recessive trait, although some females with the disorder have been reported. *(Long:640)*

20. **(E)** The clinical feature of scabies infestation that is typical for the young child is an intensely pruritic rash with involvement of the entire skin surface including the scalp, palms, and soles with lesions that are often pustulovesicular. The eruption is caused by a hypersensitivity reaction to the proteins of the scabies mite, *Sarcoptes scabiei*. *(Long:1150; Rudolph CD:1154)*

21. **(B)** Formerly known as enterohemorrhagic *E. coli*, shiga toxin-producing strains of *E. coli* (STEC) are associated with a range of gastrointestinal symptoms from self-limited nonbloody diarrhea to hemorrhagic colitis. A triad of microangiopathic hemolytic anemia, thrombocytopenia, and acute renal dysfunction is termed hemolytic-uremic syndrome and may follow the diarrheal illness within a week in 2–20% of infected children. *(Long:825; Red Book:275–276)*

22. **(E)** In general, *T. pallidum* can be demonstrated in any mucous membrane or cutaneous lesion of congenital syphilis, especially a moist one. All these lesions are capable of spreading the organism and are highly infectious. The classical cutaneous manifestations of congenital syphilis are a copper-colored maculopapular rash and vesiculobullous lesions of the palms and soles, often referred to as pemphigus syphiliticus. *(Feigin:1561–1562; Long:955, 956)*

23. **(A)** Infants less than 2 months of age who present with undifferentiated fever are at high risk for serious bacterial infection. The standard of care for such infants is a meticulous history and physical examination with laboratory evaluation to detect urinary tract, bloodstream, or CNS infection. The most common serious bacterial infection encountered in this young infant population is urinary tract infection with 90% of infections caused by *E. coli*. *(Long:112)*

24. **(A)** There are a wide range of clinical manifestations in the congenitally infected newborn. Snuffles, mucocutaneous lesions, osteochondritis or periositis, renal involvement, anemia, and central nervous system involvement are all noted. A characteristic feature of congenital syphilis is involvement of the long bones. The most common lesions are osteochondritis, periosteal new bone formation, and osteomyelitic lesions. Since the infection is transplacental, a primary chancre and the associated regional lymphadenopathy are absent. Cardiovascular involvement is rare in the congenital form of infection. Late manifestations may include interstitial keratitis, eighth nerve deafness, and Hutchinson teeth (peg-shaped, notched central incisors). The presence of these findings is referred to as Hutchinson's triad. *(Red Book:595; Long:956)*

25. **(E)** Vaginitis is the most common form of gonococcal infection in the prepubertal female. The unestrogenized, alkaline vaginal mucosa of the prepubertal girl is especially vulnerable to colonization and infection with *N. gonorrhoeae*. One study confirmed the diagnosis of gonorrhea in 9% of prepubertal children presenting with a chief complaint of vaginal discharge; sexual abuse must be considered in such patients. Ascending infection (salpingitis, peritonitis) occurs, but only rarely in prepubertal children. Arthritis is uncommon, and conjunctivitis is essentially restricted to the newborn period. *(Long:758; Red Book:287)*

26. **(B)** Gonococcal infection in the female adolescent is often asymptomatic; clinical infection usually manifests as urethritis, endocervicitis, and salpingitis. The incubation period is 2–10 days. Complications can include bartholinitis, PID, and perihepatitis. *(Red Book:285; Long:758)*

27. **(D)** Staphylococcal food poisoning is caused by a toxin elaborated in the spoiled food before ingestion. Bacteremia does not occur, since this is not an infection. Fever is uncommon. Symptoms—vomiting, abdominal cramps, and diarrhea—usually begin within 2–4 h of ingestion of the toxin. *(Red Book:561; Long:702)*

28. **(E)** Group A streptococcal infection in young children is commonly manifested by persistent fever and mucoserous nasal discharge. This syndrome has been referred to as "streptococcosis." Localized pharyngeal involvement is uncommon in the first year of life. Meningitis caused by this organism is very uncommon at all ages. The clinical picture of scarlet fever is rarely seen in the first year of life and acute rheumatic fever is rare before 4 or 5 years of age. *(Long:716; Feigin:1079)*

29. **(C)** In temperate climates, summer and late fall outbreaks of enteroviral infection are common with many thousands of cases of meningitis reported each year, the vast majority caused by entero viruses. Fever, headache, and photophobia are commonly reported in children with enteroviral meningitis. CSF pleocytosis is usually noted with white blood cell counts typically between 100 and 1000. While neutrophil predominance can be seen early on, lymphocytes predominate between 8 and 48 h of onset. Definitive diagnosis is made by culture although PCR detection is faster, more sensitive and 100% specific. *(Long:288)*

30. **(B)** Pharyngotonsillitis is the typical clinical manifestation of group A streptococcal infection. Scarlet fever is a syndrome of tonsillitis, fever, and rash caused by an erythrogenic toxin-producing *Streptococcus* in a patient lacking antitoxic immunity. Streptococcal respiratory tract infections generally peak in children of age 5–11 years and winter predominance is generally noted. Patients younger than 3 years of age with exudative pharyngitis are more likely to have viral disease as are adolescents who present with sore throat, croupy cough, and/or rhinorrhea. *(Red Book:576; Long:180)*

31. **(D)** Pneumococcal pneumonia is the most common acute bacterial pneumonia of infants (excluding the neonate) and children. It usually occurs in association with, or as a complication of, a viral upper respiratory illness. The onset of clinical manifestations is usually rapid and abrupt, and although fever is a prominent feature, respiratory signs and symptoms are

common and usually are present early. *(Long:741)*

32. **(A)** Staphylococcal scalded skin syndrome is mediated by exfoliative toxins A and B. Infants are most commonly affected and clinically present with tender, generalized erythroderma followed by generalized appearance of flaccid bullae which rupture. *(Long:704; Red Book:561)*

33. **(B)** Rotaviruses are recognized as the major cause of severe gastroenteritis in children. Most cases in the United States occur during the winter months. The most prominent clinical manifestations of rotavirus infection include nonbloody diarrhea often preceded by fever and vomiting. Approximately 10% of infected infants are hospitalized to correct dehydration. *(Long:1107; Red Book:535)*

34. **(D)** The rash of Rocky Mountain spotted fever begins as irregular pink macules that appear first on the extremities. The rash then spreads to the face and trunk and becomes petechial and purpuric. There are no papules or vesicles, and the rash is not evanescent. *(Red Book:532; Long:943)*

35. **(D)** Pertussis classically begins with a catarrhal stage indistinguishable from a common cold and lasts up to a week. This is followed by gradual worsening of the cough, finally reaching the paroxysmal stage, characterized by thick, tenacious secretions and fits of forceful coughing that often end in a whoop as the child is finally able to take a full breath. Fever is usually mild or absent. *(Red Book:472; Long:882)*

36. **(B)** Pertussis usually is associated with a marked absolute lymphocytosis. Peripheral white blood cell counts in the range of 20,000–30,000/mm^3 with a majority of lymphocytes are characteristic of this infection. This is a useful and important diagnostic feature. *(Long:883)*

37. **(B)** Typhoid fever (infection with *Salmonella typhi*) is characterized by an incubation period of 6–21 days, followed by fever, malaise, and, in some cases, rose spots. These are small,

palpable erythematous lesions on the trunk. (Petechiae are smaller and not palpable.) Diarrhea, if present, usually clears and often is followed by constipation. *(Long:115; Red Book:542)*

38. **(D)** Aseptic meningitis is one of the most common complications of mumps virus infection. In fact, it occurs so frequently that it might be considered a part of the disease rather than a complication. CSF pleocytosis often occurs in mumps infection, even in the absence of signs of meningeal irritation. Infection with mumps virus is generalized, and other target areas besides the parotid gland and the CSF include the heart, kidneys, pancreas, and testicles in males and breasts in females. *(Long;284–287; Feigin:2078–2079)*

39. **(D)** Photophobia is a relatively common finding in meningitis, both bacterial and viral. Although photophobia also occurs in other neurologic conditions, such as brain tumor and subarachnoid hemorrhage, these are less common than meningitis. In this patient, the acute onset in association with fever and headache also favors the diagnosis of meningitis. *(Long:265, 284–287)*

40. **(A)** Although the combination of fever, hemorrhagic eruption, and shock can be seen with bacteremic infection caused by a wide variety of organisms including *H. influenzae*, *S. pneumoniae*, *S. aureus*, and β-hemolytic *Streptococcus*, this combination of findings is most commonly seen with meningococcal (*N. meningitidis*) infection. The hemorrhagic skin lesions (purpura) suggest disseminated intravascular coagulation, an ominous prognostic sign. *(Long:750)*

41. **(E)** Subdural effusions are a common complication of acute bacterial meningitis, occurring in 30–50% of cases. The exact pathogenesis is unknown, but the effusions are more frequent in young infants, usually sterile, and not related either to inadequate therapy or to a bleeding disorder. They are frequently asymptomatic and rarely fatal. *(Pediatrics 86:163–170)*

42. **(D)** Infectious mononucleosis is generally caused by Epstein-Barr virus infection and

patients present with a typical clinical picture of lymphadenopathy, splenomegaly, and atypical (reactive) lymphocytes on peripheral blood smear. The monospot test is a measure of heterophile antibodies that develop in 90% of older children with Epstein-Barr virus infection. The results of monospot testing are often negative in children less than 4 years. *(Red Book:272; Rudolph CD:1037–1038)*

43. **(A)** Household contacts of those with meningococcal disease are at 500–1000 greater risk for acquisition of meningococcal infection than the general population. Although several drug regimens for prophylaxis of contacts of meningococcal disease are acceptable, the primary regimens recommended at this time are rifampin, 10 mg/kg every 12 h (q12h) for a total of four doses for children and a single dose of ciprofloxacin for those >18 years. *(Red Book:432; Long:753)*

44. **(A)** The group B *Streptococcus* is the leading bacterial cause of neonatal infection in most medical centers in the United States. Two clinical syndromes, early onset and late onset, have been described, although some features do overlap both groups. The early-onset picture is most frequent in high-risk infants (e.g., premature, prolonged rupture of membranes) and usually presents as a severe, rapidly progressive illness in the first day or even hours of life. Pneumonia and bacteremia are the most common manifestations, but meningitis occurs in about one-third of cases. Manifestations of late-onset infection are often indolent and include bacteremia and meningitis as well as other focal infections such as osteomyelitis, septic arthritis, omphalitis, and breast abscess. *(Red Book:584–585; Long:726–727)*

45. **(C)** *Listeria monocytogenes* meningitis is uncommon in childhood except for the newborn period, where in some series it accounts for up to 10% of cases of bacterial meningitis. A few pediatric cases occur in immunodeficient children, and a rare case in the otherwise normal child. There is no geographic preference and no relation to otitis media, the use of antibiotics, or

to the presence of a ventriculoperitoneal shunt. *(Red Book:405; Long:784)*

46. **(C)** Active immunization with live measles vaccine at the time of contact is too late to assure protection. Additionally, children should not receive the vaccine before the age of 6 months to assure an adequate immunologic response. The recommended management of susceptible siblings of a contact case is the use of a preventive dose of gammaglobulin (0.25 mg/kg) and later immunization with the live-virus vaccine. In the past, when most women had had natural measles infection, maternal IgG levels of measles antibody were very high, and transplacental IgG afforded the young infant relatively strong protection. Cases of measles infection in this age group were often milder than in older children. Such is not the case now. Many mothers have low levels of measles antibody (from immunization rather than natural infection), and their infants are susceptible to severe measles infection. *(Red Book:422)*

47. **(B)** The dog ascarid, *Toxocara canis*, cannot complete its life cycle in the human, and, therefore, eggs or worms are not discharged in the stool. The clinical picture of toxocariasis (often referred to as visceral larva migrans) is characterized by fever, hepatomegaly, and eosinophilia. Less frequently there may be involvement of the lung, central nervous system, heart, or retina. None of the other parasites listed characteristically causes hepatomegaly. *(Red Book:630; Long:1340–1342)*

48. **(C)** *Ascaris* is the largest intestinal roundworm, and occasionally intestinal obstruction may result from heavy infection. The incidence of this complication has been estimated at 2 per 1000 infected children per year. Intestinal obstruction has not been observed with any of the other parasites listed. *(Red Book:206; Long:1332)*

49. **(B)** Kawasaki syndrome is a multisystem vasculitis which typically manifests with high, spiking fever for 5 or more days along with conjunctival injection, mucositis, polymorphous

rash, changes in peripheral extremities, and single cervical lymph node swelling. Treatment with aspirin and intravenous immune globulin is indicated; without treatment, 20% of children develop coronary artery aneurysms. *(Red Book:392; Long:1015–1016)*

50. **(C)** The clinical manifestations of human parvovirus B-19 include erythema infectiosum (healthy child), polyarthropathy syndrome (adults especially women), chronic anemia/ pure red cell aplasia (immunocompromised hosts), transient aplastic crisis (sicklemics), and hydrops fetalis/congenital anemia (fetus). Erythema infectiosum is most commonly diagnosed and easily recognized. A distinctive rash featuring a "slapped cheek" appearance is noted that is often associated with circumoral pallor. *(Feigin:1623–1626; Red Book:459)*

51. **(A)** Salpingitis is the most common complication of gonorrhea in the adolescent female. Arthritis is the second most frequent complication and is, by far, the most common distal or extragenital complication and the most common of the choices listed in the question. The other complications listed are infrequent in adults and rare in children and adolescents. *(Red Book:285; Long:477)*

52. **(A)** The most common etiologic agents of bacterial meningitis in children beyond the newborn period are *N. meningitidis* and *S. pneumoniae*. It is possible that the relatively recently introduced vaccine against *S. pneumoniae* will impact this organism, but it is unlikely it will be completely eradicated. *(Long:264)*

53. **(B)** Neonatal herpes simplex virus infection is typically transmitted in infants when mothers experience primary infection at the time of delivery and typically manifests in the first 1–4 weeks of life. There are three forms of disease, though clinical overlap is often noted. Disease may be localized to the skin, eyes, and mouth, it may be disseminated with prominent involvement of lungs and liver, or localized central nervous system involvement may occur. HSV DNA can be detected by polymerase chain reaction assay in patients with

central nervous system disease and is the diagnostic test of choice for such patients. *(Long:1036; Red Book:344)*

54. **(C)** The typical clinical manifestations of hepatitis A virus infection is fever, malaise, jaundice, and anorexia; however, only about one-third of patients <6 years will have symptomatic infection. Fulminant, life-threatening hepatitis in the pediatric patient usually is caused by hepatitis B, rarely hepatitis A. *(Red Book:309)*

55. **(D)** Arthralgia or arthritis is common during the preicteric phase of hepatitis, especially type B. This is usually part of an immune-complex, serum-sickness-like syndrome. Extrahepatic manifestations may also include a papular acrodermatitis (Gianotti-Crosti syndrome) which may precede the icteric phase of infection. *(Red Book:318; Rudolph CD:1224)*

56. **(B)** Chronic infection with hepatitis B virus (HBV) occurs in over 90% of perinatally infected infants, 25–50% of those infected between ages 1 and 5 years, and between 6 and 10% of older children and adults. Those patients with detectable HBeAg are more likely to transmit infection as they have higher blood concentrations of HBV DNA. *(Red Book:319)*

57. **(B)** High fever without other signs and clearing of the fever on appearance of a rash are characteristic of roseola and is the defining clinical expression of primary infection with human herpes virus 6. In measles infection, fever continues for several days after the appearance of the rash. The same is true for the several types of typhus. In infection with echovirus, the rash and fever usually appear together. The rash of scarlet fever often appears at the time of temperature elevation. *(Red Book:357)*

58. **(D)** Immunization against the gonococcus has not been achieved. Currently, there is no effective vaccine (live or killed) against gonorrhea and no effective preparation of serum immune globulin. The organism is not a very potent antigen, and even naturally acquired infection

does not confer immunity against subsequent infection. *(Long:756–757)*

59. **(B)** Herpangina is a syndrome characterized by small vesicles or punched-out ulcers on the tonsils and fauces, uvula, pharynx, and edge of soft palate. The remainder of the mouth and throat usually appear normal on examination. *(Long:1182)*

60. **(D)** Hand-foot-and-mouth syndrome is a specific syndrome that can be caused by a variety of viral agents. It was originally described in association with coxsackievirus A16, but enterovirus 71 can cause an identical clinical picture. *(Red Book:269; Long:1182)*

61. **(A)** Meningococcal meningitis is one of the most common causes of bacterial meningitis in children along with *Streptococcus pneumoniae*. Chemoprophylaxis of household contacts is routine as the risk of secondary transmission is 100–1000 times that of the general population. *(Red Book:433)*

62. **(C)** Most cases of pharyngitis are caused by viruses though the finding of an exudative pharyngitis often leads the practitioner to consider the diagnosis of group A streptococcal infection. However, there are a number of pathogens which may produce exudative changes in children with pharyngeal infection including adenovirus, Epstein-Barr virus, *Corynebacterium diphtheriae*, and *Neisseria gonorrhoeae*. *(Red Book:180)*

63. **(D)** The clinical and laboratory findings described are most suggestive of infectious mononucleosis from Epstein-Barr virus. Hepatic involvement evidenced by elevated serum transaminase levels is common. *(Red Book:271)*

64. **(D)** The clinical picture described is typical of herpes simplex keratoconjunctivitis. The associated vesicular lesions on the skin and the dendritic corneal ulcers are almost pathognomonic of this infection. It is important to diagnose herpes keratitis correctly because infection can be recurrent and lead to loss of vision, and

because therapy is available. Topical trifluorothymidine is generally considered the drug of choice but iododeoxyuridine and 3% vidarabine are also used for superficial keratitis. *(Red Book:349)*

65. **(A)** Infants with perinatally acquired HIV infection often present with nonspecific symptoms and signs including lymphadenopathy, hepatosplenomegaly, failure to thrive, oral candidiasis, and recurrent diarrhea. Among the diseases listed, Pneumocystis pneumonia (PCP) is the most commonly encountered opportunistic infection in infants with perinatally acquired HIV infection. *(Red Book:360)*

66. **(B)** Infants with congenitally acquired cytomegalovirus infection are generally asymptomatic, though 10% present with a syndrome that includes intrauterine growth retardation, thrombocytopenia, jaundice, hepatosplenomegaly, microcephaly, intracerebral calcifications, and retinitis. EBV infection is not associated with congenital infection. Perinatal coxsackie infection may manifest with myocarditis and encephalitis, and human parvovirus B-19 as congenital anemia or hydrops fetalis. Infants infected perinatally with HIV are generally asymptomatic at birth. *(Red Book:259, 269, 360, 460)*

67. **(B)** Upper lobe cavity disease is characteristic of reinfection or reactivation tuberculosis and is seen primarily in adults, occasionally in adolescents. Although progressive primary disease with cavitation can occur in children, it is rather uncommon and is randomly distributed with no predilection for the upper lobes. Fever, hilar adenopathy, and tuberculin hypersensitivity manifested by a positive tuberculin skin test are common findings in children with primary tuberculosis. *(Red Book:642; Long:793)*

68. **(C)** Ehrlichia infection is an acute systemic febrile illness seen most commonly in the south central, southeastern Uinetd States with infection caused by *Ehrlichia chaffeensis* and transmitted via the bite of the lone star tick (*Amblyomma americanum*). A clinical picture

similar to Rocky Mountain spotted fever (though associated less commonly with rash) is reported with prominent CNS and gastrointestinal symptoms; hyponatremia, leukopenia, anemia, and elevated liver transaminases are commonly reported laboratory manifestations. Doxycycline is the drug of choice and should be used even in young patients, as severe and fatal disease has been confirmed. *(Red Book: 267–268; Long:914)*

69. **(B)** In the asplenic patient, there is an increased risk for fulminant life-threatening infection caused by *Streptococcus pneumoniae*. Life-threatening infection occurs in those with post-traumatic asplenia, HIV infection, congenital asplenia, polysplenia syndromes, or those who undergo splenectomy in the course of treatment for malignancy as well as sicklemic patients. *(Long:651; Red Book:492)*

70. **(E)** The rash of varicella follows an incubation period of 12–16 days. There is the onset of a very pruritic rash, with crops of lesions that begin as papules and progress to vesicles and finally crusted scabs. Typically, all three stages of skin lesions are identified on clinical examination. Fever usually is mild to moderate. While a generally self-limited and benign course is noted, severe disease may occur occasionally in the otherwise healthy, especially adolescents and adults. A progressive and severe disease with visceral dissemination is seen in 30–50% of children with lymphoproliferative malignancies, solid tumors, or post-transplantation with the development of hepatitis, encephalitis, and pneumonia. Fatal disease has also been reported in those treated with high dose corticosteroids and in those with other defects of T-cell function. *(Long:1044; Rudolph CD:1043–1044)*

71. **(A)** Congenital malformations, stillborns, and abortions all have been reported with rubella infection during pregnancy. The congenital rubella syndrome consists of ophthalmologic, cardiac, auditory, and neurologic abnormalities with rates as high as 85% if infection occurs in the first 4 weeks of gestation, decreasing to 20–30% during the second month and 5%

during the third or fourth month. These infants may continue to excrete rubella virus for 1 year or more after birth and pose a risk of infection for susceptible hosts. *(Red Book:536–537)*

72. **(E)** Infectious mononucleosis syndrome generally presents with exudative pharyngitis that may be associated with petechiae or erythematous macules on the palate. A rash occurs occasionally and splenomegaly may be noted. Airway obstruction secondary to markedly enlarged tonsils is an infrequent but important complication. *(Long:1061)*

73. **(A)** Adenovirus infection is characterized by upper respiratory tract manifestations that may include common cold, pharyngotonsillitis, otitis media, and pharyngoconjunctival fever. Severe disease may be seen in the immunocompromised. *(Red Book:190)*

74. **(A)** Pharyngitis caused by *Arcanobacterium haemolyticum* infection is hard to differentiate from that of streptococcal infection. It should be suspected in the adolescent who presents with pharyngeal exudates and a scarlatiniform rash and in whom streptococcal infection has been excluded. *(Red Book:205)*

75. **(D)** *S. aureus*-mediated TSS is caused by certain strains of staphylococci that produce one or more exotoxins and/or staphylococcal enterotoxin. These toxins can cause an acute illness characterized by fever, rapid onset hypotension, and multisystem organ involvement. The characteristic skin involvement is a diffuse macular erythema which is most prominent on the trunk. This is typically followed by desquamation 1–2 weeks after the initial onset, particularly on palms, soles, fingers, and toes. *(Red Book:561, 625; Long:99–100)*

76. **(A)** Brucellosis is a zoonotic disease in which children are an accidental host, most commonly contracting infection by ingesting unpasteurized milk. Onset of illness can be acute or insidious. Symptoms of disease are usually nonspecific and include fever, malaise, anorexia, joint pains, headache, and night sweats. Physical findings include lymphadenopathy,

hepatosplenomegaly, and occasionally arthritis. Meningitis, endocarditis, and osteomyelitis are rare complications of disease. Glaucoma is not reported. *(Red Book:222; Long:877–878)*

77. **(A)** Campylobacter infection is characterized by watery diarrhea possibly followed by blood streaked stools, fever, abdominal pain, and malaise. It is usually self-limited, but may have immunoreactive complications (Guillain-Barré syndrome, reactive arthritis, Reiter syndrome, and erythema nodosum) that occur during convalescence. It is estimated that in 30–40% of cases Guillain-Barré syndrome occurred within 2 weeks of *Campylobacter* infection. *(Red Book:227, Long:893)*

78. **(C)** Cat-scratch disease (CSD) is caused by *Bartonella henselae*. The most common manifestation is unilateral regional lymphadenopathy. Small erythematous papules can occur at the inoculation site and precede the lymphadenopathy by 1–2 weeks. The typical patient lacks constitutional symptoms, but 30% may have mild fever, malaise, headache, and anorexia. Systemic CSD is rare. *(Red Book:232; Long:874)*

79. **(A)** Respiratory syncytial virus (RSV) is the most important cause of bronchiolitis in infants and young children and causes acute respiratory tract illness in patients of all ages. Typical roentgenographic findings include hyperinflation, peribronchial thickening, and atelectasis especially involving the right upper lobe. Infiltrates typically are associated with bacterial pneumonia. Pleural effusions and hilar adenopathy are findings not typically associated with bronchiolitis. *(Long:215–216)*

80. **(A)** *Giardia lamblia* infection can cause a broad spectrum of clinical manifestations. Findings from asymptomatic secretion of organisms to chronic diarrhea and failure to thrive are seen. Most commonly, children either are asymptomatic or have an acute episode of watery diarrhea. Low-grade fever, abdominal pain, nausea, and anorexia may occur with the acute process. Protracted illness is usually associated with passage of foul smelling stools,

abdominal distention, and malabsorption. These can lead to failure to thrive. Bloody diarrhea and cough are not associated with giardiasis. *(Red Book:283; Long:1276–1277)*

81. **(D)** Tuberculous meningitis is the most serious complication of tuberculosis in children. It usually occurs within 2–6 months of initial infection. It is difficult to diagnose rapidly as skin testing may be negative and chest films may be normal. Culture results can take anywhere from 1 to 10 weeks to yield a positive result. CSF findings can give clues of the diagnosis. CSF white cell counts range from 10 to 500/mm^3 with usual lymphocytic predomination. Glucose is low normal during the early part of the second stage (when signs of increased intracranial pressure are present) and falls about 5 mg each day until the third stage at which it is very low. Protein concentration is elevated, often markedly. Blood tinged CSF is not associated with tuberculous meningitis. *(Feigin:1210–1211; Long:796)*

82. **(C)** Echovirus is a subclass of the genus enterovirus. Also included are group A and B coxsackie viruses, and newer enteroviruses. The nonpolio enteroviruses are responsible for many different illnesses in infants and children. These can include cold symptoms, herpangina, exanthem, gastrointestinal symptoms, conjunctivitis, and myopericarditis. Echovirus, in particular, commonly causes febrile illness with a nonspecific rash and aseptic meningitis. Infection is most common in summer and early fall. *(Red Book:269; Long:1181–1182)*

83. **(E)** Patients with increased availability of free iron such as those with sickle cell anemia, B-thalassemia, G6PD, etc. are at increased risk of infection with *Yersinia enterocolitica* bacteremia. Children less than 1 year of age are also at risk. This is thought to be the result of bacterial iron scavenging systems which increase virulence. The most common manifestation of *Yersinia enterocolitica* is enterocolitis with fever and bloody, mucous-filled diarrhea, not bacteremia. Patients with sickle cell anemia also have functional asplenia and are more

susceptible to infections caused by encapsulated organisms. *(Red Book:690; Long:653)*

84. **(A)** Pelvic inflammatory disease (PID) is a syndrome associated with ascending infection from the vagina through the uterus, fallopian tubes, and into the pelvic peritoneum. Symptoms include inflammation and/or abscess of the involved structures. The most common pathogens associated are *Chlamydia trachomatis* and *Neisseria gonorrhoeae*. Perihepatitis (inflammation of the capsule of the liver or Fitz-Hugh–Curtis syndrome) occurs in 5–15% of patients and is a direct result of the ascending infection. These patients typically present with right upper quadrant pain which can be deceiving. *(Long:351–354)*

85. **(C)** Kawasaki syndrome is an acute, self-limited vasculitis of unknown etiology. It is of importance because as many as 20% of untreated cases will develop coronary artery abnormalities. The diagnostic criteria include fever for at least 5 days plus four of the following: (1) bilateral conjunctival injection; (2) mucositis with cracked lips and strawberry tongue; (3) erythema and swelling of the hands and feet with periungual desquamation; (4) erythematous rash; (5) cervical lymph node enlargement to >1.5 cm. *(Long:1015–1016)*

86. **(A)** The exanthem associated with Rocky Mountain spotted fever is usually absent until the third to fifth day of illness. It initially appears on the wrists and ankles and spreads to the trunk within hours. Palms and soles are typically involved. It is characteristically erythematous and macular and progresses to maculopapular and often petechial. *(Red Book:532; Long:943)*

87. **(D)** The exanthem associated with cutaneous herpes simplex virus is characteristically deep, painful vesicles on an erythematous base. They can occur singly, but are often grouped. The groups coalesce, ulcerate, and crust over several days. The virus can affect any area of the skin, but most commonly affects the fingers (herpetic whitlow), lips (cold sore), and genital area. *(Long:1034–1035)*

88. **(B)** Koplik spots are characteristic of measles. They are white dots or specks that can appear anywhere on the buccal mucosa but usually are found opposite the lower premolars. They appear within 2–3 days of initial symptoms (cough, coryza, and fever). They eventually coalesce and spread throughout the buccal mucosa. *(Feigin:725; Long:1150)*

89. **(C)** *Necator americanus* is a common hookworm found in the Western hemisphere, sub-Saharan Africa, southeast Asia, and some Pacific Islands. Hookworm infection is currently the leading cause of iron deficiency anemia in developing countries. The larvae penetrate the skin and migrate via lymphatics and venules to the lungs and up to the GI tract where they are swallowed. The larvae continue to develop to adult worms. The worms attach to the intestinal mucosa to feed, thus causing anemia. *(Long:1333)*

90. **(A)** *Toxocara canis* infection (visceral larva migrans or ocular larva migrans) occurs when humans ingest soil containing the infective egg of the parasite. *Toxocara* species are common roundworms of dogs and cats. After ingestion, the larvae hatch in the small intestine and migrate to all organs through the bloodstream. Characteristic manifestations include fever, eosinophilia, hepatomegaly, leukocytosis, and hypergammaglobulinemia. *(Long:1340–1341; Red Book:630)*

91. **(D)** *Trichuris trichiura* is a whipworm named for its characteristic shape. Infection occurs after the ingestion of fertilized eggs which then hatch into adults in the intestine. Most infections are asymptomatic, however heavy worm load is responsible for trichuris dysentery or chronic colitis. Trichuris dysentery is an acute diarrheal illness that includes passage of blood and mucous in stool. The profound mucosal edema that occurs from inflammation leads to tenesmus and in severe cases, rectal prolapse. *(Long:1335–1336)*

92. **(E)** Infection with the pinworm, *Enterobius vermicularis*, is very common in the United States and developed countries. There are high rates of transmission in schools and daycare centers.

Ingestion of eggs leads to development of adult worm in the intestine. Adult female worms live mostly in the colon where they migrate out and lay eggs on the perianal skin. This causes intense pruritus likely secondary to allergic response. *(Long:1336)*

93. **(C)** Rat-bite fever is caused by *Spirillum minus* or *Streptobacillus moniliformis*. *S. moniliformis* infection is characterized by fever, a petechial rash on the extremities, and, occasionally, adenopathy; migratory polyarthritis follows in approximately half of patients. *(Red Book: 521–522)*

94. **(A)** *Pasteurella multocida* is a common oropharyngeal flora of many animals, especially cats and dogs. Infection occurs most commonly after an animal bite; in up to 75% of cat bites and up to 50% of dog bites. Characteristic wound infections occur with erythema swelling and purulent discharge from the site. Fever and regional lymphadenopathy are common. *(Long:853)*

95. **(D)** Birds are the major reservoir for *Chlamydia psittaci*. Psittacosis is an acute febrile respiratory illness. It can include systemic symptoms such as nonproductive cough, malaise, and headache. People in the environment of infected birds are at greatest risk of infections. Common infected birds include psittacine birds (parakeets, parrots, and macaws) as well as pigeons and turkeys. *(Red Book:237)*

96. **(D)** Respiratory syncytial virus (RSV) is the most common cause of bronchiolitis in infants. Other causes include parainfluenza viruses, adenovirus, influenza A or B, metapneumovirus, or rhinovirus. *(Long:214; Pediatrics 111:1407–1410)*

97. **(C)** Influenza virus can cause many different clinical syndromes. It is usually associated with high fever, chills or rigors, malaise, myalgia, headache, and nonproductive cough. Sore throat, nasal congestion, rhinitis, and cough may also be prominent. It can also cause croup, bronchiolitis, pneumonia, and a sepsis-like picture in young infants. *(Red Book:382)*

98. **(D)** Conditions that increase the risk of severe or fatal RSV infection include cyanotic heart disease, prematurity with underlying pulmonary disease, and immunodeficiency or immune suppression. *(Red Book:523)*

99. **(C)** Congenital cytomegalovirus (CMV) is difficult to diagnose as initial infection may be asymptomatic. Proof of congenital infection requires a positive viral culture obtained from body fluid within the first 3 weeks of life. Urine and oral cultures are usually used because of ease of collection. After 3 weeks, culture does not prove congenital infection. *(Red Book:260; Long:1055)*

100. **(B)** HSV encephalitis can be detected by polymerase chain reaction on CSF from infected neonates. It is now the gold standard for the laboratory diagnosis of HSV encephalitis. PCR has sensitivity and specificity that exceed 90% and leads to a more rapid diagnosis. *(Long:1036–1037; Red Book:46–47)*

101. **(B)** Detecting HIV in an infant or child less than 18 months of age is complicated as these children can carry maternal antibody to HIV and not be infected. PCR assay is the preferred diagnostic test. Infants born to HIV infected mothers should be tested by HIV PCR in the first 48 h of life. These infants need follow-up tests at 1–2 months of age and again at 2–4 months of age. Infection is confirmed with two separate positive tests. Infection is excluded if two PCR tests performed beyond 1 month of age and a third performed at or beyond 4 months of age are all negative. *(Red Book:366–367)*

102. **(C)** The diagnosis of group B streptococcal meningitis should always be confirmed by culture of the CSF. Gram-positive cocci seen on staining techniques provide presumptive evidence, especially if the history correlates, but culture needs to confirm the diagnosis. *(Red Book:586; Long:728)*

103. **(D)** Serologic testing is the primary means of diagnosing toxoplasmosis infection. Congenital infection is confirmed by demonstration of

toxoplasma specific antibodies in the CSF. Tests to detect IgA and IgE antibodies, which decrease to undetectable levels sooner than IgM antibodies, are useful in detecting congenital infections. *(Red Book:633; Long:1313)*

104. **(A)** The clinical manifestations of tetanus include four patterns: generalized, localized, cephalic, and neonatal. Generalized tetanus is the most common pattern. Trismus (lock jaw) is usually the presenting symptom with progression to other muscle groups. Fortunately, tetanus is almost never encountered in a fully immunized child. *(Long:982; Fiegin:1580–1581)*

105. **(C)** Diphtheria typically presents as membranous nasopharyngitis or obstructive laryngotracheitis. Serious complications include toxic myocarditis, toxic neuropathy, and upper airway obstruction. Toxic myocarditis occurs in 10–25% of patients and carries significant mortality. *(Red Book:263; Long:773)*

106. **(D)** *Streptococcus pneumoniae (Pneumococcus)* is the most common cause of invasive bacterial infections in children, including pneumonia and bacteremia with or without a focus. It is also one of the two most common causes of bacterial meningitis (along with *Neisseria meningitidis*) in children. *(Red Book:490; Long:740–741)*

107. **(B)** Infection with rabies is a four-phase process. The first phase is the incubation period, which generally lasts from 10 to 90 days. The second phase is 2–10 days and is when the virus attacks the CNS. The third phase includes encephalitis when the virus has caused widespread infection in the brain. This usually includes alterations in normal behavior. The fourth phase is coma. Death usually ensues within 7 days of coma. *(Long:1156–1157; Red Book:514)*

108. **(A)** In the United States, most cases of tetanus occur in inadequately immunized individuals after puncture wounds, farming or gardening activities, or in association with illicit drug use. *(Long:82)*

109. **(A)** Cough, coryza, conjunctivitis, and Koplik spots are the hallmark characteristics of measles infection. *(Red Book:419)*

110. **(D)** Necrotizing fasciitis and other invasive group A *Streptococcus* infections often occur as complications of varicella infection. *(Red Book:574)*

111. **(C)** Orchitis is a common complication of mumps virus, especially after puberty. It occurs in 14–35% of male cases. It is usually unilateral and resolves in 3–7 days. *(Red Book:439; Long:1137)*

112. **(B)** There are several described anomalies with congenital rubella syndrome. Findings include ophthalmologic: cataracts, retinopathy, and congenital glaucoma; cardiac: patent ductus arteriosis and peripheral pulmonary artery stenosis; and neurologic: meningoencephalitis, behavioral disorders, sensorineural hearing impairment, and mental retardation. *(Red Book:536)*

113. **(C)** CSF pleocytosis is a common finding in mumps infection. Symptoms of aseptic meningitis only occur in 1–10% of patients with mumps infection. Symptomatic disease occurs 3–10 days after the onset of parotitis and is generally self-limited. Encephalitis occurs in approximately 0.1% of patients with measles. *(Long:1136)*

114. **(D)** Reye syndrome is uncommon but severe complication of varicella or influenza infection. There has been a significant decrease in the incidence of Reye syndrome with the diminished use of aspirin in children. It is characterized by encephalitis and fatty infiltration of the liver. It usually presents with repetitive vomiting and altered mental status. Mortality is about 30% even with aggressive supportive care and management. *(Long:320–322)*

115. **(A)** Subacute sclerosing panencephalitis (SSPE) is a rare degenerative central nervous system process that occurs as a result of persistent measles virus infection. It is characterized by behavioral and intellectual deteriorization as well as seizures. It generally occurs years after

original infection and is ultimately fatal. *(Red Book:420; Long:1151)*

116. (A) Studies in the United States have confirmed low levels of vitamin A in children with measles. Administration of vitamin A to children with active measles in regions that are known to be vitamin A deficient, or where measles mortality is 1% or greater, has significantly reduced the complications such as diarrhea and pneumonia. *(Long:1150; Red Book:421)*

117. (B) Group B *Streptococcus* infection in young infants is characterized in two groups. Early onset occurs within the first 6 days of life (usually within 24 h) and manifests as respiratory distress, apnea, shock, and less commonly meningitis. Late onset disease occurs at 3–4 weeks of age and commonly manifests as occult bacteremia or meningitis. It is the most common cause of meningitis in the neonate (typically defined as a baby up to 4 weeks of age). *(Red Book:585–586)*

118. (C) *Streptococcus pneumoniae* (*Pneumococcus*) is the most common cause of invasive bacterial infections in children. Meningitis in children under 5 years of age most commonly is caused by *N. meningitidis* (4–5/100,000) and *S. pneumoniae* (2.5/100,000). *(Long:264; Red Book:490)*

119. (D) Isolation of coagulase-negative staphylococci (CoNS) generally represents contamination of skin culture material as it is a common skin flora. However, CoNS is the major cause of CNS infection in patients with intraventricular shunts or ventriculostomy catheters. Seventy percent of these infections occur within 2 months of placement of the catheter. *(Long:710)*

120. (C) Children with a basilar skull fracture or a cribriform plate fracture and CSF leak are at high risk for pneumococcal meningitis. *(Long: 264; Red Book:492)*

121. (C) Children with asplenia, such as those with sickle cell anemia, are at greater risk for infection with encapsulated organisms. *Pneumococcus* (another name for *Streptococcus pneumoniae*) is therefore the most common cause of meningitis

in children with sickle cell anemia. *(Long:264, Red Book:492)*

122. (A) Chronic diarrhea and malabsorption are commonly seen in X linked agammaglobulinemia and are often associated with infections with rotavirus and *Giardia lamblia*. *(Long:626)*

123. (A) In addition to the greater susceptibility to bacterial infections, patients with XLA are also predisposed to chronic and severe enteroviral infections. This includes encephalitis. Chronic enteroviral and pulmonary infections remain the most common causes of death in XLA patients. *(Long:626–627)*

124. (B) Severe combined immune deficiency (SCID) is an inherited deficiency of T and B lymphocyte function that occurs in about 1/50,000 live births. Fungal infections, such as PCP, are suggestive of severe CD4 lymphocyte deficiency. PCP is a common infection associated with SCID. *(Long:643)*

125. (B) Adenosine deaminase deficiency is an autosomal recessive form of SCID. It causes increased thymocyte and immature B-cell death from accumulation of purine metabolites. *(Long:643–644)*

126. (C) Chronic granulomatous disease is caused from a defective or absent phagocyte respiratory burst. The result is reduced ability to overcome catalase-positive bacteria and fungi. The result is recurrent infections with these organisms. Liver abscesses and lymphadenitis are the most common manifestations of infection. *(Long:638–640)*

127. (D) Common variable immunodeficiency (CVID) is a group of disorders characterized by abnormal antibody production. Recurrent sinopulmonary infections are common. Antibody replacement with intravenous immune globulin and prophylactic antibiotics are beneficial for survival. *(Long:628–629)*

128. (B) DTaP vaccine should be given as a primary series at 2, 4, and 6 months of age followed by a dose at 12–15 months and 4–6 years. *(Red Book:24)*

129. **(A)** MMR vaccine should be given at 12–15 months of age followed by a dose at 4–6 years. *(Red Book:24)*

130. **(A)** Primary varicella vaccine should be given at 12–15 months of age. Studies are ongoing to assess the need for additional doses. *(Red Book:24)*

131. **(B)** Pneumococcal conjugate vaccine (PCV) should be given as a primary series at 2, 4, and 6 months of age followed by a fourth dose at 12–15 months. *(Red Book:24)*

132. **(D)** Hepatitis A vaccine series should be given at age of 24 months or older. *(Red Book:24)*

133. **(C)** Tetanus-diphtheria vaccine (Td) should be given at age of 11–12 years (if at least 5 years have elapsed since the last administered dose of tetanus and diphtheria toxoid-containing vaccine) with routine subsequent boosters every 10 years. *(Red Book:24–25)*

BIBLIOGRAPHY

American Academy of Pediatrics. 2003 Red Book, *Report of the Committee on Infectious Diseases*, 26th ed. Elk Grove Village, IL: American Academy of Pediatrics, 2003.

Esper F, Boucher D, Weibel C, Martinello RA, Kahn JS. Human metapneumovirus infection in the United States: clinical manifestations associated with a newly emerging respiratory infection in children. *Pediatrics* 2003;111(6 Pt 1):1407–1410.

Feigin RD, Cherry JD. *Textbook of Pediatric Infectious Diseases*, 4th ed. Philadelphia, PA: W.B. Saunders, 1998.

Long SS, Pickering LK, Prober CG (eds.). *Principles and Practice of Pediatric Infectious Diseases*, 2nd ed. New York, NY: Churchill Livingstone, 2003.

Rudolph CD, Rudolph AM, Hostetter MK, et al. *Rudolph's Pediatrics*, 21st ed. New York, NY: McGraw-Hill, 2003.

Snedeker JD, Kaplan SL, Dodge PR, Holmes SJ, Feigin RD. Subdural effusion and its relationship with neurologic sequelae of bacterial meningitis in infancy: a prospective study. *Pediatrics* 1990;86(2):163–170.

CHAPTER 8

General Pediatrics

Catalina Kersten, MD

This chapter is designed to include topics not covered in other chapters, and to reinforce some important previously mentioned concepts.

Questions

1. The highest death rate in the pediatric age group occurs

   (A) in the first month of life
   (B) between 2 and 12 months of life
   (C) between 2 and 4 years of life
   (D) just before puberty
   (E) during adolescence

2. The diagnosis of Werdnig-Hoffmann disease is most likely in an infant with severe hypotonia and

   (A) normal deep tendon reflexes
   (B) seizures
   (C) fasciculations of the tongue
   (D) recurrent fevers
   (E) atrophy of the optic nerve

3. Early diagnosis of cerebral palsy is important because it permits

   (A) genetic counseling to prevent subsequent cases
   (B) treatment of the underlying lesion and prevention of progression
   (C) guidance that may minimize or prevent secondary physical and emotional problems

   (D) prophylactic anticonvulsant treatment before the onset of seizures
   (E) avoidance of unrealistic expectations

4. Congenital malformations, other than those of the head and face, most commonly seen in association with craniosynostosis involve the

   (A) trachea and esophagus
   (B) heart
   (C) umbilicus
   (D) extremities
   (E) spine

5. The arthritis of acute rheumatic fever usually

   (A) is monoarticular
   (B) heals without deformity
   (C) appears after the fever subsides
   (D) is seen only in patients with concurrent carditis
   (E) involves large and small joints equally

6. A 2-month-old infant has severe dyspnea and cyanosis. Chest roentgenogram reveals minimal cardiomegaly and a diffuse reticular pattern of the lung fields. Which of the following best explains these findings?

   (A) acute viral myocarditis
   (B) hypoplastic left heart
   (C) pulmonary artery atresia
   (D) total anomalous pulmonary drainage with venous obstruction
   (E) transposition of the great arteries

7. Which of the following statements regarding brain tumors in childhood is true?

    (A) Most are located in the midline and/or below the tentorium cerebri.

    (B) Brain tumors are a rare type of cancer in childhood.

    (C) Signs of increased intracranial pressure are rare.

    (D) Seizures are the presenting complaint in most cases.

    (E) Most cases occur in the first year of life.

8. An 8-month-old child has vomiting and screaming episodes for 12 h. Physical examination reveals a sausage-shaped mass in the right upper quadrant. Which of the following would be most useful?

    (A) passage of nasogastric tube

    (B) examination of a stool specimen for ova and parasites

    (C) blood culture

    (D) abdominal ultrasound

    (E) barium enema study

9. Most cases of pancreatic insufficiency in childhood are caused by

    (A) hyperthyroidism

    (B) biliary atresia

    (C) carcinoma

    (D) congenital absence of the pancreas

    (E) cystic fibrosis

10. Which of the following conditions is associated with an increased risk of brain abscess?

    (A) chronic renal failure

    (B) idiopathic or familial epilepsy

    (C) congenital cyanotic heart disease

    (D) chronic or recurrent tonsillitis

    (E) Langerhans cell histiocytosis

11. A positive serum rheumatoid factor is uncommon in children with rheumatoid disease other than systemic lupus erythematosus. When it does occur, it is most likely in a girl with

    (A) the acute systemic form of juvenile rheumatoid arthritis

    (B) the pauciarticular form of juvenile rheumatoid arthritis

    (C) the polyarticular form of juvenile rheumatoid arthritis

    (D) psoriatic arthritis

    (E) ankylosing spondylitis

12. A 2-year-old Black child presents with anemia and painful swelling of the hands and feet. The most likely diagnosis is

    (A) child abuse

    (B) congenital syphilis

    (C) leukemia

    (D) sickle cell disease

    (E) vitamin D deficiency

13. Which of the following is most likely to occur as an isolated manifestation of acute rheumatic fever?

    (A) arthritis

    (B) carditis

    (C) chorea

    (D) erythema marginatum

    (E) fever

14. Which of the following is most frequently an important factor in the etiology of iron deficiency anemia in a 2-year-old child?

    (A) pica

    (B) lack of fresh vegetables in the diet

    (C) intake of inadequate amounts of fruit juice

    (D) intake of excessive amounts of vitamin C

    (E) intake of large amounts of unmodified cow milk

15. Bone marrow aspiration is most likely to confirm the diagnosis in a patient with which one of the following malignancies?

    (A) hepatoblastoma

    (B) neuroblastoma

    (C) retinoblastoma

    (D) rhabdomyosarcoma

    (E) Wilms tumor

16. Intestinal lactase deficiency in infancy

    (A) may be either genetic or acquired
    (B) often is associated with pancreatitis
    (C) causes a strongly alkaline pH of the stool
    (D) is a recognized cause of intestinal obstruction
    (E) usually leads to malabsorption without clinically evident diarrhea

17. Features of the McCune-Albright syndrome include polyosteotic fibrous dysplasia of bone, abnormal skin pigmentation, and

    (A) anemia
    (B) deafness
    (C) precocious puberty
    (D) multiple neurofibromas
    (E) chronic glomerulonephritis

18. A patent ductus arteriosus in an otherwise normal 6-month-old infant is likely to be associated with

    (A) a right-to-left shunt
    (B) a continuous cardiac murmur
    (C) a narrow pulse
    (D) bacterial endocarditis
    (E) right ventricular hypertrophy

19. The most common presentation of congenital aganglionic megacolon (Hirschsprung disease) in the newborn is

    (A) an abdominal mass
    (B) diarrhea
    (C) intestinal obstruction
    (D) peritonitis
    (E) sepsis

20. Complex partial (psychomotor) seizures are characterized by

    (A) lack of alterations in mental state, consciousness, or responsiveness
    (B) a brief tonic-clonic phase
    (C) automatisms

    (D) three-per-second spike-and-wave pattern on EEG
    (E) lack of postictal phenomenon

21. Increased intracranial pressure may be seen with

    (A) achondroplasia
    (B) glycogen storage disease
    (C) hypervitaminosis C
    (D) galactosemia
    (E) juvenile rheumatoid arthritis

22. The most common ophthalmologic complication in children with juvenile rheumatoid arthritis is

    (A) cataracts
    (B) ptosis
    (C) glaucoma
    (D) corneal ulcerations
    (E) iridocyclitis

23. Which of the following carries the most unfavorable prognosis in children with systemic lupus erythematosus?

    (A) fever and leukocytosis
    (B) anti-DNA antibodies
    (C) polyserositis
    (D) nephritis
    (E) seizures

24. Which malignancy is uncommon in children under the age of 5 years?

    (A) retinoblastoma
    (B) neuroblastoma
    (C) osteosarcoma
    (D) leukemia
    (E) Wilms tumor

25. Wilms tumor has been associated with

    (A) aniridia
    (B) hemihypertrophy
    (C) Beckwith-Wiedemann syndrome
    (D) Denys-Drash syndrome
    (E) all the above

26. A 12-year-old girl develops jaundice, progressive tremors, and emotional lability. You are most likely to find which of the following during physical examination?

    (A) head circumference greater than 95th percentile
    (B) brown discoloration of the limbic region of the cornea
    (C) bilateral conductive hearing loss
    (D) generalized lymphadenopathy
    (E) sacral hair tuft and dimple

27. A 12-month-old infant is unable to sit by herself and parents have noticed an exaggerated startle response. What are you most likely to find on physical examination?

    (A) holosystolic murmur
    (B) absent knee-jerk reflex
    (C) syndactily
    (D) cherry red macular spot
    (E) bilateral inguinal hernias

28. An infant has been diagnosed with congenital hypoparathyroidism. What are you most likely to find on evaluation?

    (A) microcephaly
    (B) hyponatremia
    (C) hyperkalemia
    (D) goiter
    (E) candidiasis

29. A little boy has severe eczema, recurrent sinus and ear infections, and thrombocytopenia. Inheritance of this disorder is most likely from

    (A) father
    (B) mother
    (C) both parents
    (D) random mutation
    (E) multifactorial

30. A 12-year-old girl has had progressive muscle weakness over the past weeks. She has also developed an erythematous, scaly rash on the face, arms and thighs, and a lacy rash on her upper eyelids. The next best laboratory study is

    (A) rheumatoid factor
    (B) erythrocyte sedimentation rate (ESR)
    (C) urine analysis
    (D) serum creatinine kinase
    (E) antinuclear antibody (ANA) panel

31. Which of the following is true of both congenital pure red cell aplasia (Diamond-Blackfan syndrome) and transient erythroblastopenia of childhood (TEC)?

    (A) Corticosteroid treatment is usually beneficial.
    (B) Red blood cell transfusions may be necessary.
    (C) Hepatosplenomegaly is usually present.
    (D) Spontaneous recovery is common.
    (E) Parvovirus infection has been associated with both diseases.

32. A 2-year-old White girl is listless and pale. You obtain a complete blood count and find that the patient has severe megaloblastic anemia. What additional history explains this?

    (A) eats only organically grown products
    (B) drinks exclusively goat milk
    (C) required phototherapy in neonatal period
    (D) has required multiple antibiotics for middle ear infections
    (E) mother had gestational diabetes during pregnancy

33. A 12-month-old child has had poor weight gain. The child started to have loose stools at the age of 8 months and has a very poor appetite. On examination, you see a clingy, irritable child with very little subcutaneous fat and a protuberant abdomen. The next best test is

    (A) IgA-endomysial antibody
    (B) urine analysis
    (C) sweat chloride
    (D) quantitative immunoglobulins
    (E) fecal blood

34. The best initial study for a child with secondary nocturnal enuresis is

    (A) renal ultrasound
    (B) voiding cystourethrogram
    (C) abdominal radiograph
    (D) urine analysis
    (E) creatinine clearance

35. A 5-year-old girl suffers from a second episode with meningococcal meningitis. What is the best next laboratory study?

    (A) quantitative immunoglobulin levels
    (B) T-cell subset analysis
    (C) CH_{50}
    (D) quantitative nitroblue tetrazolium test
    (E) delayed hypersensitivity skin testing

36. A 2-year-old child is referred to you for evaluation of child abuse. On physical examination, you find a pale child with diffuse petechiae. HEENT examination reveals bilateral proptosis with periorbital ecchymoses. Which of the following statements is true about this condition?

    (A) Age at presentation does not affect the prognosis.
    (B) A full skeletal survey should be obtained next.
    (C) Hematuria is a common finding.
    (D) It usually presents between 4 and 8 years of age.
    (E) Spontaneous regression has occurred in some children.

37. Which study is the most important to obtain in a 2-year-old child with Beckwith-Wiedemann syndrome and an abdominal mass?

    (A) hepatobiliary scintigraphy
    (B) upper gastrointestinal endoscopy
    (C) urine catecholamine levels
    (D) serum α-fetoprotein level
    (E) voiding cystourethrogram

38. A 9-year-old African American child presents with anemia and stroke. The most likely finding with hemoglobin electrophoresis is

    (A) HbS 45%
    (B) HbA 65%
    (C) HbA_2 15%
    (D) HbF 15%
    (E) HbC 45%

39. Finding of what organisms in the stool would best support your diagnosis of AIDS?

    (A) rotavirus
    (B) *Salmonella*
    (C) *Mycobacterium avium*
    (D) *Giardia*
    (E) *Yersinia enterocolitica*

40. Each of the following is associated with group A beta-hemolytic streptococcal infections, either pharyngeal, skin or both. Which of the following is associated only with pharyngeal infections?

    (A) scarlatina
    (B) toxic shock syndrome
    (C) rheumatic fever
    (D) necrotizing fasciitis
    (E) glomerulonephritis

41. A 7-year-old child has abdominal pain and a rash that started several days ago. On examination, you notice a palpable purpuric rash over his calves and buttocks with swelling of both ankles. Abdominal examination is unremarkable. You most likely will find

    (A) decreased platelet count
    (B) hypochromic microcytic anemia
    (C) elevated blood urea nitrogen and creatinine
    (D) low C3 complement levels
    (E) normal clotting parameters

42. A true statement about fragile X syndrome is

    (A) premutation carriers generally have phenotypic manifestations
    (B) inheritance is autosomal dominant
    (C) it is the most common form of inherited mental retardation

(D) affected males typically have microorchidism

(E) a single gene point mutation is the cause of this syndrome

43. Which of the following abnormalities is the most common in Down syndrome?

(A) leukemia

(B) patent ductus arteriosus

(C) seizure disorder

(D) hearing loss

(E) gastrointestinal tract anomalies

44. The most important test in a 14-year-old girl with primary amenorrhea, short stature, and an ejection click heard over the right sternal border is

(A) sweat chloride testing

(B) karyotyping

(C) fluorescent in situ hybridization (FISH) of chromosome 22q11

(D) antiendomysial antibodies

(E) blood antineutrophil cytoplasmic antibodies

45. What are the blood requirements for transfusion of a patient with hypocalcemia, heart defect, and recurrent infections?

(A) leucocyte depleted

(B) HLA matched

(C) CMV negative

(D) O negative

(E) irradiated

46. What hematologic abnormality should you suspect in a newborn with bilateral absence of radius?

(A) thrombocytopenia

(B) anemia

(C) neutropenia

(D) pancytopenia

(E) lymphopenia

47. What laboratory abnormality do you expect to find in a 3-year-old child with severe mental retardation, coarse facies, hazy corneas, hepatosplenomegaly, and multiple skeletal x-ray abnormalities?

(A) increased serum homocystine

(B) deficiency of leucocyte hexosaminidase A

(C) urinary excretion of dermatan sulfate and heparan sulfate

(D) deficiency of liver glucose-6-phosphatase activity

(E) increased serum uric acid

48. Which statement about serum rheumatoid factor (RF) in children is true?

(A) RF is often positive in young children at onset of diagnosis.

(B) Presence of RF implicates a good prognosis.

(C) RF is more frequently found in older children with later onset of disease.

(D) Presence of RF is associated with development of uveitis.

(E) RF is a helpful diagnostic tool in a child with acute arthritis.

49. The major contributor to nephrotic syndrome related mortality is

(A) bacterial peritonitis

(B) acute renal failure

(C) hyperlipidemia

(D) congestive heart failure

(E) hypertension

50. The most common infectious organism causing chronic malabsorption is

(A) human immunodeficiency virus

(B) rotavirus

(C) *Salmonella*

(D) *Cryptosporidium*

(E) *Giardia*

51. The most common cause for pulmonary insufficiency in obese children is

    (A) pneumothorax
    (B) gastric esophageal reflux disease
    (C) congestive heart failure
    (D) asthma
    (E) sleep apnea

52. The single most critical factor in evaluating the growth of a child is

    (A) body mass index
    (B) upper-to-lower body segment ratio
    (C) bone age
    (D) height velocity
    (E) arm span width

53. The most common explanation for childhood constipation is

    (A) Hirschsprung disease
    (B) functional fecal retention
    (C) hypothyroidism
    (D) lead poisoning
    (E) iron therapy

54. A 6-month-old boy is found to have very low levels of IgG, IgM, and IgA. Which of the following organisms is most likely to cause problems in this patient?

    (A) enterovirus
    (B) herpesvirus
    (C) *Shigella*
    (D) *Escherichia coli*
    (E) *Mycobacterium tuberculosis*

55. Which of the following statements about children's growth is true?

    (A) Term infants usually lose 10–15% of their birth weight immediately after birth.
    (B) Term infants double their birth weight in 4–5 months and triple it by 1 year of age.
    (C) A child's height doubles from that at birth by 2 years of age.

    (D) The average size of a 4-year-old is 50 in and 45 lb
    (E) From 3 to 10 years of age, children grow an average of 1.5 in per year

56. Which statement about hypertension is correct?

    (A) Coarctation of the aorta is a rare cause for hypertension in infancy.
    (B) Essential hypertension is the most common cause among adolescents.
    (C) The incidence in White adolescents is twice that of African American adolescents.
    (D) Most pediatric patients with hypertension are symptomatic.
    (E) An adolescent with hypertension should not participate in sports.

57. The most common cause of dysfunctional uterine bleeding in adolescents is

    (A) immature hypothalamic-pituitary-ovarian axis
    (B) polycystic ovarian syndrome
    (C) blood dyscrasia
    (D) systemic illness
    (E) sexually transmitted disease

58. Which statement about systemic onset juvenile rheumatoid arthritis (JRA) is true?

    (A) The diagnosis is often one of exclusion.
    (B) Fever spikes are unpredictable and temperature does not return to baseline.
    (C) Antinuclear antibodies (ANAs) and rheumatoid factor (RF) are often positive.
    (D) Fever responds well to nonsteroidal anti-inflammatory drugs.
    (E) Rash is often present for days.

59. The most common cause of acute, painful scrotal swelling in adolescents is

    (A) inguinal hernia
    (B) hematocele
    (C) torsion of the spermatic cord

(D) epididymitis

(E) orchitis

60. The most common cause of secondary amen-orrhea in young females who have otherwise completed their sexual development is

(A) polycystic ovaries syndrome

(B) Kallman syndrome

(C) pituitary infarct

(D) hypothyroidism

(E) imperforate hymen

61. Which of the following studies is most useful for establishing the diagnosis of ankylosing spondylitis?

(A) erythrocyte sedimentation rate (ESR)

(B) rheumatoid factor

(C) antinuclear antibodies (ANAs)

(D) HLA-B8

(E) sacroiliac radiographs

62. Rectal prolapse in an infant with failure to thrive is most suggestive of

(A) Crohn disease

(B) functional constipation

(C) Ehlers-Danlos syndrome

(D) intussusception of the colon

(E) cystic fibrosis

63. Which of the following statements regarding a Meckel diverticulum is true?

(A) Routine barium studies typically are diagnostic.

(B) It is the most common congenital gastrointestinal anomaly.

(C) Are typically located within 1 cm of the ileocecal valve.

(D) Most common presentation is partial or complete bowel obstruction.

(E) Usually become clinically apparent after 2 years of age.

64. Which of the following disorders is associated with an elevated conjugated bilirubin?

(A) Crigler-Najjar syndrome

(B) Gilbert syndrome

(C) Dubin-Johnson syndrome

(D) Lucey-Driscoll syndrome

(E) isoimmune hemolysis

65. Diagnostic criteria for Kawasaki disease include

(A) conjunctivitis, fever, cervical lym-phadenopathy

(B) meningitis, conjunctivitis, pallor

(C) cervical lymphadenopathy, hepatitis, rash

(D) fever, irritability, pancreatitis

(E) hepatosplenomegaly, rash, conjunctivitis

66. In patients with Langerhans cell histiocytosis, bony lesions occur most frequently in the

(A) ribs

(B) femur

(C) sternum

(D) skull

(E) humerus

67. Findings in Prader-Willi syndrome include

(A) hypotonia, failure to thrive, and mental retardation

(B) mental retardation, seizures, and undescended testes

(C) hypogonadism, undescended testes, and hypertonia

(D) seizures, hypotonia, and obesity

(E) obesity, mental retardation, and hypotonia

68. Thrombocytopenia is most commonly seen in association with

(A) lead poisoning

(B) hemolytic uremic syndrome

(C) Henoch-Schönlein purpura

(D) Kawasaki disease

(E) iron deficiency anemia

69. Which is the most common cause of persistent stridor during infancy?

    (A) vascular ring
    (B) laryngomalacia
    (C) tracheomalacia
    (D) laryngeal clefts
    (E) subglottic stenosis

70. Which of the following laboratory features is characteristic of hereditary spherocytosis?

    (A) decreased osmotic fragility
    (B) increased mean corpuscular volume (MCV)
    (C) decreased mean corpuscular hemoglobin concentration (MCHC)
    (D) increased relative distribution width (RDW)
    (E) decreased reticulocyte count

71. The most likely cause of hematuria and decreased serum complement (C3) level is

    A) acute poststreptococcal glomerulonephritis
    (B) IgA nephropathy
    (C) Alport syndrome
    (D) hemolytic uremic syndrome
    (E) hypercalciuria

72. The first sign of puberty in girls is the development of

    (A) menarche
    (B) axillary hair
    (C) breast buds
    (D) pubic hair
    (E) acne

73. Which statement about anorexia nervosa is true?

    (A) A hyperchloremic acidosis often occurs.
    (B) The death rate is about 2%.
    (C) The incidence has been stable over the past 20 years.
    (D) Amenorrhea is rare.
    (E) Constipation is a common problem.

74. What is the most common cause of severe obstructive uropathy in children?

    (A) urethral strictures
    (B) anterior urethral valves
    (C) prune-belly syndrome
    (D) posterior urethral valves
    (E) meatal stenosis

75. The most common cause of esophageal infection in immunocompetent children is

    (A) herpes simplex virus
    (B) candida
    (C) cytomegalovirus
    (D) group A *Streptococcus*
    (E) varicella zoster virus

76. The most common risk factor for development of bacterial tracheitis is

    (A) viral croup
    (B) laryngomalacia
    (C) necrotizing esophagitis
    (D) reactive airway disease
    (E) cystic fibrosis

77. The most likely diagnosis in a 4-week-old male infant with vomiting and a hypochloremic metabolic alkalosis is

    (A) maple syrup urine disease
    (B) adrenal insufficiency
    (C) gastroenteritis
    (D) pyloric stenosis
    (E) homocystinuria

78. What combination of findings is characteristic for prune-belly syndrome?

    (A) imperforate anus, urinary tract abnormalities, and mental retardation
    (B) deficient abdominal muscles, undescended testes, and urinary tract abnormalities
    (C) mental retardation, undescended testes, and cleft lip

(D) ovarian dysgenesis, renal agenesis, and congenital heart disease

(E) ectopic bladder, undescended testes, and congenital heart disease

79. What is the most helpful finding to differentiate Crohn disease from ulcerative colitis?

(A) rectal bleeding
(B) crypt abscesses
(C) ileal involvement
(D) erythema nodosum
(E) cholangitis

80. A previously healthy 4-month-old infant develops generalized weakness with difficulty in sucking, swallowing, crying, and breathing. No fever is present. Which is the most likely diagnosis?

(A) botulism
(B) hypocalcemia
(C) hypothyroidism
(D) poliomyelitis
(E) encephalitis

81. A previously healthy 5-year-old child develops a limp and complains of hip pain. The most likely cause is

(A) septic arthritis
(B) slipped capital femoral epiphysis
(C) transient synovitis
(D) osteosarcoma
(E) juvenile rheumatoid arthritis

82. You have followed a 7-month-old infant that has had failure to gain weight. Birth weight was 3250 g; the child weighs 5.5 kg right now. In your office, the baby takes an 8-oz bottle with ease and does not vomit. The next best step is

(A) placement of nasogastric feeding tube
(B) hospitalization of the child with unlimited feedings
(C) contact child protective services for placement in foster care
(D) a barium swallowing study
(E) scheduled return visit in 1 month

83. A patient with streptococcal pharyngitis develops tender red bumps along her entire tibia. The most likely diagnosis is

(A) sarcoidosis
(B) cellulitis
(C) thrombophlebitis
(D) insect bites
(E) erythema nodosum

84. A 2-year-old child develops apnea, cyanosis, and loss of consciousness with repeated generalized clonic jerks after being scolded by his mother. On examination, the child appears completely normal. The best treatment option is

(A) tegretol
(B) valproic acid
(C) antiarrhythmics
(D) cardiac pacemaker
(E) counseling of parents

85. A 16-year-old high school soccer player complains of chronic knee pain that has not been associated with an injury. The pain is worse upon going up stairs and after sitting for prolonged periods. The only abnormal finding on examination is peripatellar tenderness. The most likely diagnosis is

(A) meniscal tear
(B) patellofemoral pain syndrome
(C) shin splints
(D) stress fracture
(E) anterior cruciate ligament sprain

86. Which of the following manifestations is required to make a diagnosis of attention-deficit hyperactivity disorder?

(A) occurrence before the age of 10 years
(B) concurrent learning disability
(C) impulsivity
(D) history of birth trauma
(E) a sibling with the diagnosis of ADHD

87. What statement about neonatal circumcision is true?

    (A) There is clearly an increased risk for penile cancer in uncircumcised males.

    (B) Urinary tract infections are 10–15 times more common in uncircumcised infants.

    (C) Circumcision reduces the risk of sexually transmitted diseases.

    (D) Complications following circumcision are very rare.

    (E) Circumcision can be safely done in infants with hypospadias.

88. A true statement about the ethical concept of competence is that

    (A) adolescents cannot be viewed as competent individuals in health-care decision making

    (B) parents have full authority to make health care–related decisions for their children

    (C) competent individuals have an almost absolute right to determine what shall be done with their own bodies

    (D) competent individuals only have absolute right in health care–related decisions if their health is not harmed by these decisions

    (E) autonomy is not related to competence

DIRECTIONS (Questions 89 through 113): Each set of matching questions in this section consists of a list of five to eight lettered options followed by several numbered items. For each numbered item select the ONE lettered option with which it is most closely associated. Each lettered option may be selected once, more than once, or not at all.

Questions 89 through 94

    (A) ventricular septal defect
    (B) atrial septal defect
    (C) bicuspid aortic valves
    (D) coronary aneurysm
    (E) third degree heart block
    (F) aortic aneurysm

    (G) supravalvular aortic stenosis
    (H) pulmonary stenosis

89. Williams syndrome

90. Neonatal lupus

91. Noonan syndrome

92. Kawasaki disease

93. Turner syndrome

94. Marfan syndrome

Questions 95 through 99

    (A) 6 weeks of age
    (B) 8 weeks of age
    (C) 12 weeks of age
    (D) 16 weeks of age
    (E) 6 months of age
    (F) 8 months of age
    (G) 12 months of age

95. Sits without support

96. Hands together in midline

97. Bangs two cubes

98. Thumb–finger grasp

99. Disappearance of Moro reflex

Questions 100 through 105

    (A) Hb 12 g/dL; WBC 11,500/mm^3; platelets 160,000/mm^3; reticulocytes 1%

    (B) Hb 12 g/dL; WBC 11,500/mm^3; platelets 25,000/mm^3; reticulocytes 1%

    (C) Hb 5.5 g/dL; WBC 3000/mm^3; platelets 35,000/mm^3; reticulocytes 0.5%

    (D) Hb 5.5 g/dL; WBD 8000/mm^3; platelets 400,000/mm^3; reticulocytes 0.5%

    (E) Hb 8 g/dL; WBC 19,500/mm^3; platelets 17,000/mm^3; reticulocytes 14%

100. Idiopathic thrombocytopenic purpura

101. Normal 2-year-old child

102. Sickle cell disease, not in crisis

103. Iron deficiency anemia

104. Acute lymphoblastic leukemia

105. Acquired aplastic pancytopenia

Questions 106 through 108

    (A) Congenital aganglionic megacolon
    (B) Duodenal atresia
    (C) Jejunoileal atresia
    (D) Intestinal malrotation
    (E) Meconium ileus

106. Cystic fibrosis

107. Midgut volvulus

108. Enterocolitis

Questions 109 through 114

    (A) sensorineural deafness
    (B) limb abnormalities
    (C) short stature
    (D) glaucoma
    (E) hydrocephalus
    (F) tram-track calcifications
    (G) saddle nose
    (H) skin, eye, mouth infection

109. Neonatal herpes

110. Congenital cytomegalovirus infection

111. Congenital toxoplasmosis

112. Congenital syphilis

113. Congenital varicella

Answers and Explanations

1. **(A)** The highest pediatric death rate is in the first month of life. Mortality then decreases steadily with increasing age until adolescence, when the death rate rises, primarily from an increase in injuries including those sustained in homicide and suicide. More than half of the deaths in the first year of life occur during the first 28 days. *(Behrman:1–2)*

2. **(C)** Werdnig-Hoffmann disease is an autosomal recessive disorder affecting the anterior horn cells and the motor nuclei of the brainstem. Loss of motor function begins in infancy and progresses fairly rapidly, leading to ventilatory failure within the first 2 years of life. Clinical features include hypotonia, weakness or paralysis, hyporeflexia and muscle fasciculations, which are most readily noted in the tongue. Seizures, optic atrophy, and fever are not features of this disorder. There also is a rare, late-onset, more slowly progressive degenerative disorder of the anterior horn cells referred to as Kugelberg-Welander disease. *(Behrman: 1887–1888)*

3. **(C)** The term cerebral palsy refers to a static, nonprogressive abnormality of the central nervous system affecting motor function and resulting from a perinatal (before or during birth or in early infancy) insult. By definition, this is a nonprogressive disorder, and, therefore, treatment can be aimed only at preventing secondary problems rather than preventing progression of the disorder itself. The underlying lesion is the end result of a perinatal injury and as such is not treatable. Since the causes of cerebral palsy are so varied, and since so few cases are related to recognizable genetic disorders, effective genetic counseling to prevent subsequent cases is difficult. Although the risk of developing epilepsy is significantly greater for these children than for the general population, only 25–35% will eventually do so, and administration of anticonvulsant drugs prior to the onset of seizures is not indicated. Thus, the importance of early diagnosis is to help the parents understand the infant or child and his or her problem and to minimize or prevent secondary physical or emotional problems. *(Behrman:1843–1845)*

4. **(D)** Craniosynostosis is the condition of premature fusion of one or more of the cranial sutures and occurs both as an isolated abnormality and in association with a wide variety of congenital malformations, syndromes, and chromosomal abnormalities. Excluding abnormalities of the head and face, the extremities are the organs most frequently involved with associated defects. The most common and best known such syndrome is the autosomal dominant Apert syndrome—craniosynostosis plus extensive syndactyly of the fingers and toes. *(Behrman:1812–1813)*

5. **(B)** The arthritis of acute rheumatic fever is a painful acute migratory polyarthritis. Although any joint can be involved, it is primarily the large joints of the extremities that are affected in most cases. Pain and swelling in one joint subsides as another joint becomes symptomatic. Eventually, all joints heal without deformity or other permanent sequelae. Fever and arthritis usually occur concomitantly but may occur in the presence or absence of carditis. *(Behrman:807)*

6. **(D)** The clinical findings described are classic for the entity of total anomalous pulmonary venous return with obstruction of the veins. In this condition, the pulmonary veins drain to the right rather than the left atrium. After mixing with systemic venous return in the right atrium, some of the oxygenated pulmonary venous blood shunts across the foramen ovale (which is kept open by the increased right atrial pressure), providing a right-to-left shunt of partially oxygenated blood into the systemic circulation. In many cases, the pulmonary venous return is not directly into the right atrium but rather takes a devious route, often coursing below the diaphragm before reaching the right atrium. In such instances, venous obstruction is the rule, and cyanosis results both from the right-to-left shunt and from wet, congested lungs. A diffuse reticular pattern to the lung fields is characteristically seen on roentgenogram. Although the heart may be considerably enlarged in patients without venous obstruction, it is characteristically normal or only minimally enlarged in those with obstruction. *(Behrman:1399–1400)*

7. **(A)** Brain tumors, although rare in the first year of life, are the second most common type of cancer in childhood, exceeded only by leukemia. More than half of the tumors in children are located below the tentorium, and about three-quarters are in the midline. For this reason, increased intracranial pressure from obstruction of the third or fourth ventricle is a common finding. Seizures can be the presenting complaint but are not in the majority of cases. *(Behrman: 1858–1862)*

8. **(E)** The infant described most likely has an intussusception of the intestine. This condition is most frequent in the second half of the first year of life and involves the telescoping of one segment of bowel into another, most frequently the ileum into the colon (ileocolic intussusception). Intermittent abdominal pain and vomiting are common features. Mild fever and leukocytosis are frequent. Very often the intussusceptum can be palpated as a sausage-shaped mass. Circulation to the intussuscepted bowel can be impaired, resulting in discharge

of a bloody, mucous stool—the so-called "currant jelly" stool. Barium enema is the procedure of choice and can be therapeutic as well as diagnostic. Under fluoroscopic visualization, the radiologist usually is able to employ the hydrostatic pressure of the enema to reduce the intussuscepted bowel. *(Behrman:1142–1143)*

9. **(E)** Cystic fibrosis is the most common cause of pancreatic insufficiency in childhood, accounting for almost all cases. Biliary atresia is not associated with pancreatic insufficiency, and carcinoma of the pancreas is not seen in childhood. Congenital hypoplasia or absence of the pancreas is recognized but rare. Schwachman syndrome is a rare condition of unknown cause characterized by pancreatic insufficiency and neutropenia. *(Behrman:1190)*

10. **(C)** Brain abscess is an infrequent but not rare disorder of childhood. It has been estimated that almost one-third of all brain abscesses occur in pediatric-age patients. Recognized predisposing conditions include penetrating head injury, brain surgery, immunodeficiency, cystic fibrosis, and infection of the middle ear, mastoid, or facial sinuses. Right-to-left intracardiac shunts in children with cyanotic congenital heart disease bypass the macrophage-filtering mechanism of the lungs and increase the access of bacteria to the brain. In these children, cerebral hypoxia and focal encephalomalacia also may predispose to infection. *(Behrman:1857–1858)*

11. **(C)** There are three classic clinical presentations of juvenile rheumatoid arthritis (JRA)—acute systemic, pauciarticular, and polyarticular. A positive rheumatoid factor (RF) is uncommon in JRA, occurring only in some patients, usually females, with the polyarticular form. Those patients with polyarticular JRA who are RF positive tend to be older and to have more severe joint involvement than those who are RF negative. Neither ankylosing spondylitis nor psoriatic arthritis is associated with RF. *(Cassidy:233–234)*

12. **(D)** The child described has the classic hand-foot syndrome seen in infants and toddlers with sickle cell disease. Dactylitis, presumably

secondary to infarction of the small bones, causes painful swelling of the hands and feet. *(Behrman:1479)*

13. **(C)** The interval between the streptococcal infection and the onset of manifestation is much greater for chorea (months) than for any of the other signs or symptoms of acute rheumatic fever (1–2 weeks). As a result, rheumatic chorea often occurs in the absence of any other clinical or laboratory manifestations of acute rheumatic fever and frequently in the absence of evidence of recent streptococcal infection. *(Behrman:807, 1840–1841)*

14. **(E)** Inadequate dietary iron is the leading cause of iron deficiency anemia in children. Milk has low iron content, and the iron in cow milk is not well absorbed. If a large percentage of dietary calories come from milk, the diet is apt to be low in iron. Additionally, microscopic gastrointestinal blood loss associated with the intake of unmodified cow milk is an important contributing factor to iron deficiency. *(Behrman: 1469–1470)*

15. **(B)** Although rhabdomyosarcoma and, infrequently, hepatoblastoma can metastasize to bone, few solid cancers of childhood spread to bone as regularly as neuroblastoma. Additionally, whereas bone metastases of other tumors tend to be focal, involvement by neuroblastoma frequently is diffuse. In some series of neuroblastoma, bone marrow involvement has exceeded 50% of cases. Thus, bone marrow aspiration, even in the absence of radiographic evidence of osseous involvement, is more likely to be diagnostic in neuroblastoma than in any other solid cancer of childhood. *(Behrman:1552; Pizzo:904–905)*

16. **(A)** Intestinal lactase deficiency in infancy may be either genetic (rare) or acquired (common) secondary to damage to the intestinal mucosa. Watery diarrhea is a prominent feature of these disorders. The stool is strongly acidic because of lactic and other acids produced by the action of bowel bacteria on the undigested sugars. Neither pancreatitis nor intestinal obstruction has been reported as associated

with disaccharidase deficiency. There is also a late-onset lactase deficiency that occurs secondary to a regulatory gene that turns off lactase activity after lactation. This is most common in nonwhite individuals. *(Behrman:1168)*

17. **(C)** The McCune-Albright syndrome consists of fibrous dysplasia of bone, multiple large pigmented nevi (generally on only one side of the trunk), and precocious puberty, which is more common in females than in males. Other endocrine disorders occur less frequently and include hyperthyroidism and hyperadrenalism (Cushing syndrome). *(Behrman:1692–1693)*

18. **(B)** Since aortic pressure is significantly greater than pulmonary artery pressure throughout the cardiac cycle, a patent ductus arteriosus (PDA) characteristically results in a continuous left-to-right shunt and a continuous murmur. The increased left ventricular output, coupled with runoff from the aorta through the ductus, produces a widened pulse pressure and a bounding or collapsing pulse. The increased flow to the lungs and back to the left ventricle causes hypertrophy of that chamber rather than of the right ventricle. Manifestations of a PDA in a premature infant would be quite different from those in a 6-month-old. These infants are relatively intolerant of left-to-right shunts and are more likely to develop congestive heart failure. Also, the high pulmonary vascular resistance results in a systolic-only murmur rather than the classical continuous murmur. *(Behrman:1372–1373)*

19. **(C)** Congenital megacolon (Hirschsprung disease) is the result of congenital absence of ganglion cells in a segment of large bowel. Absent or deficient peristalsis in the affected segment results in functional obstruction. This causes constipation and distention of bowel proximal to the aganglionic area. It is this chronically distended bowel that has led to the name megacolon. Severe cases present as neonatal intestinal obstruction. Enterocolitis with diarrhea is a well-recognized complication, especially in older, undiagnosed, and untreated infants, but certainly is not the most common presentation. *(Behrman:1139–1141)*

20. **(C)** Complex partial seizures is the current name for what had previously been termed temporal lobe or psychomotor seizures. Complex partial seizures are characterized by alterations of mental status, consciousness, or responsiveness. During the seizure, there may be confusion, emotional reactions, feelings of detachment, and hallucinations. Automatisms (semipurposeful but inappropriate motor acts) are frequent. There is no tonic or clonic component. Postictal confusion is common. The usual EEG finding is spike-wave activity over one or both temporal lobe regions. A three-per-second spike-and-wave pattern on EEG is characteristic of absence seizures. *(Behrman:1815)*

21. **(A)** The head is large in achondroplasia, not just relative to the small body. Although this is not associated directly with increased intracranial pressure, achondroplasia also is associated with platybasia of the skull, which often results in obstructive hydrocephalus and increased intracranial pressure. Overdoses of vitamin A have been associated with pseudotumor cerebri, but overdoses of vitamin C do not have this effect. *(Behrman:2121)*

22. **(E)** Iridocyclitis (anterior uveitis) is the only ophthalmologic complication seen in children with juvenile rheumatoid arthritis (JRA). It usually occurs in those with the ANA-positive, pauciarticular form of the disease. Iridocyclitis may be insidious yet severe, resulting in permanent blindness. Corneal ulcerations, ptosis, glaucoma, and cataracts are not recognized complications of JRA. *(Cassidy:250–251)*

23. **(D)** The prognosis in children with systemic lupus erythematosus is determined primarily by the extent of renal involvement. The major causes of death are renal failure and opportunistic infection. The latter usually is secondary to immunosuppressive therapy of kidney disease. None of the other items listed (fever, leukocytosis, anti-DNA antibodies, polyserositis, or seizures) is prognostic of a bad outcome. *(Cassidy:436–438)*

24. **(C)** Retinoblastoma, neuroblastoma, and Wilms tumor all are most common in the first few

years of life. The peak incidence of childhood leukemia is between 2 and 6 years of age. Osteosarcoma, in contrast, is quite rare in the first half-decade of life. *(Behrman:1531–1532)*

25. **(E)** Wilms tumor is the most common primary renal malignancy in children. It has been associated with many congenital anomalies such as the WAGR syndrome (Wilms tumor, aniridia, genitourinary malformations, and mental retardation), Denys-Drash syndrome, Beckwith-Wiedemann syndrome, and hemi-hypertrophy. It usually presents in toddlers as an asymptomatic flank mass. The combined approach of surgery and combination chemotherapy has improved the survival significantly. *(Behrman: 1554–1556; Pizzo:865–893)*

26. **(B)** The patient most likely has Wilson disease. Wilson disease or hepatolenticular degeneration is an autosomal recessive disorder of copper metabolism. Copper accumulates in the brain, liver, and cornea where deposits are visible as brown rings (Kayser-Fleischer). Untreated, this disorder ultimately leads to death secondary to hepatic, neurologic, renal, or hematologic complications. Chelation therapy with oral penicillamine should start as early as possible. *(Behrman:1209–1210)*

27. **(D)** The patient most likely has the infantile form of Tay-Sachs disease. Tay-Sachs is a member of the family of lipid storage diseases. These diseases have a deficiency of a lysosomal hydrolase enzyme leading to the lysosomal accumulation of specific sphingolipids. Common features of these disorders are neurodegeneration and organomegaly. Tay-Sachs disease is caused by deficiency of β-hexosaminidase A and is inherited as an autosomal trait with a carrier frequency of 1/25 in the Ashkenazi Jewish population. The infantile form of this disease will often become manifest in early childhood with loss of milestones, increased startle reaction (hyperacusis), and cherry-red spot on retinoscopy. *(Behrman:1850)*

28. **(E)** The DiGeorge sequence is characterized by aplasia or hypoplasia of the thymus and parathyroid glands. During early embryogenesis there

is dysmorphogenesis of the third and fourth pharyngeal pouches. Other organs that are formed during the same time period are frequently affected as well. Facial abnormalities, esophageal atresia, bifid uvula, and congenital heart disease are some of the anomalies associated with this syndrome. Patients with complete DiGeorge sequence have problems early in life with increased susceptibility to infections such as viruses and fungi. Microcephaly, hyponatremia, hyperkalemia, and goiter are not associated with this syndrome. *(Behrman: 599–560, 1716)*

29. **(B)** The patient described most likely has Wiskott-Aldrich syndrome. This syndrome is characterized by thrombocytopenia, atopic dermatitis, and severe immunodeficiency. The inheritance pattern is X-linked and affects boys only. Severe atopic dermatitis and recurrent infections usually become manifest during the first year of life. Patients are susceptible to infections with bacteria with polysaccharide capsules, such as pneumococci resulting in frequent otitis media, sinusitis, pneumonia, and sepsis. Infections with *Pneumocystis carinii*, herpes- and cytomegalovirus can also become a problem. The only curable treatment is bone marrow transplantation. *(Behrman:624)*

30. **(D)** The patient has the classical symptoms of juvenile dermatomyositis (JDM). Patients with this disorder usually present with a combination of malaise, fever, fatigue, muscle weakness, and rash. Determination of serum levels of muscle enzymes is important for diagnosis and monitoring the disease course once therapy has been instituted. Rheumatoid factor tests in children with JDM are almost always negative. Antinuclear antibodies (ANAs) can be positive in JDM, however, this would not be the first test of choice. Erythrocyte sedimentation rate is a nonspecific indicator of inflammation and of little help in making a diagnosis of JDM. Renal abnormalities are rare in JDM. *(Cassidy:468–471)*

31. **(B)** Corticosteroid therapy is frequently beneficial in the treatment of Diamond-Blackfan syndrome but does not appear to have any

value in the treatment of TEC. Whereas TEC is a transient disorder and usually resolves spontaneously by 1–2 months, Diamond-Blackfan syndrome does not resolve spontaneously and may become a chronic disease if the response to prednisone is poor. Hepatosplenomegaly is not a feature of either disease. Red blood cell transfusions may be necessary for both disorders. Parvovirus infection has not been associated with either disease. *(Behrman:1463–1464)*

32. **(B)** Megaloblastic anemia in children almost always results from a deficiency of folic acid, vitamin B_{12}, or both. In the peripheral blood, red blood cells are large and frequently hypersegmented neutrophils appear. Folic acid is abundant in many foods, including green vegetables, fruits, and animal organs. Human and cow milk provide adequate amounts of folic acid, but goat milk is clearly deficient in folic acid. Vitamin B_{12} is present in many foods and dietary deficiency is therefore rare. It can be seen in vegans who do not consume any animal products. *(Behrman:157)*

33. **(A)** The child described most likely has celiac disease or gluten-sensitive enteropathy. This disorder is the result of small bowel mucosal damage caused by sensitivity to dietary gluten and has an incidence in the United States of approximately 1:10,000. The incidence appears higher in Europe. Symptoms typically start after gluten is introduced in the diet. The clinical spectrum of this disease is wide but failure to thrive, diarrhea, irritability, vomiting, and anorexia are common. The sensitivity and specificity of serum IgA-endomysial antibody testing is very high but histologic findings on small bowel biopsy remain the standard for making the diagnosis. *(Behrman:1165–1167)*

34. **(D)** Secondary nocturnal enuresis is defined by the occurrence of night time bedwetting after being dry for a minimum of 6 months. An organic cause can only be found in 2–3% of patients with nocturnal enuresis. Any organic factors or disease should be ruled out during the office visit. Every child with enuresis should have a urine analysis. Diabetes mellitus, diabetes insipidus, or urinary tract infections can

be quickly diagnosed or ruled out. *(Pediatr Rev 18:183–190, 1997)*

35. **(C)** A defect in complement function should be suspected in any patient with recurrent pyogenic infections or recurrent *Neisseria meningitidis* or *Neisseria gonorrhea* infections. Testing for total hemolytic complement activity (CH_{50}) is a good screening tool for complement abnormalities. *(Behrman:631)*

36. **(E)** The child presented most likely has metastatic neuroblastoma. The median age at diagnosis is 2 years. Age, stage of disease at diagnosis, and biology of the tumor are prognostic factors in neuroblastoma. Children under the age of 1 year with limited disease and without *mycn* gene amplification have a 95% survival. Imaging with CT scan or MRI, bone scans and bone marrow biopsy are part of the staging for this disease. Bone radiographs may be abnormal but are not used for staging purposes. Hematuria is not a common feature of this tumor. There are a number of well-documented cases in infants that have had complete regression of their tumor without medical intervention. *(Behrman:1552–1554; Pizzo:897)*

37. **(D)** Beckwith-Wiedemann syndrome is characterized by neonatal overgrowth. Infants are large for gestational age, have macroglossia, hepatosplenomegaly and often difficult to control hypoglycemia. Children with this disorder are at increased risk for development of Wilms tumor, hepatoblastoma and adrenocortical carcinoma. Serum α-fetoprotein is elevated in about 90% of patients with hepatoblastoma. *(Behrman:445)*

38. **(D)** The presented patient most likely has sickle cell disease. As many as 10% of patients with sickle cell anemia will exhibit sequelae of strokes. The diagnosis of sickle cell disease can be made by hemoglobin electrophoresis. A patient who is homozygous for the sickle cell gene has no normal hemoglobin (HbA_1), will have a high amount of sickle hemoglobin (HbS), and an increased amount of fetal hemoglobin (HbF). A carrier of the sickle cell gene

will have about 50% HbA_1 and less than 50% HbS. *(Behrman:1479–1481)*

39. **(C)** With the exception of cervical adenitis, infections with nontuberculous *Mycobacterium* species are relatively rare in healthy children. However, widespread *Mycobacterium avium* infection is common in patients with terminal acquired immunodeficiency syndrome (AIDS). Blood cultures in AIDS patients with disseminated infection are 90–95% sensitive. Recovery of *M. avium* in the stool of a patient with suspected human immunodeficiency virus (HIV) infection is not predictive of the development of widespread infection. Rotavirus, *Giardia, Salmonella,* and *Yersinia* have all been associated with gastroenteritis in healthy children and recovery of these organisms would not support a diagnosis of HIV infection. *(Behrman: 901–902, 1026)*

40. **(C)** The incidence of group A streptococcal disease depends on the age group, the season, the climate, and degree of contact with infected individuals. Suppurative and nonsuppurative complications from group A streptococcal disease have increased. Streptococcal skin infections can cause impetigo, cellulitis, erysipelas, and necrotizing fasciitis. Nonsuppurative complications from streptococcal skin infections include scarlatina, poststreptococcal glomerulonephritis, and toxic shock syndrome. Acute rheumatic fever is a nonsuppurative complication from streptococcal pharyngitis but is not associated with streptococcal skin infections. *(Behrman:802–805)*

41. **(E)** The child described most likely has Henoch-Schönlein purpura (HSP). HSP typically develops in a previously healthy child with a distinctive rash that often involves the extensor surfaces of the lower extremities. Arthritis or arthralgia develops in 75% of cases and most patients have some gastrointestinal symptoms. Intussusception can be a serious complication occurring in about 5% of patients. Renal involvement is detected in about half of the patients and can range from mild to very severe. One percent of patients will develop end-stage renal disease. The diagnosis can be difficult to make when gastrointestinal symptoms or arthritis precede the rash. Laboratory studies are typically not helpful in making the diagnosis. Clotting functions are generally normal and platelet counts in these patients are normal or elevated. *(Behrman: 728–729; Zitelli: 248–250)*

42. **(C)** Fragile X syndrome is the most frequent cause of hereditary mental retardation. This syndrome is caused by amplification of CGC triplets on the X chromosome. Both male and female premutation carriers of this syndrome typically have no phenotypic manifestations. Premutations can expand to full mutations only in female meiotic transmission. Affected males typically develop testicular enlargement after puberty. *(Behrman:331, 1751–1752; Jones: 1550–1553)*

43. **(D)** The occurrence of trisomy 21 or Down syndrome increases with advancing maternal age. There is no single physical finding that makes a diagnosis of Down syndrome; rather, the combination of minor and major anomalies often leads to a diagnosis. All the listed anomalies are more common in Down syndrome, however, hearing loss affecting more than 60% of patients is the most common. About 40% of patients have cardiac abnormalities with the endocardial cushion defect being the most common. *(Jones:8–13)*

44. **(B)** The patient described most likely has Turner syndrome. Patients with this syndrome have an XO karyotype. Short stature is the cardinal finding in all girls with Turner syndrome. Ovarian dysgenesis is present and sexual maturation usually fails to occur, although a small percentage of girls may have spontaneous breast development and menstrual periods. Other clinical features that may be present are webbed neck, low hairline, and wide spaced nipples. Cardiac defects occur in about half of the patients and bicuspid aortic valves are the most commonly found abnormality. Renal abnormalities, such as horseshoe kidney, occur in a majority of patients. *(Behrman:1753–1755; Jones:81–83)*

45. **(E)** The patient described most likely has DiGeorge sequence. Dysmorphogenesis of the third and fourth pharyngeal pouches during early embryogenesis leads to thymic and hypoparathyroid aplasia in varying degrees of severity. When absence of the thymus is complete, patients suffer from a severe combined immunodeficiency (SCID) with abnormalities of both B lymphocyte and T lymphocyte functions. These infants are at risk for graft versus host disease (GVHD) from nonirradiated blood products and may actually develop GVHD from maternal derived cells in their circulation. DiGeorge sequence can be part of the CATCH 22 syndrome (cardiac, abnormal facies, thymic hypoplasia, cleft palate, hypocalcemia), which includes the broad clinical spectrum of conditions with chromosome 22q11.2 deletions. *(Behrman:599–560)*

46. **(A)** Thrombocytopenia absent radius (TAR) syndrome is one of the congenital thrombocytopenia syndromes. The thrombocytopenia severity usually lessens with advancing age. Patients may occasionally have other congenital abnormalities. Wiskott-Aldrich syndrome (WAS) is another congenital thrombocytopenia syndrome in which boys are affected with thrombocytopenia, eczema, and severe immunodeficiencies. Congenital amegakaryocytic thrombocytopenia usually presents in the first weeks of life with petechiae and purpura. *(Jones:322; Behrman:1523)*

47. **(C)** The patient described has all the features of mucopolysaccharidosis I (MPS I). The MPS are inherited disorders characterized by deficiency of lysosomal enzymes needed to break down glycosaminoglycans, the intralysosomal accumulation of glycosaminoglycans and excessive urinary excretion of glycosaminoglycans such as dermatan sulfate, heparan sulfate, or keratan sulfate. The MPS disorders share many clinical features although in varying degrees of severity. The course is often chronic and progressive, many organs are involved, and typically organomegaly and abnormal facial features and dysostosis multiplex on skeletal radiographs are present. Hurler syndrome is the most severe in this group of disorders and is due to a deficiency of α-L-iduronidase. *(Behrman:420–423; Jones:456–471)*

48. (C) Rheumatoid factors are IgM antibodies against IgG. RF are only positive in a small percentage of children with JRA and rarely aid in making diagnosis at onset. RF are most commonly found in children with later onset of arthritis, in older children with subcutaneous nodules and patients with more severe disease. *(Cassidy:259–260)*

49. (A) About 75% of nephrotic syndrome in children 1–12 years of age is due to minimal-change disease. The mortality in minimal-change nephrotic syndrome is about 1–2%. Most of the mortality is related to an increased susceptibility for infections, with bacterial peritonitis being the most serious one. The majority of the remainder of deaths is due to thromboembolic events. Hyperlipidemia is associated with nephrotic syndrome but is generally not associated with clinical complications. Acute renal failure can occur with intravascular volume depletion and decreased renal perfusion but is easily treatable. *(Pediatr Rev 23:237–247, 2002)*

50. (E) *Giardia* occurs worldwide and is endemic in developing countries where sanitation is poor. *Giardia* is the most common parasite identified in stool specimens in the United States. It causes significant morbidity in child-care centers and chronic residential institutions. The clinical manifestations of giardiasis can range from asymptomatic colonization to acute or chronic diarrhea and malabsorption. *(Behrman: 1036–1037)*

51. (E) Obesity in children is on the rise and is reaching epidemic proportions in the United States. Current estimates indicate that 20–25% of children between the age of 6–19 years old are obese. Obesity is a significant risk factor for many serious medical problems. These patients are at risk for psychologic problems, pulmonary insufficiency, skeletal abnormalities, metabolic diseases, cardiovascular diseases, and malignancies. Sleep apnea resulting from upper airway obstruction can be a dangerous complication and is the most common cause for pulmonary insufficiency in obese patients. *(Pediatr Rev 19:312–315, 1998)*

52. (D) Following a child's growth is an important tool to assess the general health of the child. Standard growth curves from growth data of different ethnic groups are available. However, the distinction between normal and abnormal growth is not always easy to make. The single most critical factor to determine whether the growth of a child is normal is to determine the height velocity. An easy way to decide if the height velocity is normal is by observing whether a height is crossing percentiles on the linear growth curve. *(Pediatr Rev 19:92–99, 1998)*

53. (B) Constipation is a source of frustration for patients, families, and healthcare workers. Hard stools, pain with defecation, or failure to pass three stools per week are usually labeled as constipation. There are functional and non-functional etiologies of constipation. Functional fecal retention is the most common explanation for childhood constipation. This can first start around potty training time or as a normal avoidance technique in the context of painful anal inflammation. It may be accompanied by early satiety, increasing irritability, and abdominal pain. Unabated functional fecal retention eventually leads to encopresis. *(Pediatr Rev 19:23–31, 1998)*

54. (A) The patient most likely has X-linked agammaglobulinemia. Patients with this immunodeficiency typically have no symptoms during the first 6–9 months of life because of passive transfer of maternal antibodies. Thereafter, they are susceptible for severe infections with extracellular pyogenic organisms such as *Streptococcus pneumoniae* and *Haemophilus influenzae*. Fungal infections typically do not occur and viral infections are generally handled well with the exception of hepatitis viruses and enteroviruses. *(Behrman:596–597)*

55. (B) The CDC published the revised growth charts for children in 2002 to replace those published in 1977. Term infants usually lose 5–10% of their birth weight immediately after birth, but gain back to birth weight by 2 weeks of age. Term infants typically double their birth weight by 4–5 months of age and triple it by

1 year. A child's height doubles from that at birth by 3–4 years of age and the average size of 4-year-old children is 40 in and 35 lb. From 3 to 10 years of age, children grow an average of 3.5 in per year. *(Pediatrics 109:45–60, 2002)*

56. **(B)** Hypertension is classified as primary (essential) or secondary. Essential hypertension is a diagnosis of exclusion. Essential hypertension is the most common cause of hypertension in adults but is a significant pediatric diagnosis only in the adolescent age group. The younger the patient and the more severe the hypertension, the more likely a secondary cause will be found. Coarctation of the aorta is responsible for about a third of the cases of neonatal hypertension. As in adults, hypertension in African American adolescents is about twice as common as in White adolescents. Most pediatric patients with hypertension are asymptomatic. Sports participation should not be limited on the basis of hypertension alone. Regular exercise should be part of life-style recommendations, especially if the hypertension is associated with obesity. *(Pediatr Rev 23:197–208, 2002)*

57. **(A)** Dysfunctional uterine bleeding (DUB) is most common in the first 2 years after menarche. Almost all cases of DUB during adolescence are due to anovulatory cycles. The most common reason for anovulatory cycles at this age group is immaturity of the hypothalamic-pituitary-ovarian axis. There are other causes for anovulation that must be ruled out. Polycystic ovarian syndrome (PCOS) affects about 5–10% of women and is associated with irregular menses and physical signs of hyperandrogenism. Systemic illness, especially if associated with significant weight loss, can lead to anovulation. The most common endocrine disorder associated with anovulation is hypothyroidism but hyperprolactinemia and Cushing syndrome are also associated. Abnormal uterine bleeding can sometimes be the first presenting symptom of a blood dyscrasia. These disorders most often present as regular but heavy menses. Sexually transmitted diseases as well as complications of pregnancy can present with irregular and/or painful menses. *(Pediatr Rev 23:227–232, 2002)*

58. **(A)** Juvenile rheumatoid arthritis presents with severe systemic symptoms in about 10% of children. The fevers typically have a quotidian pattern and respond poorly to the usual nonsteroidal anti-inflammatory drugs. The intermittent fevers are often accompanied by the classic salmon rash, which tends to be migratory and evanescent. The diagnosis can be difficult to make in children at the onset of disease, especially when the child has high spiking fevers with signs of systemic inflammation but no signs of arthritis. *(Cassidy:236–239)*

59. **(C)** Testicular torsion is the most common cause of testicular pain and swelling in adolescent boys. It rarely occurs under the age of 10 years. It is caused by excessive mobility of the testis because of inadequate fixation within the scrotum. After several hours ischemia to the testis will occur and spermatogenesis is lost. Rapid surgical exploration is indicated when there is suspicion of testicular torsion to preserve function. *(Behrman:1651–1652)*

60. **(A)** Obesity, hirsutism, and secondary amenorrhea are the classical features of PCOS but not all these manifestations need be present. There is still uncertainty about the cause of PCOS. Patients typically have an elevated LH/FSH ratio. PCOS is the most common cause of anovulatory infertility during the reproductive years. *(Behrman:1757–1758)*

61. **(E)** Juvenile ankylosing spondylitis (JAS) occurs most frequently in older boys, adolescents, and young adults. Oligoarthritis and pain around insertion sites of tendons and ligaments are the first manifestations of early onset JAS. Involvement of the sacroiliac joints usually does not occur until later in the disease. Unfortunately there are no specific diagnostic laboratory tests. The histocompatibility antigen HLA-B27 is present in more than 90% of patients but is not diagnostic. Rheumatoid factor and antinuclear antibodies are not present. The erythrocyte sedimentation rate may be elevated but is a nonspecific indicator of inflammation. Radiographs may document involvement of the sacroiliac joints within 3–4 years following the onset of symptoms. The

destruction of the joints is progressive with eventual joint obliteration. *(Behrman:710–711)*

62. **(E)** Rectal prolapse can occur with many disorders such as acute diarrhea, Ehlers-Danlos syndrome, chronic constipation, ulcerative colitis, and cystic fibrosis. For an infant with failure to thrive the most common diagnosis is cystic fibrosis. However, most cases of rectal prolapse are idiopathic. Usually the protruding rectal mucosa can be reduced by gentle pressure. Controlling the pancreatic steatorrhea with pancreatic enzyme replacement provides adequate treatment in cystic fibrosis. Surgical intervention is occasionally required. *(Behrman:1182)*

63. **(B)** Meckel diverticulum is a remnant of the omphalomesenteric duct or the vitelline duct. In the fetus this duct connects the gut to the yolk sac. Meckel diverticulum is the most common congenital gastrointestinal anomaly and occurs in 2–3% of all infants. They are located within 100 cm of the ileocecal valve. Most of the symptomatic Meckel diverticula are lined with acid-secreting mucosa. The most common symptom is painless rectal bleeding caused by ulceration of the adjacent normal ileal mucosa. Symptoms usually arise in the first 2 years of life but can occur throughout the first decade. Confirmation of a Meckel diverticulum can be difficult. Plain abdominal radiographs and routine barium studies are usually not helpful. The most sensitive study is a scan with technetium-99m pertechnetate, which is taken up by the mucus secreting cells of the ectopic gastric mucosa. Surgical excision is the treatment for symptomatic Meckel diverticula. *(Behrman:1137–1138)*

64. **(C)** The differential diagnosis of jaundice is extensive, but may be divided by elevation of unconjugated (indirect) or conjugated (direct) bilirubin. Gilbert syndrome patients have mild unconjugated hyperbilirubinemia secondary to decreased hepatic bilirubin uptake, the exact mechanism of which remains to be understood. No treatment is necessary. Crigler-Najjar syndrome is characterized by absent (type I) or deficient (type II) hepatic glucuronyl transferase activity and consequent unconjugated hyperbilirubinemia. Liver transplant may be necessary in these patients. Lucy-Driscoll syndrome, or transient familial neonatal unconjugated hyperbilirubinemia, is thought to be caused by the transient presence of a glucuronyl transferase inhibitory factor. Dubin-Johnson syndrome is an inherited defect in hepatocyte secretion of bilirubin glucuronide excretion, resulting in conjugated hyperbilirubinemia. Isoimmune hemolysis is a cause of unconjugated hyperbilirubinemia. *(Behrman: 1199, 1208–1209)*

65. **(A)** Kawasaki disease, also known as mucocutaneous lymph node syndrome, is the most common cause of acquired heart disease in pediatrics. Criteria for diagnosis are fever for greater than 5 days *plus* four of the following five features: conjunctivitis, cervical adenitis, mucous membrane changes, a polymorphous rash of the trunks and extremities, and distal extremity changes. The illness can be divided into three phases. The acute phase is characterized by fever, conjunctivitis, cervical adenopathy, rash, mucous membrane changes, extremity swelling, and erythema which are seen in the first 10 days. The subacute phase occurs over the next 14 days and is manifested by a decrease in fever, thrombocytosis, and distal extremity skin desquamation. The convalescent phase is characterized by coronary artery aneurysms, which occur in approximately 40% of untreated patients. Early treatment with intravenous gamma-globin and salicylates reduces the risk of developing coronary artery aneurysms. *(Behrman:725–727)*

66. **(D)** Three classes of childhood histiocytosis are recognized. They all have in common a prominent accumulation of cells of the monocyte-macrophage lineage. Accumulation can occur in different organs. Eosinophil granuloma, Hand-Schuller-Christian disease and Letterer-Siwe disease are all included in the Class I histiocytoses and are commonly described as Langerhans cell histiocytoses (LCH). LCH can present as localized or generalized disease. The skeleton is involved in 80% of the patients and bony lesions are most commonly seen in the skull. *(Behrman:1570–1571)*

67. (E) Prader-Willi syndrome is characterized by hypotonia, hypogonadism, obesity, mental retardation, and undescended testis in males. Although there may be feeding difficulties in infancy, these children eventually develop excessive appetites and obesity. The obesity accentuates the appearance of a micropenis. Hypotonia becomes less marked with time. Seizures are not a feature of the Prader-Willi syndrome. Approximately 70% of affected individuals have a microdeletion of the long arm of the paternal derived chromosome 15. The majority of the remainder are due to two maternal copies of the long arm of chromosome 15 and no paternal copy. (Jones:202–205)

68. (B) Thrombocytopenia is part of the diagnostic criteria for hemolytic uremic syndrome, an acute microangiopathic hemolytic anemia. Hemolytic uremic syndrome typically follows a gastrointestinal infection and is characterized by hemolytic anemia, acute renal failure, and thrombocytopenia. Enterohemorrhagic *Escherichia coli* (0157:H7) has been most frequently associated with hemolytic uremic syndrome but other organisms have been found as well. Lead poisoning, Henoch-Schönlein purpura, Kawasaki disease, and iron deficiency anemia do not cause thrombocytopenia. (Behrman: 1586–1587)

69. (B) Stridor is a musical inspiratory sound of a single pitch produced by narrowing of the extrathoracic airway. Laryngomalacia is the most common cause of persistent stridor in infants, and is usually present by 6 weeks of age. Laryngomalacia is caused by underdevelopment of the cartilaginous support of the supraglottic airway structures. It generally is a benign disorder, which resolves as the cartilaginous support develops, usually by the age of 2 years. Diagnosis is confirmed by direct visualization of the larynx during an endoscopic procedure. (Behrman:1271–1272)

70. (D) Hereditary spherocytosis is the most common inherited disorder of red blood cell membranes. It occurs in all ethnic groups but is most frequently found in those of northern European descent. One of several membrane protein defects may cause hereditary spherocytosis. Defects in spectrin are the most common. The patient typically has a mild to moderate chronic hemolytic anemia. Red cell indices demonstrate a decreased MCV, an increased MCHC (cellular dehydration), and an elevated RDW (presence of microspherocytes and reticulocytes). The reticulocyte count is elevated in response to chronic hemolysis. The osmotic fragility test is the diagnostic test of choice, as the spherocytes will display increased fragility in hypotonic solutions. (Behrman:1475–1477)

71. (A) The differential diagnosis of hematuria in children includes glomerular diseases, extraglomerular renal diseases, and various nonrenal diseases. The glomerular diseases include acute or chronic glomerulonephritis, IgA nephropathy, benign familial hematuria, Alport syndrome, systemic vasculitis, and hemolytic uremic syndrome. Hypercalciuria can also cause hematuria. Serum complement, both total and C3, is decreased in conditions such as poststreptococcal glomerulonephritis, systemic lupus erythematosus, and bacterial endocarditis. Serum complement is normal in the other diseases listed. (Behrman:1577–1582)

72. (C) The first physical sign of puberty in girls is the development of breast buds. Menarche usually occurs 2–2.5 years later. Adrenal production of testosterone leads to the development of acne, axillary sweating, and axillary and pubic hair growth. This usually occurs right after the development of breast buds. (Behrman 53–54)

73. (E) The incidence of anorexia nervosa (AN) has steadily risen over the past 20 years and current estimates indicate the occurrence of 1 in every 100 females. To make a diagnosis of AN the DSM-IV criteria should be met. These include fear of becoming obese, disturbance in body image perception, body weight 15% below expected, and in females the absence of at least three consecutive menstrual cycles. Disturbances in almost any organ can be seen. Congestive heart failure, electrolyte disturbances, and cardiac arrhythmias contribute to the mortality, which is about 10%. Diuretic and laxative abuse combined with vomiting and

excessive water intake often lead to the development of a hypochloremic alkalosis. Constipation is very common among patients with anorexia nervosa. *(Behrman:562–563)*

74. **(D)** Posterior urethral valves are the most common cause of severe obstructive uropathy. They only occur in boys and in about 30% of patients will lead to end-stage renal disease or chronic renal insufficiency. If the obstruction is very severe the diagnosis is sometimes made in utero and these infants carry the worst prognosis because they often have associated oligohydramnios and pulmonary hypoplasia. Urethral strictures in males are usually the result of trauma and they are exceptional in females. Anterior urethral valves are very rare. Meatal stenosis is an acquired condition that can occur after circumcision and almost never leads to obstructive uropathy. *(Behrman: 1636–1637)*

75. **(B)** The most common cause of infection of the esophagus in immunocompetent children is candidiasis. Oral candidiasis is usually not present. Viral esophagitis can be caused by herpes simplex, cytomegalovirus, and occasionally by varicella zoster virus. The latter two are only cause of disease in immunocompromised patients. *(Behrman:1126)*

76. **(A)** Bacterial tracheitis can cause life-threatening obstruction of the airway. It is typically caused by *Staphylococcus aureus*. It is most commonly seen during the cold seasons in conjunction with viral croup. Most likely the tracheitis is a complication of a viral disease and not a primary bacterial infection. Laryngomalacia, necrotizing esophagitis, reactive airway disease, and cystic fibrosis are not associated with bacterial tracheitis. *(Behrman: 1279)*

77. **(D)** The infant presented most likely has pyloric stenosis. Pyloric stenosis is four times as common in boys as in girls. There is a genetic predisposition; infants of mothers with pyloric stenosis have a much higher incidence of pyloric stenosis than the general population. It often presents as nonbilious vomiting in the first weeks of life. The vomiting may become projectile and classically a hypochloremic metabolic alkalosis will develop. The infants generally appear hungry and experienced examiners can feel the thickened pyloric muscle (olive) in most of the cases. After the alkalosis has been corrected pyloromyotomy can be performed. Maple syrup urine disease is an organic acidemia and would not lead to alkalosis. Adrenal insufficiency may cause persistent vomiting but would not cause alkalosis. Homocystinuria usually is asymptomatic in childhood and does not present with vomiting. Children with gastroenteritis typically have diarrhea and are more prone to develop a metabolic acidosis. *(Behrman:1130–1131)*

78. **(B)** This syndrome occurs mostly in males; only 5% of the patients are females. It is characterized by a deficiency in abdominal muscles, undescended testes, and urinary tract abnormalities. Imperforate anus, mental retardation, cleft lip, renal agenesis, and ectopic bladder are not associated with this syndrome. *(Behrman:1635)*

79. **(C)** Although Crohn disease and ulcerative colitis (UC) have many similar symptoms a diagnosis can usually be made based on the clinical presentation, radiologic, endoscopic, and histopathologic findings. Rectal bleeding is more common in UC but can occur in Crohn disease. Cholangitis occurs more commonly in UC but can occur in Crohn disease as well. Abdominal pain can be present in both diseases. Crypt abscesses are more commonly seen in UC whereas granulomas are more commonly seen in Crohn disease but neither one is pathognomonic. Ileal involvement occurs only in Crohn disease and is not seen in UC. *(Behrman:1150)*

80. **(A)** The infant most likely suffers from botulism. Infant botulism is a life-threatening condition that often is misdiagnosed at onset. In the majority of cases suspected sepsis is the reason for admission. Botulinum toxin is neurotoxic; it binds irreversibly at cholinergic synapses, blocks the release of acetylcholine and causes impaired neuromuscular and autonomic transmission. Sensory nerves are not

affected and bulbar involvement is severe. In infants, inhalation and subsequent swallowing of airborne clostridial spores most likely cause the disease and prevention is therefore difficult. The only avoidable source of botulinum spores is honey. Honey should not be given to children under the age of 1 year. *(Behrman: 875–878)*

81. **(C)** Transient synovitis is the most common cause for limping in a healthy child at this age. Transient synovitis classically occurs 1–2 weeks after a nonspecific upper respiratory tract infection. Transient synovitis is a diagnosis of exclusion. Osteomyelitis and septic arthritis must be excluded. Patients with transient synovitis are usually afebrile or may have a low-grade fever. Laboratory studies are usually normal although a mild elevation in the erythrocyte sedimentation rate may be seen. Ultrasound of the hip can demonstrate a hip joint effusion. Treatment of this disorder is symptomatic with bedrest and analgesics. *(Behrman:2079–2080)*

82. **(B)** This child most likely has nonorganic (no known medical condition) failure to thrive (FTT) which is far more common than organic (marked by an underlying medical condition) FTT. Nonorganic FTT is due to lack of adequate caloric intake. Typically there is an abnormality in the infant–mother relationship. The best-offered option for this child with a weight of 5.5 kg (far below the 5th percentile) is to hospitalize the infant. Unlimited amount of calories should be given, weight should be followed closely and the mother–child interaction should be carefully observed. Typically children with nonorganic FTT who are in a controlled healthy environment will gain more than 2 oz per day for the first week. It is reasonable and practical to avoid laboratory studies as long as the child is showing good weight gain with this approach. None of the other offered choices are valid options at this point in time. *(Behrman: 117–118)*

83. **(E)** The patient most likely has erythema nodosum, which is characterized by pretibial tender erythematous nodules. Common infectious diseases that have been associated with

erythema nodosum are streptococcal pharyngitis, tuberculosis, *Yersinia*, histoplasmosis, and coccidioidomycosis. Other associated noninfectious diseases are inflammatory bowel disease, sarcoidosis, or spondyloarthropathy. *(Behrman: 699)*

84. **(E)** The patient most likely had a breath-holding spell. These are always provoked by upsetting or scolding a child. The peak age for occurrence is 2 years. The child typically has a brief shrill followed by apnea, cyanosis, and loss of consciousness. Posturing and generalized clonic jerks may occur during an episode. The clinical setting and the occurrence of apnea and cyanosis usually differentiate breath-holding spells from seizure disorders. The best approach is to do a thorough examination followed by an explanation to the parents of the mechanism of breath-holding spells. Breath-holding spells can recur and it is important for parents not to reinforce the child's behavior. *(Behrman:1829–1830)*

85. **(B)** Patellofemoral pain syndrome is the most common cause of chronic anterior knee pain. As in this patient, it typically worsens upon going up the stairs, after sitting for prolonged periods, or after squatting or running. The finding of peripatellar tenderness on examination confirms the diagnosis. Intensity of treatment is based on the severity of the symptoms and is focused on improving strength and flexibility of the vastus medialis muscle. *(Behrman:2106)*

86. **(C)** Attention-deficit hyperactivity disorder (ADHD) is characterized by problems with task attendance, motoric overactivity, and impulsivity. According to DSM-IV criteria, the symptoms must be evident before the age of 7 years and must be present in at least two different settings, such as school and home. They must also impair the child's functioning. The prevalence of comorbidities is high. Oppositional and aggressive behaviors, anxiety, mood disorders, and concurrent learning difficulties are some of the more common ones. Comorbidities do not have to be present to meet the diagnostic criteria for ADHD. The presence of another child in the family with ADHD or a history of

birth trauma are also not part of the diagnostic criteria. *(Behrman:100–103)*

87. **(B)** There are many controversies around the subject of circumcision in newborn boys. The American Academy of Pediatrics issued a circumcision policy statement in 1999. The only solid evidence regarding the benefit of circumcision is that urinary tract infections (UTI) are much less common in circumcised infants than in uncircumcised infants. The increased risk for UTI in uncircumcised infants is primarily in the first 6 months, although the risk remains increased at least through the age of 5 years. There is no solid evidence that circumcision significantly lowers the risk for sexually transmitted diseases or penile cancer. Boys with hypospadias should not be circumcised. *(Behrman:1647; Pediatrics 103:686–693, 1999)*

88. **(C)** Autonomy and competence are closely linked since only competent patients have the complete autonomy to decide what shall be done or not done with their bodies. Whether the patient's decisions are rational or not does not change this. Adolescents can often be viewed as competent patients and should have a major role in such decision making. However, younger pediatric patients are not competent to make such decisions and traditionally parents have made such decisions on behalf of their children without much controversy. The limits of this parental autonomy are increasingly questioned, especially when a child's health could be potentially harmed by parental decisions. *(Behrman:5–6)*

89. **(G)** Supravalvular aortic stenosis is the least common type of aortic stenosis. It may be sporadic, familial, or associated with Williams syndrome. Other features of Williams syndrome include mental retardation, elfin facies, and idiopathic hypercalcemia of infancy. *(Behrman: 1377)*

90. **(E)** An infant born to a mother with lupus may develop the neonatal lupus syndrome. Associated problems are cutaneous lesions, liver disease, thrombocytopenia, neutropenia, pulmonary disease, neurologic disease, and congenital heart block. Except for the congenital heart block which often requires cardiac pacing, these associated problems usually resolve over time. *(Behrman:716)*

91. **(H)** Noonan syndrome is characterized by short stature, webbing of the neck, pectus excavatum, characteristic facies and cardiac defects, most commonly pulmonary valvular stenosis. *(Behrman:1747)*

92. **(D)** Kawasaki disease leads to aneurysms of the coronary or systemic arteries in approximately 25% of untreated patients. Three to four percent of patients with Kawasaki disease treated with intravenous gammaglobulin will develop aneurysms. *(Behrman:1449)*

93. **(C)** Clinical features of Turner syndrome include edema of the dorsa of the hands and feet, webbing of the neck, low posterior hairline, broad chest, and short stature. Sexual maturation fails to occur at the expected age. About one-third to half of the girls with Turner syndrome have bicuspid aortic valves. *(Behrman: 1753)*

94. **(F)** Classical features of Marfan syndrome include tall stature, ocular abnormalities, arachnodactyly, and scoliosis. Morbidity of Marfan syndrome is substantial; about 80–100% of patients will develop aortic root dilatation. *(Behrman:2131)*

95. **(E), 96. (C), 97. (F), 98. (F), 99. (C)**
Sitting without support is on average mastered at 6 months of life. Generally a 3-month-old infant can bring the hands together in the midline. An average 8-month-old child can bang two cubes and will have a thumb–finger grasp. The Moro reflex is typically gone by 12 weeks of life. *(Behrman:34–35)*

100. **(B)** In idiopathic thrombocytopenia (ITP) the platelet count is decreased, usually below 60,000/mm^3, while the remainder of the blood count is normal unless there has been significant bleeding, in which case the Hb may be decreased and the reticulocyte count increased.

Most pediatric cases of ITP occur in the first 5–6 years of life. *(Behrman:1520–1522)*

101. (A) A Hb concentration of 12 g/dL and a WBC count of 11,500/mm³ are within statistical "normal" limits for a 2-year-old child (mean 12.5; 10th percentile 11.5). *(Behrman:1457)*

102. (E) In children with sickle cell disease the Hb is usually between 7 and 10 g/dL, and the WBC count is between 15,000 and 25,000/mm³. The reticulocyte count is increased except in the presence of an aplastic crisis, when the Hb will be lower with low reticulocyte count. *(Behrman: 1480)*

103. (D) In the presence of iron deficiency anemia, the reticulocyte count typically is low. Hemoglobin values of 5 g/dL are not uncommon, and values as low as 2 g/dL are seen occasionally in very severe cases. Striking increases in platelet counts have been noted in children with iron deficiency anemia. *(Behrman:1469–1471)*

104. (C) Acute lymphoblastic leukemia (ALL) often presents with anemia and thrombocytopenia. The total WBC count may be increased, normal, or decreased. In about 10% of the cases the peripheral WBC count is below 3000/mm³ at the time of presentation. A more definitive diagnosis of ALL in the absence of increased WBC count and absence of lymphoblasts can only be made by examination of the bone marrow. *(Behrman:1543–1546)*

105. (C) As the name implies, in pancytopenia, *all* blood elements are quantitatively diminished. The low reticulocyte count reflects failure of the bone marrow, which is the usual cause of pancytopenia. *(Behrman:1497–1498)*

106. (E) Meconium ileus is intestinal obstruction in the newborn caused by impacted meconium in the small bowel, usually the ileum. The condition is essentially always associated with cystic fibrosis. In this disease, meconium is abnormally thick and sticky, partly because of abnormal glycoproteins and partly because of pancreatic insufficiency, and accumulates in the intestinal lumen, producing bowel obstruc-

tion even before birth. About 10–15% of infants with cystic fibrosis have meconium ileus at birth. *(Behrman:1318)*

107. (D) Malrotation of the intestines is an abnormality that results from a failure of counterclockwise rotation of the fetal intestine as it returns to the abdominal cavity at about week 10 of gestation. The condition often is associated with duodenal obstruction secondary to constricting peritoneal bands. However, in a small percentage of cases, obstruction results from a midgut volvulus. This is a potentially devastating complication in which the mobile, malrotated bowel twists about the superior mesenteric artery. Infarction and necrosis of major segments of bowel may occur. Midgut volvulus is a surgical emergency. *(Behrman:1136)*

108. (A) Enterocolitis is a well-recognized complication of congenital aganglionic megacolon (Hirschsprung disease) that occurs primarily in undiagnosed or inadequately managed patients. Severe recurrent diarrhea secondary to enterocolitis may be the presenting complaint in a young infant with congenital megacolon. Recognition of the underlying abnormality is important, as the mortality of secondary enterocolitis (*toxic megacolon*) can be quite high. *(Behrman:1139–1141)*

109. (H) Neonatal herpes infections are usually acquired at the time of delivery and many of the mothers do not have evidence of genital herpes lesions. The infection usually manifests within the first month of life. Three major categories exist. The localized skin, eye, and mouth infection is present in about 30–40% of infants at onset. Isolated CNS infection and disseminated infection are the other two categories. The morbidity and mortality are high, especially with the systemic form of infections. A high index of suspicion for herpes should arise when dealing with infants and sepsis unresponsive to antibiotics. *(Behrman:969)*

110. (A) Cytomegalovirus (CMV) is the most common identified etiologic agent in congenital infections. Only 5% of infants with congenital CMV have the full spectrum of hepatosplenomegaly, jaundice, petechia, purpura, and microcephaly. The majority of patients are born with subclinical but chronic CMV infections. The most common sequel of congenital CMV infection is sensorineural hearing loss. *(Behrman:982–983)*

111. **(E)** Congenital infection with *Toxoplasma gondii* can range from having completely asymptomatic infection to severe neonatal disease. As with the other congenital infections, patients can have hepatosplenomegaly, thrombocytopenia and CNS involvement. Intracranial calcifications with congenital toxoplasmosis are usually diffuse. A unique problem with congenital toxoplasmosis is the occurrence of hydrocephalus in some infants. *(Behrman: 1056–1057; Zitelli:450)*

112. **(G)** The early manifestations of congenital syphilis can involve many different organ systems. Late manifestations are the consequence of chronic inflammation of bone, teeth, and central nervous system. Hutchinson teeth and saddle nose are some of the characteristic findings that occur at later age. *(Behrman:903–905)*

113. **(B)** Most of the stigmata of congenital varicella syndrome can be attributed to viral-induced nervous system injury. Stigmata involve mainly the skin, extremities, eyes, and brain. Extremities may be shortened and malformed, often covered with zigzag scarring (cicatrix). *(Behrman: 974–975)*

BIBLIOGRAPHY

Abi-Hanna A, Lake AM. Constipation and encopresis in childhood. *Pediatr Rev* 1998;19:23–31.

American Academy of Pediatrics Task Force on Circumcision. Circumcision Policy Statement (RE9850). *Pediatrics* 1999:103:686–693.

Behrman RE, Kliegman RM, Arvin AM. *Nelson Textbook of Pediatrics*, 16th ed. Philadelphia, PA: W.B. Saunders, 2000.

Cassidy JT, Petty RE. *Textbook of Pediatric Rheumatology*, 4th ed. Philadelphia, PA: W.B. Saunders, 2001.

Jones KL. *Smith's Recognizable Patterns of Human Malformation*, 5th ed. Philadelphia, PA: W.B. Saunders, 1997.

Klish WJ. Childhood obesity. *Pediatr Rev* 1998; 19:312–315.

Norwood VF. Hypertension. *Pediatr Rev* 2002; 23:197–208.

Pizzo PA, Poplack DG. *Principles and Practice of Pediatric Oncology*, 4th ed. Philadelphia, PA: JB Lippincott, 2002.

Rimsza ME. Dysfunctional uterine bleeding. *Pediatr Rev* 2002;23:227–232.

Roth KS, Amaker BH, Chan JCM. Nephrotic syndrome: pathogenesis and management. *Pediatr Rev* 2002;23: 237–247.

Schmitt BD. Nocturnal enuresis. *Pediatr Rev* 1997;18: 183–191.

Vogiatzi MG, Copeland KC. The short child. *Pediatr Rev* 1996;19:92–99.

Zitelli BJ, Davis HW. *Atlas of Pediatric Physical Diagnosis*, 4th ed. Philadelphia, PA: Mosby, 2002.

CHAPTER 9

Therapeutics

Joseph D. Tobias, MD

Sara S. Viessman, MD

Pediatric therapeutics is challenging on many fronts. You probably have heard, "Children are not simply small adults." The basic principles are the same as those used in adult therapeutics, but with more than a few twists! Disease processes and therapies vary with age. For the pediatric patient, age, body weight, and/or surface area are necessary in calculating caloric requirements, fluid requirements, and specific drug dosages. Practical issues such as the mode of delivery for medicines, the complex social situations, and the impact of behavioral problems in therapy become obvious with clinical experience.

Many drugs have unique kinetics or side effects in certain age groups and may be contraindicated in those age groups. For example, chloramphenicol is so poorly metabolized by the newborn infant's liver that the drug can rapidly accumulate to lethal blood levels. Tetracyclines deposit in growing bones and developing teeth, and thus generally are contraindicated in young children.

Some agents generally safe in adults proved to be lethal in our youngest patients. Prior to 1972, hexachlorophene was widely used as a nonprescription topical antiseptic. A 1972 disaster involving the topical use of talcum powder containing very high levels of hexachlorophene resulted in the death of 36 infants and prompted the FDA to restrict hexachlorophene to prescription status.

Propylene glycol is a second agent generally safe in adults but found to be toxic in our youngest patients. This basically inert ingredient used as a solvent or stabilizer in many medications was found to cause intoxication, hypoglycemia, and seizures in young children. In premature infants it induced hyperosmolality and renal failure. The discovery of these problems and others led to the 1997 FDA Modernization Act. This Act allows the FDA to ensure that all ingredients, including alcohol and "inactive" ingredients be identified in nonprescription and prescription drugs.

Physicians caring for children know the stakes are especially high. Meeting the challenge of appropriately diagnosing and treating age-specific childhood illnesses requires a solid foundation of knowledge, practical experience, ongoing self-education, and a good heart.

Questions

DIRECTIONS: Each of the numbered items or incomplete statements in this section is followed by answers or by completions of the statement. Select the ONE lettered answer or completion that is BEST in each case.

1. A 5-year-old boy with classic hemophilia A presents to the emergency center with hemarthrosis of the right knee. The most important aspect of care for this child would be

   (A) intravenous administration of factor IX concentrate
   (B) intravenous administration of cryoprecipitate
   (C) injection of factor VIII concentrate into the joint
   (D) intravenous administration of factor VIII concentrate
   (E) intravenous administration of a vasopressin analog DDAVP

2. Which of the following is categorized as a depolarizing neuromuscular blocking agent?

   (A) pancuronium
   (B) vecuronium
   (C) atracurium
   (D) succinylcholine
   (E) tubocurare

3. A 6-month-old infant with bronchopulmonary dysplasia (BPD) on home oxygen and caloric supplementation presents with slow growth. You consider starting a thiazide diuretic to decrease airway resistance and improve lung compliance. Which of the following electrolyte abnormalities may result from the use of thiazide type diuretics?

   (A) hypoglycemia
   (B) hyperuricemia
   (C) hyperkalemia
   (D) hypernatremia
   (E) hypocalciuria

4. Methylphenidate is most commonly prescribed in the management of children with

   (A) poor appetites
   (B) temper tantrums
   (C) seizure disorders
   (D) breath-holding spells
   (E) attention-deficit hyperactivity disorders

5. A 1-year-old male with Beckwith-Wiedemann syndrome presents with an abdominal mass confirmed by studies to be a hepatoblastoma. The initial treatment of choice is

   (A) radiation therapy
   (B) chemotherapy
   (C) chemotherapy and surgery
   (D) vitamin B_{12}
   (E) a combination of radiation and chemotherapy

6. Which of the following is true concerning magnesium?

   (A) The adverse effects of hypermagnesemia can be reversed by the administration of potassium.
   (B) High levels may occur in patients chronically receiving diuretics.

(C) It is the most abundant intracellular cation.

(D) It may be of therapeutic benefit in patients with status asthmaticus.

(E) High levels can cause neuromuscular excitation.

7. A 2-month-old male presents with failure to thrive and dehydration. Laboratory evaluation reveals a serum sodium of 164 meq/L and a urine specific gravity of 1.001. The urine was negative for glucose. Which of the following may be most beneficial in the long-term management of this patient's condition?

(A) antidiuretic hormone
(B) extra salt in the diet or formula
(C) fluid restriction
(D) oral bicarbonate
(E) thiazide diuretics

8. Which of the following drugs can decrease the rate of recurrence of febrile seizures?

(A) carbamazepine
(B) clonapin
(C) phenobarbital
(D) phenytoin
(E) felbamate

9. A child with Graves disease treated with propyl-thiouracil presents with a febrile illness. Which of the following is most likely related to the medical therapy?

(A) agranulocytosis
(B) acute renal failure
(C) hypoglycemia
(D) pseudotumor cerebri
(E) seizures

10. A 6-year-old Black female with nephrotic syndrome is receiving steroids. Which of the following is the rationale for using alternate-day prednisone therapy?

(A) It is more effective.
(B) It is more convenient.
(C) There is less adrenal suppression.

(D) It permits use of a lower total dose.
(E) There is less suppression of the immunologic system.

11. A 14-year-old White female presents to the emergency room 20 h following ingestion of 8.5 g of acetaminophen. Therapy with which of the following should be initiated?

(A) deferoxamine
(B) physostigmine
(C) N-acetylcysteine
(D) glutathione
(E) no therapy is indicated

12. Which of the following antibiotics would be most appropriate for prophylaxis against bacterial endocarditis in a 10-year-old child with mild congenital aortic stenosis undergoing an invasive dental procedure?

(A) amoxicillin
(B) clindamycin
(C) erythromycin
(D) oxacillin
(E) vancomycin

13. Which of the following is most appropriate for the treatment of *Mycoplasma pneumoniae* infection in a 4-year-old child?

(A) cefuroxime
(B) chloramphenicol
(C) erythromycin
(D) penicillin
(E) tetracycline

14. Cyanide is produced in the metabolism of

(A) sodium nitroprusside
(B) nitroglycerin
(C) labetalol
(D) dobutamine
(E) amrinone

15. An 8-year-old male presents following a syncopal episode. His mother is concerned because an uncle had episodes of syncope prior to his sudden death at the age of 35. After a complete history and physical examination you obtain an ECG which reveals a prolonged QT interval. Which of the following drugs would be most beneficial in the management of this condition?

    (A) atropine
    (B) digitalis
    (C) lidocaine
    (D) phenylephrine
    (E) propranolol

16. Normal saline contains

    (A) no sodium
    (B) 34 meq/L sodium
    (C) 77 meq/L sodium
    (D) 104 meq/L sodium
    (E) 154 meq/L sodium

17. Palliative surgery for the small infant with severe tetralogy of Fallot, deep cyanosis, and paroxysmal dyspnea would be

    (A) pulmonary artery banding
    (B) atrial septostomy
    (C) aorta-to-pulmonary artery anastomosis
    (D) ductal ligation
    (E) implantation of a pacemaker

18. Ethosuximide (Zarontin) is most useful in the treatment of

    (A) phenobarbital overdosage
    (B) absence (petit mal) seizures
    (C) akinetic seizures
    (D) tonic-clonic seizures
    (E) complex partial seizures

19. A 6-day-old male infant is brought to the emergency center with complaints of poor feeding and lethargy for 2 days. On physical examination, the infant is hypotonic and responds poorly to painful stimuli. The initial Dextrostix is 30 mg%. Two mL/kg of $D_{25}W$ are administered in addition to 20 mL/kg of normal saline. Initial laboratory evaluation includes sodium 128 meq/L, potassium 8.4 meq/L, bicarbonate 8 meq/L, and chloride 104 meq/L. The next intervention should be to

    (A) obtain plasma for 17-OH progesterone level and administer 10 mg/kg hydrocortisone
    (B) start prostaglandin E
    (C) administer 3 mL/kg of hypertonic saline
    (D) obtain a urine metabolic screen
    (E) check serum ammonia and liver function tests

20. A 14-month-old male is admitted to the PICU for bleeding from his nose and gums. There is no family history of bleeding tendency. On further history you determine the family has a problem with mice and rats and have rodenticides around the house. Which of the following should be included in initial treatment?

    (A) vitamin C
    (B) vitamin K
    (C) copper sulfate
    (D) a phenothiazine
    (E) atropine

21. A 16-year-old girl is referred to the dentist for removal of an infected first molar. The past history is positive for type I von Willebrand disease that has required treatment only twice in the past following minor surgical procedures. Appropriate therapy includes

    (A) administration of factor VIII concentrate
    (B) administration of factor IX concentrate
    (C) administration of DDAVP 1–2 h prior to the procedure
    (D) 3 units of platelets 1 h prior to the procedure
    (E) 20 units of cryoprecipitate 1 h prior to the procedure

22. Treatment of acute nitrite poisoning may require the administration of

    (A) hydralazine
    (B) morphine
    (C) methylene blue

(D) corticosteroids

(E) thiosulfate

23. A 6-month-old day care–attending female presents with fever, vomiting, and lethargy. On physical examination, you confirm the lethargy and note a full fontanel despite signs of dehydration. Which of the following would be the initial antibiotic(s) of choice?

(A) cefuroxime + vancomycin

(B) ceftriaxone + vancomycin

(C) clindamycin

(D) vancomycin

(E) amoxicillin

24. Which of the following doses of dexamethasone is equivalent to 5 mg of prednisone in glucocorticoid effect?

(A) 0.1 mg

(B) 0.75 mg

(C) 1.5 mg

(D) 2.5 mg

(E) 5.0 mg

25. A 2-day-old male was born at home and has been a poor feeder. His parents bring him to the ER because he has become very pale and listless over a matter of hours. On examination, you note a lethargic newborn in shock with a large liver and a gallop. Chest x-ray reveals increased pulmonary vasculature and cardiomegaly. You begin antibiotic therapy but suspect congenital cardiac disease. Which of the following is the drug of choice?

(A) dobutamine

(B) digoxin

(C) prostaglandin E_1

(D) amrinone

(E) nicardipine

26. Which of the following is true concerning lidocaine?

(A) It is a class II antiarrhythmic agent.

(B) It is useful in the treatment of atrial arrhythmias.

(C) It has similar electrocardiographic effects as mexiletine.

(D) It is available in oral form.

(E) It can be administered safely only as a continuous drip.

27. A 13-year-old female is referred for 18 mm indurated reaction to a tuberculin skin test. Her grandfather is undergoing therapy for tuberculosis and his infecting organism is isoniazid-susceptible. Because her examination and chest x-ray are normal, you diagnose latent tuberculosis infection (LTBI) and start isoniazid. Which of the following statements regarding isoniazid is true?

(A) Administration in adolescent patients should be supplemented with vitamin B_6.

(B) It should be given in divided daily dosage, at least twice a day.

(C) It should be taken with milk or an antacid.

(D) The most common toxic effect is renal injury with proteinuria.

(E) Use in conjunction with rifampin is contraindicated.

28. A 10-kg, 2-year-old child has ingested an unknown amount of methadone. In the emergency room the child is comatose. After stabilizing the airway, you should administer

(A) intravenous physostigmine

(B) intravenous naloxone

(C) subcutaneous adrenalin

(D) intravenous atropine

(E) intravenous flumazenil

29. A 7-year-old male adopted from Romania presents with hematemesis. He is known to have severe chronic hepatitis. An upper endoscopy reveals esophageal variceal bleeding. Which of the following agents is most likely to be beneficial in controlling the esophageal blood loss?

(A) octreotide

(B) PGE_1

(C) nitric oxide

(D) prostacyclin

(E) dexamethasone

30. Which of the following would be indicated for a child with Sydenham (rheumatic) chorea?

    (A) aspirin
    (B) bed rest
    (C) diphenylhydantoin
    (D) injections of Bicillin every 4 weeks
    (E) promethazine

31. The use of oral pancreatic enzyme replacement therapy is most helpful in patients with

    (A) protein-losing enteropathy
    (B) celiac disease
    (C) ulcerative colitis
    (D) alpha$_1$-antitrypsin deficiency
    (E) cystic fibrosis

32. Which of the following agents is effective against central nervous system (CNS) leukemia when administered systemically?

    (A) methotrexate
    (B) prednisone
    (C) vincristine
    (D) cyclophosphamide
    (E) daunorubicin

33. Following an injection of succinylcholine for intubation and induction of anesthesia, a 5-year-old child is noted to remain apneic and paralyzed for an extended period of time. The child most likely

    (A) received an excessive dose of the drug
    (B) has been receiving aminoglycosides
    (C) has impaired renal function
    (D) has pseudocholinesterase deficiency
    (E) had an allergic reaction to the succinyl-choline

34. Hyperuricemia is seen in which of the following inherited disorders?

    (A) Lesch-Nyhan syndrome
    (B) Gaucher's disease
    (C) Tay-Sachs disease
    (D) cystic fibrosis
    (E) galactosemia

35. The clinical feature common to both classic galactosemia and galactokinase deficiency is

    (A) hypotonia
    (B) hyperbilirubinemia
    (C) cataracts
    (D) seizures
    (E) metabolic acidosis

36. A 2-week-old neonate presents with lethargy, hypothermia, and poor feeding. Evaluation of the cerebrospinal fluid reveals a white blood cell count of 1200 cells/mm^3 (95% polymorphonucleocytes) with an elevated protein and decreased glucose. The initial antibiotic regimen of choice is

    (A) ampicillin
    (B) ceftriaxone
    (C) cefotaxime
    (D) cefuroxime + ampicillin
    (E) gentamicin + ampicillin

37. One tablespoon contains about

    (A) 5 mL
    (B) 10 mL
    (C) 15 mL
    (D) 20 mL
    (E) 30 mL

38. A 6-month-old infant presents with a weak cry, decreased activity, and poor feeding that has progressed over a couple of weeks. Prior to that he had been very healthy, but constipated. On examination he is generally weak and hypotonic, with a diminished gag reflex and subtle ocular palsies. There are no glossal fasciculations. Which of the following statements concerning this self-limited condition is true?

    (A) It is X-linked in inheritance.
    (B) Initial symptoms include hyperactivity and fever.
    (C) It has been associated with feeding honey to infants.

(D) CSF examination will reveal a predominance of lymphocytes with a high protein.

(E) It generally results from ingestion of the preformed toxin.

39. Use of the gluteal area for intramuscular injections in infants and young children should be avoided because

(A) the area is too vascular

(B) hematomas may dissect into the spine or rectum

(C) such injections may injure the sciatic nerve

(D) it is psychologically undesirable

(E) absorption from this site is poor

40. Acquired primary syphilis is best treated by

(A) ampicillin, 3.5 g orally, plus 1 g of probenecid

(B) procaine penicillin G, 4.8 million units IM as a single dose plus 1 g of probenecid

(C) benzathine penicillin G, 2.4 million units IM as a single dose

(D) spectinomycin, 2 g IM as a single dose

(E) cefuroxime, 4 g IV as a single dose

41. A 2-year-old male presents with a rash that is macular and predominantly located on the trunk. Three days prior he was diagnosed with otitis media and placed on amoxicillin. He is otherwise healthy. This rash

(A) indicates too high a dosage of amoxicillin

(B) is unrelated to the amoxicillin

(C) typically resolves in 1–3 days

(D) places the patient at considerable risk for a severe immediate hypersensitivity reaction if the drug is given again

(E) mandates that the medication be stopped immediately

42. Hemorrhagic cystitis is associated most closely with large doses of

(A) cyclophosphamide

(B) methotrexate

(C) actinomycin D

(D) L-asparaginase

(E) prednisone

43. Which of the following agents is contraindicated as the sole agent to treat hypertension associated with cocaine ingestion?

(A) labetalol

(B) sodium nitroprusside

(C) nicardipine

(D) hydralazine

(E) propranolol

44. Administration of which agent is recommended in patients with methanol ingestion?

(A) N-acetylcysteine

(B) amyl nitrite

(C) sodium thiosulfate

(D) ethanol

(E) vitamin B_{12}

45. A 2-month-old female presents with a 4-day history of coughing spells that last at least 30 s. After the coughing spells she vomits. She is otherwise well. Laboratory evaluation reveals a peripheral white blood cell count of $42,000/mm^3$ with 86% lymphocytes. Family and day care contacts of this child should receive prophylaxis with

(A) rifampin

(B) erythromycin

(C) gentamicin

(D) penicillin

(E) trimethoprim-sulfamethoxazole

46. The drug of choice for the treatment of meningococcal meningitis is

(A) cefotaxime

(B) ceftriaxone

(C) vancomycin

(D) chloramphenicol

(E) penicillin

47. Complications related to the administration of beta-adrenergic agonists such as albuterol or terbutaline in the treatment of status asthmaticus include

    (A) bradycardia
    (B) constipation
    (C) hypotonia
    (D) hyperkalemia
    (E) myocardial ischemia

48. Reducing agents such as methylene blue are used in the treatment of methemoglobinemia. Methemoglobin is

    (A) hemoglobin that has bound cyanide
    (B) hemoglobin in which the iron moiety has been oxidized from the ferrous (2+) state to the ferric (3+) state
    (C) hemoglobin that contains two alpha and two gamma chains
    (D) hemoglobin with an extra iron moiety
    (E) hemoglobin with an abnormal alpha chain

49. A 3-year-old male was discovered at his grandparents holding an empty bottle of iron tablets. At 4 h postingestion, his serum iron level is 550 µg/dL. Which of the following should be administered?

    (A) dimercaprol (BAL)
    (B) deferoxamine (Desferal)
    (C) versenate (EDTA)
    (D) penicillamine
    (E) sodium bicarbonate

50. A child has been poisoned by an anticholinesterase-containing (carbamate) insecticide. The nicotinic effects (paralysis) of the poison likely would be diminished or reversed by the prompt administration of

    (A) atropine
    (B) N-acetylcysteine
    (C) pralidoxime
    (D) bicarbonate
    (E) physostigmine

51. With proper therapy, which of the following childhood malignancies has the highest cure rate?

    (A) Wilms tumor
    (B) neuroblastoma
    (C) medulloblastoma
    (D) rhabdomyosarcoma
    (E) non-Hodgkin lymphoma

52. Which of the following is a useful agent for the treatment of intestinal infection with *Entamoeba histolytica*?

    (A) ampicillin
    (B) rifampin
    (C) aztreonam
    (D) cefotaxime
    (E) metronidazole

53. Fluoride supplementation is recommended for

    (A) all infants and young children
    (B) young children living in areas where the water supply contains less than 0.6 ppm of fluoride
    (C) infants and young children living in geographic areas of limited sunlight
    (D) infants and young children who consume less than a quart of milk per day
    (E) adolescents

54. Pulmonary fibrosis may be caused by

    (A) bleomycin
    (B) doxorubicin
    (C) daunomycin
    (D) etoposide
    (E) vincristine

55. Neurotoxicity is a common adverse effect of which chemotherapeutic agent?

    (A) methotrexate
    (B) cyclophosphamide
    (C) chlorambucil
    (D) procarbazine
    (E) vincristine

56. A 10-year-old male is admitted to the hospital with a 4-day history of nausea, vomiting, and abdominal pain. The pain is located in the epigastrium and radiates to the back. Recent history includes a 10-day course of corticosteroids for reactive airway disease. The next most appropriate step is to

   (A) administer morphine
   (B) obtain liver function tests and hepatitis titers
   (C) obtain a surgical consult
   (D) obtain serum amylase, lipase
   (E) order stool cultures for bacterial pathogens

57. A toddler known to have Wolff-Parkinson-White syndrome presents with pallor, lethargy, and a heart rate of 240/min. He is obtunded and in shock. The treatment of choice is

   (A) digoxin
   (B) bretylium
   (C) synchronized cardioversion
   (D) propranolol
   (E) adenosine

58. Which agent is most likely to decrease systemic vascular resistance in patients with tetralogy of Fallot?

   (A) morphine
   (B) propranolol
   (C) esmolol
   (D) sodium nitroprusside
   (E) phenylephrine

59. An adolescent male presents with a urethral discharge. Gram stain of the exudate reveals intracellular gram-negative diplococci. The initial treatment of choice is

   (A) ampicillin, 1 g a day orally for 3 days
   (B) doxycycline, 100 mg twice a day for 7 days
   (C) procaine penicillin G, 1.2 million units IM once
   (D) benzathine penicillin G, 2.4 million units IM once
   (E) ceftriaxone, 250 mg IM once

60. Which of the following statements is true regarding the toxicity of acetaminophen overdose?

   (A) primarily involves the liver
   (B) primarily involves the central nervous system
   (C) is most severe in patients less than 2 years of age
   (D) is best treated with beta-blockers
   (E) is best treated with intravenous methylene blue to reverse the methemoglobinemia

61. Which of the following drugs in toxic amounts is resistant to reversal of effects by Naloxone (Narcan)?

   (A) codeine
   (B) dextropropoxyphene (Darvon)
   (C) pentazocine (Talwin)
   (D) phenobarbital
   (E) methadone

62. Naloxone may be of therapeutic benefit in patients that have ingested

   (A) clonidine
   (B) ethanol
   (C) midazolam (Versed)
   (D) acetaminophen
   (E) methanol

63. Side effects of corticosteroids include

   (A) peripheral obesity
   (B) gigantism
   (C) cataracts
   (D) hypoglycemia
   (E) hypotension

64. Which of the following drugs has an ability to alter the cardiac action potential?

   (A) propranolol
   (B) metoprolol
   (C) esmolol
   (D) atenolol
   (C) sotalol

65. A neonate is receiving intravenous ampicillin and gentamicin for sepsis. A blood culture reveals group B *Streptococcus*. The antibiotic of choice is

    (A) clindamycin
    (B) penicillin
    (C) cefuroxime
    (D) vancomycin
    (E) tobramycin

66. A 6-year-old girl is brought to the emergency room with obtundation and urinary incontinence following an 8-week history of headaches and blurred vision. Her heart rate is 52 bpm, the blood pressure is 160/100 mmHg, with a respiratory rate of 8 bpm. The left pupil is larger than the right and minimally reactive to light. The left eye is deviated medially. The decision is made to intubate her trachea and provide controlled ventilation. Which of the following sedative agents could cause worsening of her condition?

    (A) sodium thiopental
    (B) propofol
    (C) midazolam
    (D) etomidate
    (E) ketamine

67. A 14-year-old boy presents to the emergency room with a 48-h history of upper respiratory symptoms and 6-h history of "difficulty breathing." Physical examination reveals a respiratory rate of 30 bpm, diffuse inspiratory and expiratory wheezes. Which of the following has the slowest onset of clinical results?

    (A) subcutaneous epinephrine
    (B) subcutaneous albuterol
    (C) inhaled albuterol
    (D) inhaled sodium cromolyn
    (E) inhaled ipratropium bromide

68. Which agent is effective in treating a malignant hyperthermia crisis?

    (A) ethanol
    (B) succinylcholine
    (C) halothane
    (D) potassium
    (E) dantrolene

69. Which compound functions as a transport vehicle for fatty acids across the mitochondrial membrane?

    (A) branched chain amino acids
    (B) carnitine
    (C) cytochrome *c*
    (D) coenzyme Q
    (E) albumin

70. Which agent is indicated in newborns with tricuspid atresia?

    (A) phenylephrine
    (B) norepinephrine
    (C) PGE$_1$
    (D) prostacyclin
    (E) nitric oxide

71. Which agent is known as endothelial derived relaxing factor (EDRF)?

    (A) prostacyclin
    (B) arachidonic acid
    (C) leukotriene C
    (D) nitric oxide
    E) adenosine

72. Alkalinization of the urine increases the excretion of which drug?

    (A) morphine
    (B) acetaminophen
    (C) diazepam
    (D) cocaine
    (E) salicylate

73. The spectrum of activity of aztreonam most closely resembles that of

    (A) vancomycin
    (B) oxacillin
    (C) gentamicin

(D) cefazolin

(E) clindamycin

74. A 14-year-old girl is admitted to the emergency department with an acute change in mental status. She recently had a fight with her parents and threatened to kill herself. Initial vital signs are stable. She is placed on a cardiac monitor and an electrocardiogram is obtained which shows prolongation of the QRS interval. The most likely agent ingested is

(A) nortriptyline

(B) phenobarbital

(C) acetaminophen

(D) cocaine

(E) phencyclidine

75. Minutes later the QRS complex abruptly widens. Treatment should include the immediate administration of

(A) *N*-acetylcysteine

(B) sodium bicarbonate

(C) sodium nitroprusside

(D) amyl nitrite

(E) lidocaine

76. Midline facial defects have been described with the maternal ingestion of

(A) cocaine

(B) acetaminophen

(C) methotrexate

(D) phenytoin

(E) ethanol

77. A 5-year-old boy is admitted to the hospital for treatment of *H. influenzae* meningitis. His 3-year-old incompletely immunized sibling should receive prophylaxis with

(A) intravenous ceftriaxone

(B) intravenous cefotaxime

(C) oral rifampin

(D) oral erythromycin

(E) oral amoxicillin

78. Which of the following opioids has the longest plasma half-life?

(A) fentanyl

(B) morphine

(C) hydromorphone (Dilaudid)

(D) meperidine

(E) methadone

79. A 4-year-old child develops lymphadenopathy, fever, and generalized fatigue 7 days after hunting with his father. During the hunting trip, the father and son shot and skinned several rabbits. The initial treatment of choice is

(A) streptomycin

(B) ceftriaxone

(C) oxacillin

(D) vancomycin

(E) ciprofloxacin

80. Which of the following clotting factors are contained in cryoprecipitate?

(A) VII, VIII

(B) VIII, IX

(C) I, VIII, XIII

(D) X

(E) I, II

81. A 12-year-old boy with Duchenne muscular dystrophy is admitted to the pediatric ICU with a history of progressive fatigue, shortness of breath, and exercise intolerance. The blood pressure is 130/69 mmHg, the heart rate is 120 bpm, and the respiratory rate is 24 bpm. Chest x-ray reveals a large cardiac silhouette. Echocardiography reveals diminished left ventricular contractility. A pulmonary artery catheter is placed and demonstrates decreased cardiac index with a high systemic vascular resistance. The most appropriate inotropic agent to administer is

(A) dopamine

(B) dobutamine

(C) digoxin

(D) norepinephrine

(E) nitroglycerin

82. Accepted therapy for hemolytic uremic syndrome includes

    (A) exchange transfusion
    (B) antibiotics to cover gram-negative organisms
    (C) peritoneal dialysis
    (D) streptokinase
    (E) fresh frozen plasma

83. Which antihypertensive agent decreases central sympathetic outflow?

    (A) alpha-methyldopa (Aldomet)
    (B) phentolamine
    (C) sodium nitroprusside
    (D) nicardipine
    (E) nitroglycerin

84. A 5-year-old boy is admitted to the burn unit following an immersion hot water injury with resultant second degree burns covering 20% of the body surface area. Fluids are started at maintenance plus 4 mL/kg/%BSA burned according to the Parkland formula with half of the fluid administered over the first 8 h and the remainder over the following 16 h. A Foley catheter is placed to monitor urine output. Six hours after admission, the urine output has decreased to 0.5 mL/kg/h for the past 2 h. The most appropriate therapy would be

    (A) continue to observe the urine output
    (B) furosemide 1 mg/kg intravenously
    (C) furosemide 2 mg/kg orally
    (D) mannitol 0.5 g/kg intravenously
    (E) fluid bolus of 20 mL/kg of normal saline

85. Sodium overload can be seen with the administration of

    (A) ciprofloxacin
    (B) ticarcillin
    (C) gentamicin
    (D) cefotaxime
    (E) vancomycin

86. A 3.8 kg term infant presents at 6 days of age with poor feeding, lethargy, and cyanosis. Physical examination reveals stable heart rate and blood pressure with a respiratory rate of 44 bpm. Oxygen saturation by pulse oximetry is 72% and increases to 76% with an FiO_2 of 1.0. The ECG reveals left-axis deviation. The most likely diagnosis is

    (A) tetralogy of Fallot
    (B) tricuspid atresia
    (C) transposition of the great vessels
    (D) total anomalous pulmonary venous return
    (E) truncus arteriosus

87. Which of the following antibiotics likely will be useful in the treatment of infections due to *P. aeruginosa*?

    (A) penicillin
    (B) erythromycin
    (C) cefuroxime
    (D) ticarcillin
    (E) ceftriaxone

88. A normal anion gap is expected in

    (A) diabetic ketoacidosis
    (B) proximal renal tubular acidosis
    (C) lactic acidosis
    (D) methanol ingestion
    (E) methylmalonic aciduria

89. Nephrogenic diabetes insipidus may occur with the therapeutic use of which cation?

    (A) calcium
    (B) magnesium
    (C) lithium
    (D) copper
    (E) zinc

90. Allopurinol is useful in the management of acute leukemia of childhood

    (A) to induce remission
    (B) to maintain remission
    (C) both to induce and to maintain remission
    (D) to prevent vomiting from chemotherapy
    (E) to prevent hyperuricemia associated with chemotherapy and the tumor lysis syndrome

91. Propranolol may be indicated for the treatment of

    (A) asthma
    (B) allergic rhinitis
    (C) cardiogenic shock
    (D) tonic-clonic seizures
    (E) paroxysmal supraventricular tachycardia

92. A 6-month-old male presents with a history of mild cold symptoms for 2 days. Overnight he developed inspiratory stridor which alarmed the parents. On examination he is afebrile, happy, and drooling but has mild inspiratory stridor. His lung fields otherwise are clear. You carefully instruct the parents regarding this condition. The most appropriate drug to administer is

    (A) albuterol
    (B) amoxicillin-clavulanate
    (C) dexamethasone
    (D) amoxicillin
    (E) acetaminophen

Answers and Explanations

1. **(D)** The most important aspect of treatment of hemarthrosis in children with classic hemophilia A (factor VIII deficiency) is to increase the plasma activity of factor VIII in the patient. This is accomplished with intravenous administration of factor VIII concentrate. Intravenous administration of DDAVP (a synthetic arginine vasopressin that causes the release of stores of factor VIII) typically results in a threefold rise in factor VIII levels. Therefore, DDAVP is helpful only for patients with *mild* hemophilia A who have higher baseline factor VIII levels. DDAVP must be given parenterally, not into the joint. *(Rudolph CD:1572)*

2. **(D)** Neuromuscular blocking agents are classified as either nondepolarizing or depolarizing agents. Nondepolarizing agents act as competitive antagonists for acetylcholine at the acetylcholine receptor of the neuromuscular junction. By blocking the receptor without stimulating it, they stop neuromuscular transmission from occurring. The depolarizing agents such as succinylcholine interact with the receptor and cause the muscle end-plate to depolarize. Unlike acetylcholine, succinylcholine is resistant to degradation by acetylcholinesterase and as such continues to occupy the receptor preventing the muscle from repolarizing. It must be degraded by pseudocholinesterase which is present in the serum. This accounts for its duration of action of 45 min. *(Pediatr Ann 25:317–328, 1996)*

3. **(B)** Long-term therapy with thiazide diuretics has been shown to be beneficial in the management of BPD-associated pulmonary edema. The thiazides act by blocking the reabsorption of sodium and chloride in the thin portion of the ascending limb of the loop of Henle. In addition, they block the reabsorption of calcium leading to hypercalciuria, which can lead to the production of nephrocalcinosis and eventual renal failure. Increased urinary excretion of potassium can result in hypokalemia. The thiazides block the excretion of uric acid and can lead to hyperuricemia with symptomatic gout in susceptible patients. *(Rudolph CD:1965; Tobias:198)*

4. **(E)** Stimulant drugs such as methylphenidate (Ritalin), amphetamines, and pemoline (Cylert) have been shown to have a beneficial effect in many children with attention-deficit hyperactivity disorder. The seemingly paradoxical calming action of stimulant drugs in these children may be related to increased awareness of, and therefore response to, external stimuli, permitting sustained attention. The drugs have no role in the management of seizure disorders, temper tantrums, or breath-holding spells. Appetite *suppression* often is a side effect of these drugs. *(Rudolph CD:431–433; Pediatrics 105:1158–1170, 2000)*

5. **(C)** Hepatoblastomas in childhood tend to metastasize later than those in adults. Surgery (partial hepatectomy) and chemotherapy is the treatment regimen of choice and carries a 30–50% 5-year cure rate. Hepatoblastomas are associated with congenital anomalies including genitourinary abnormalities, Beckwith-Wiedemann syndrome, and hemihypertrophy. They are also seen in higher frequency in patients with germline mutation of the adenomatous polyposis coli gene. *(Rudolph CD:1621)*

6. **(D)** Therapeutic applications of magnesium include the treatment of preeclampsia, prevention of cardiac arrhythmias, and treatment of status

asthmaticus. Adverse effects of magnesium relate to its ability to block the release of acetylcholine at the neuromuscular junction. This leads to muscle weakness and respiratory failure when levels exceed 8–10 mg/dL. Treatment of such problems includes the administration of calcium which antagonizes magnesium's effects at the neuromuscular junction. Potassium is the most abundant intracellular cation. (*Tobias:48–49, 301–302; Hay:375*)

7. **(E)** Congenital nephrogenic diabetes insipidus is a genetically determined (X-linked dominant with variable penetrance in women) abnormality of renal tubular response to antidiuretic hormone (ADH). Infants with this disorder do not concentrate urine well because of an insensitivity of the collecting tubule to ADH. Symptoms generally begin shortly after birth and include fever, vomiting, constipation, dehydration, hypernatremia, polyuria, polydipsia, and failure to thrive. There is no response to even large doses of ADH or its analogs. The seemingly paradoxical response to chronic administration of thiazides is believed to result from total body sodium depletion and enhanced proximal reabsorption of glomerular filtrate. Dietary salt restriction is also helpful, but water intake must be generous. Central diabetes insipidus is unlikely at this age. (*Rudolph CD:1774*)

8. **(C)** Daily administration of phenobarbital reduces by two-thirds the recurrence rate for febrile seizures. However, in most cases of febrile seizures, the continuous administration of phenobarbital is not necessary or recommended. The therapy does not prevent the development of epilepsy and prevents febrile seizures which in the overwhelming majority of patients are benign. The undesirable side effects (rashes, hyperactivity, irritability, lethargy) are found in at least 20% of patients taking continuous phenobarbital. Phenytoin has not been shown to be effective. Although valproic acid is effective, the potential toxicities outweigh the benefit and prevent its routine use. Intermittent therapy with phenobarbital is ineffective. (*Rudolph CD: 2270–2271*)

9. **(A)** Toxic reactions to propylthiouracil are fairly common. Granulocytopenia may occur after 4–8 weeks of therapy and usually resolves with discontinuation of medication. Agranulocytosis is one of the most important toxic side effects of propylthiouracil. Patients should be informed about this possibility and advised to obtain a blood count with every febrile illness. Other side effects include hepatitis, purpura, dermatitis, and lymphadenopathy. (*Rudolph CD:2075–2076*)

10. **(C)** The major advantage of administering the total 48-h dose of prednisone at one time (*alternate-day therapy*) is that it results in less adrenal suppression than is seen with daily administration. Although this dosage is not effective in all diseases for which corticosteroids are used, it is effective for many cases of asthma or nephrotic syndrome. (*Rudolph CD:2052–2053*)

11. **(C)** Ingestion of toxic doses of acetaminophen (greater than 140 mg/kg) results in the depletion of hepatic glutathione stores and the production of the toxic intermediate metabolite, *n*-acetyl-benxoquinoneimine. The toxic intermediate metabolite covalently binds to hepatocytes and leads to cellular death. *N*-acetylcysteine acts as a surrogate glutathione or sulfate donor and thereby prevents the binding of the toxic intermediary to the hepatocyte. Therapy is indicated based on the acetaminophen level obtained 4 h postingestion. *N*-acetylcysteine is most effective if administered within 12–24 h postingestion. (*Rudolph CD: 360–362*)

12. **(A)** Although many organisms can cause endocarditis following a dental procedure, *Streptococcus viridans* remains the most common. Penicillin is highly effective against this organism, but amoxicillin, with a longer half-life, is the drug of choice. Patients with rheumatic heart disease who are receiving continuous prophylaxis with penicillin may harbor strains of *S. viridans* that are relatively resistant to penicillin. Therefore, for patients receiving continuous penicillin, an alternate antibiotic regimen (e.g., erythromycin) may be advisable for prophylaxis against endocarditis. (*Rudolph CD:911*)

13. **(C)** Penicillins and cephalosporins are ineffective against *Mycoplasma*. Erythromycin and tetracycline are effective, but the former is preferred in young children because tetracycline is

deposited in growing bone and teeth. Although such deposition has not been shown to have significant pathophysiologic effects, it does cause staining of the teeth that is cosmetically unacceptable. Chloramphenicol is effective; however, the infrequent but lethal side effect of aplastic anemia restricts use of this drug to certain serious infections. *(Rudolph CD:965–966)*

14. **(A)** The sodium nitroprusside molecule contains cyanide which is released following the metabolism of the parent compound. Cyanide normally is converted by the rhodanase enzyme of the liver to thiocyanate which is then excreted by the kidneys. The risk of cyanide toxicity increases with the dose and the duration of administration of sodium nitroprusside. Cyanide binds to cytochrome oxidase and inhibits oxidative phosphorylation leading to a metabolic acidosis. Cyanide also increases the effects of catecholamines on the smooth muscle of the arterioles leading to an increase in blood pressure and a need to increase the dose of nitroprusside (tachyphylaxis). Treatment of cyanide toxicity includes discontinuation of sodium nitroprusside and administration of thiosulfate. Thiosulfate provides a sulfur donor for the rhodanase enzyme to convert cyanide to thiocyanate. In extreme cases, amyl nitrite or sodium nitrite is administered to induce methemoglobinemia since cyanide will bind to the methemoglobin instead of the cytochrome oxidase. *(Tobias:427; Rudolph CD:1875)*

15. **(E)** Hereditary prolongation of the QT interval occurs either with deafness (Jervell-Lange-Nielsen syndrome) or without deafness (Romano-Ward syndrome). Both syndromes have been associated with syncope and sudden death. Although propranolol does not alter the electrocardiographic findings, the drug has been helpful in preventing episodes of ventricular fibrillation and death in patients with either syndrome. *(Rudolph CD:1762, 1858)*

16. **(E)** Normal saline contains 154 meq/L of both sodium and chloride. The sodium concentration is somewhat higher than that of normal plasma (135–145 meq/L) while the chloride concentration is significantly higher. *(Tobias:23)*

17. **(C)** Tetralogy of Fallot is characterized by ventricular outflow tract stenosis, ventricular septal defect, dextroposition of the aorta, and right ventricular hypertrophy. The major problem in tetralogy is that too little blood reaches the lungs. Palliation consists of establishing a shunt from the systemic circulation to the pulmonary artery, increasing pulmonary blood flow. In small infants an aorta-to-pulmonary artery anastomosis may be used. In larger infants or children a subclavian-pulmonary anastomosis is preferred. Although total intracardiac surgical correction is feasible for most patients, the very small infant with a hypoplastic right ventricle or pulmonary arteries will require a palliative shunt until definitive surgery can be performed at a later date. *(Rudolph CD:1822; Tobias:161–163)*

18. **(B)** Ethosuximide is one of the drugs of choice in the treatment of absence (petit mal) seizures *(Rudolph CD:2256; Hay:731)*

19. **(A)** The most likely diagnosis is congenital adrenal hyperplasia or CAH. CAH results from an enzymatic defect in the adrenal cortical production of corticosteroids. Ninety percent of cases and the one presenting as outlined above result from deficiency of the 21-hydroxylase enzyme. Without this enzyme, there is deficiency of corticosteroids resulting in an Addisonian-like state and deficiency of aldosterone resulting in hyperkalemia. The overproduction of adrenal androgens can result in virilization of female infants. Careful physical examination is necessary to be certain that the testes are palpable and that the infant in question is not a virilized female. *(Tobias:20–21; Rudolph CD:2031–2039)*

20. **(B)** Many rodent poisons contain warfarin, an anti-coagulant that inhibits the production of prothrombin by the liver, leading to hemorrhage. Symptoms typically are delayed for 12–24 h following ingestion. The degree and duration of toxicity is variable depending on the size of the child, amount of ingestion, and formulation of the rodenticide. The hepatic toxicity can be effectively counteracted by large doses of vitamin K. *(Rudolph CD:361)*

21. **(C)** von Willebrand (VW) disease is due to abnormalities of VWF, a plasma protein that is a cofactor for platelet adhesion, and that forms a complex that carries factor VIII. Type I VW disease is classified as mild disease with little or no spontaneous bleeding, but with episodes of bleeding following minor trauma. Administration of DDAVP, a synthetic posterior pituitary extract that causes the release of factor VIII antigen from the endothelial cells, is indicated prior to minor surgical procedures in patients with type I VW disease. Although cryoprecipitate contains factor VIII antigen, it carries infectious disease risks and is indicated only for severe bleeding. *(Rudolph CD:1573; Hay:457)*

22. **(C)** Nitrite poisoning can result from medication overdose or ingestion (amyl nitrate, nitroglycerin, nitrate food additives, or contaminated well water). Nitrites increase the oxidation of hemoglobin, resulting in methemoglobinemia. Methemoglobin contains oxidized iron (ferric or Fe^{3+}) as opposed to reduced iron (ferrous or Fe^{2+}) found in normal hemoglobin. Methemoglobin can be converted to hemoglobin by a reducing agent such as methylene blue, which is administered intravenously as a 1% solution. *(Tobias:429)*

23. **(B)** The increasing percentage of *Streptococcus pneumoniae* resistant to penicillin has followed widespread overuse of antibiotics. Penicillin resistance is defined as a minimum inhibitory concentration (MIC) of penicillin greater than 1 µg/mL. Meningitis or septicemia potentially caused by *S. pneumoniae* should be initially treated with a third-generation cephalosporin plus either vancomycin or rifampin. Therapy should be appropriately altered with identification and susceptibility testing of the organism isolated. Cefuroxime is a second generation cephalosporin and is not recommended in the treatment of meningitis. *(Tobias:400–402; Rudolph CD:903, 979)*

24. **(B)** Various steroid preparations have different relative potencies in regard to glucocorticoid (anti-inflammatory) and sodium retention effects. Regarding the glucocorticoid effects, equivalent doses would be: hydrocortisone 20 mg, prednisone 5 mg, methylprednisolone 4 mg, and dexamethasone 0.75 mg. *(Rudolph CD: 2049–2054)*

25. **(C)** Although a diagnosis of sepsis should not be eliminated immediately, hypoplastic left heart syndrome or other obstructive left-sided cardiac lesions are most likely given this neonate's clinical presentation. Prostaglandin E_1 maintains patency of the ductus arteriosus and thereby preserves blood flow to the systemic circulation. Although this is deoxygenated blood due to total mixing, there is adequate oxygen delivery to maintain life. Amrinone is a phosphodiesterase inhibitor whose cardiovascular effects include increased inotropy and peripheral vasodilatation. These effects are the same as those of dobutamine which acts through $beta_{1,2}$-adrenergic receptors. *(Tobias:156; Rudolph CD:292)*

26. **(C)** Lidocaine is classified as a class IB antiarrhythmic agent along with mexiletine (which can be given orally) and phenytoin. It is generally administered as a bolus dose followed by a continuous infusion for ventricular arrhythmias. It has no role in the treatment of atrial arrhythmias. *(Tobias:169–179)*

27. **(A)** Peripheral neuritis rarely is seen in young children receiving isoniazid (INH) but more commonly is a problem in adolescents and adults. This complication can be prevented by administration of 10 mg of vitamin B_6 for each 100 mg of INH. It usually is recommended that INH be given as a single daily dose, which is no less effective and no more toxic than divided doses. The major toxic effects are hepatic, not renal. Although concurrent administration of rifampin does increase the risk of drug-induced hepatitis, it is not contraindicated and is a very commonly used combination. *(Rudolph CD: 956–959)*

28. **(B)** Naloxone (Narcan) is a specific opiate antagonist that acts at the µ opioid receptor. It will reverse opioid-induced coma and respiratory depression. The drug has a wide margin of safety and may be repeated as frequently as every 5–10 min. This may be necessary since many of the commonly used opioids have half-lives of 2–3 h while naloxone has a half-life of

20–30 min. Naloxone can be given through an endotracheal tube if venous access cannot be established. *(Tobias:431–432; Rudolph CD:372)*

29. **(A)** Octreotide is a somatostatin analogue that increases the resistance in the splanchnic vasculature and reduces portal venous pressure and thereby decreases the bleeding from esophageal varices. It has replaced vasopressin in this clinical situation as octreotide has less of an effect on systemic blood pressure. *(Tobias:439–443; Rudolph CD:1515)*

30. **(D)** There is no evidence to suggest that rheumatic chorea responds to the usual antirheumatic agents such as salicylates. Bed rest per se is not necessary. The most important aspects of management are quiet sympathetic care, avoidance of emotional trauma and stress, and the judicious use of tranquilizers or phenobarbital. Drugs such as clonazepam and haloperidol appear to be useful in severe cases. Steroids have been suggested by some authors, but there are no data to document efficacy. It is most important that the patient be started on prophylactic penicillin to prevent recurrent attacks of acute rheumatic fever. *(Rudolph CD:1901–1904)*

31. **(E)** Cystic fibrosis is the most common cause of pancreatic insufficiency in childhood. Most patients with this disease have less steatorrhea and improved weight gain when receiving pancreatic replacement therapy. *(Rudolph CD:1977)*

32. **(B)** With current induction regimens for acute leukemia of childhood, the central nervous system has become a major site of relapse. Of the antileukemic agents listed, only prednisone achieves a therapeutic level in the cerebrospinal fluid when administered systemically. Methotrexate is effective when given intrathecally. Craniospinal irradiation also is very effective, but it may result in late neurologic and intellectual sequelae. *(Rudolph CD:1596–1599)*

33. **(D)** The genetically determined condition of succinylcholine sensitivity is based on an abnormality (decreased activity) of the serum enzyme pseudocholinesterase which is responsible for the breakdown of succinylcholine. Patients with

this condition may experience prolonged apnea and paralysis following administration of succinylcholine instead of the usual duration of action of 4–5 min. These findings can be reversed either by transfusion of normal plasma or by administration of a purified preparation of human pseudocholinesterase. However, the safest option generally is the continuation of mechanical ventilation until normal muscle strength returns. A similar phenomenon has been reported with children with organophosphate poisoning given succinylcholine in preparation for intubation. *(Ann Emerg Med 16:215, 1987; Arch Neurol 28:274, 1973)*

34. **(A)** The condition known as Lesch-Nyhan syndrome is a disorder of purine metabolism with deficiency of the enzyme hypoxanthine-guanine phosphoribosyl transferase (HGPRT). This X-linked genetic disease causes severe mental retardation, seizures, self-mutilation, and complications associated with hyperuricemia. Children with this condition excrete over 600 mg per day of uric acid, which is about 4x the normal rate. *(Rudolph CD:692)*

35. **(C)** The clinical finding present in both disorders of galactose metabolism is that of cataracts. *Classic galactosemia* is caused by deficiency of the enzyme galactose-1-phosphate uridyl transferase and results in a systemic disorder leading to cataracts, lethargy, hypotonia, metabolic acidosis, and liver dysfunction. The clinical problems start after milk feedings are introduced. Another interesting clinical association is an increased incidence of infection especially with *E. coli. Galactokinase deficiency* produces only cataracts without systemic manifestations. *(Rudolph CD:641:1486)*

36. **(E)** Neonatal meningitis and sepsis most commonly are caused by group B *Streptococcus*, gram-negative enteric bacilli, and *Listeria monocytogenes*. Combination therapy with ampicillin plus gentamicin or ampicillin plus cefotaxime is recommended. Neither the cephalosporins nor gentamicin provides coverage against *L. monocytogenes*. Cefuroxime is not recommended for treatment of meningitis because of reports of

delayed CSF sterilization. *(Tobias:400; Rudolph CD:899, 945)*

37. **(C)** The official tablespoon of the American Standards Association contains 14.79 mL or approximately 15 mL. Home spoons, of course, vary considerably. A teaspoon holds approximately 5 mL. Differences in the size of home teaspoons and tablespoons make this mode of administration unsatisfactory for situations in which accurate dosage is important. Many prescription drugs are dispensed with syringes or calibrated spoons or droppers, essential for drugs such as digoxin or furosemide which require precise dosing. *(Dorland's:1783, 1791)*

38. **(C)** Infantile botulism is caused by the production of toxin by the organism *Clostridium botulinum*. Unlike adult disease which is caused by ingestion of the preformed toxin, disease in infants generally is caused by ingestion of the spores which germinate in the GI tract and produce toxin. Clinical findings include lethargy, hypotonia, and fatigue with repeated motor activity. Constipation typically precedes the other symptoms. CSF examination is unremarkable. Elevated CSF white blood cell count or protein suggests another diagnosis. *(2003 Red Book:243–245; Rudolph CD:917–918)*

39. **(C)** Use of the gluteal muscle as a site for injections in the infant or young child is dangerous. Injury to the sciatic nerve may occur with resultant neuropathy, weakness, or stunting of leg growth. The anterolateral aspect of the thigh is the preferred site in children who are less than 2 years of age. *(Pediatrics 70:944–948, 1982)*

40. **(C)** Penicillin remains the drug of choice for the treatment of syphilis. Treatment requires maintenance of an effective blood level of the antibiotic for about 10 days. This is achieved conveniently with an appropriate dose of benzathine penicillin G as a single injection. *(2003 Red Book:604; Rudolph CD:1002–1005)*

41. **(C)** Most rashes occurring in children receiving ampicillin or amoxicillin do not represent an IgE-mediated immediate-type hypersensitivity reaction. These patients are not at risk of a serious immediate reaction if the medication is taken again. As a matter of fact, such nonurticarial rashes generally do not require that the drug be stopped and do not contraindicate its use again at a later date. Such rashes are especially frequent (up to 90% in some series) when children with Epstein-Barr virus infections receive ampicillin. *(Am J Dis Child 125:187–190, 1973)*.

42. **(A)** High doses of cyclophosphamide results in bladder epithelial dysplasia, hemorrhagic cystitis, and sterility. *(Hay:832)*

43. **(E)** Cocaine results in the liberation of endogenous catecholamines including epinephrine and norepinephrine. These agents increase blood pressure and heart rate via activation of both alpha and beta receptors. Hypertension should be treated with either direct acting vasodilators (sodium nitroprusside, nicardipine, hydralazine) or drugs (labetalol) that block both the alpha and beta receptors. Beta-adrenergic antagonists such as propranolol block only beta receptors leading to unopposed alpha agonism which may actually increase systemic vascular resistance. *(Rudolph CD:377; Tobias:433–436)*

44. **(D)** Methanol (found in windshield washing fluids, solvents, fuels, and paint products) and ethylene glycol (found in antifreeze) ingestions more commonly occur in young children. Methanol is metabolized via alcohol dehydrogenase to formic acid. Formic acid accounts for the majority of the toxicity related to methanol ingestions. The administration of ethanol can slow the conversion of methanol to formic acid (and thereby slow the toxic effects) by competing for the enzyme alcohol dehydrogenase. *(Rudolph CD:371–372)*

45. **(B)** Erythromycin is the drug of choice to prevent spread of pertussis. Administration to the index case generally will eradicate the organism from the tracheobronchial tree and reduce dissemination. Although erythromycin alters the clinical course of pertussis when given early in the paroxysmal stage, it does not seem to alter

the clinical course if started later in the illness. A 14-day course of erythromycin is recommended for prevention and treatment of pertussis. *(2003 Red Book:474–475)*

46. **(E)** Penicillin remains the drug of choice for the treatment of meningococcal meningitis. It is highly effective, inexpensive and, except for allergic reactions, generally free of significant side effects. It has been in clinical use for over four decades, and it is unlikely that previously unrecognized toxic effects will be found. Several of the third-generation cephalosporins are useful for the treatment of *H. influenzae* meningitis and for the treatment of bacterial meningitis prior to identification of the infecting organism. However, once *Neisseria meningitides* has been identified, penicillin becomes the antibiotic of choice. The drug of choice for prophylaxis of close contacts is rifampin, not penicillin. *(2003 Red Book:431; Rudolph CD:970–971)*

47. **(E)** Beta-adrenergic agonists such as terbutaline and albuterol used in the treatment of status asthmaticus are nonspecific agents that activate cardiac beta receptors leading to tachycardia, arrhythmias, and myocardial ischemia. Activation of cellular beta receptors leads to an intracellular shift of potassium with resultant hypokalemia. *(Pediatr Ann 25:394–399, 1996)*

48. **(B)** Methemoglobin contains iron that has been oxidized from the ferrous (2+) state to the ferric (3+) state. Many agents such as nitrites can cause this to happen. Methemoglobin cannot carry oxygen and when methemoglobin levels exceed 30%, tissue hypoxia may occur. Treatment includes the administration of reducing agents such as methylene blue that regenerate hemoglobin. *(Rudolph CD:371–372)*

49. **(B)** Deferoxamine (desferrioxamine) is the chelating agent of choice for iron poisoning. It effectively binds the metal and is excreted in the urine. Deferoxamine is indicated for severe intoxication (ingestion of more than 25 mg/kg of elemental iron or severe illness) or a serum iron concentration exceeding 350 mg/dL. Dimercaprol (BAL) actually enhances the toxicity

of iron and is contraindicated in cases of iron poisoning. *(Tobias:430–431; Rudolph CD:367–368)*

50. **(C)** Organophosphate insecticides of the carbamate class are reversible inhibitors of the enzyme acetylcholinesterase. Atropine reverses the muscarinic action and central nervous system effects of the anticholinesterases. A cholinesterase-reactivating oxime such as pralidoxime (PAM) is effective against both the nicotinic (skeletal muscle paralysis) and the muscarinic as well as the central nervous system effects of the poison. It acts to regenerate the acetylcholinesterase which is inhibited by the toxin. Physostigmine is an acetylcholinesterase inhibitor like the organophosphates and would make the patient worse rather than better. *(Tobias:426–427; Rudolph CD:373–374, 2288)*

51. **(A)** With the aggressive and coordinated use of surgery, radiotherapy and currently available chemotherapeutic agents, the outlook for Wilms tumor is the best of any of the common childhood solid tumors. Overall survival is about 80% and may be as high as 90% in patients with favorable histologic features. *(Rudolph CD: 1614–1616)*

52. **(E)** Metronidazole, chloroquine, diiodohydroxyquin, emetine, and dehydroemetine are effective amebicidal drugs useful in the treatment of enteric infection. Emetine and dehydroemetine are quite toxic (vomiting, abdominal pain, tachycardia, hypotension, and arrhythmias) and generally are indicated only when other, safer agents have failed. Iodoquinol is used for mild or asymptomatic intestinal infection. Metronidazole is employed for more severe intestinal infection and for hepatic abscesses. *(Rudolph CD:1122–1123)*

53. **(B)** Fluoride supplementation is useful from 6 months to about 8 years of age, when calcification of most of the permanent teeth is complete. Supplementation is recommended for children >3 years of age in areas where the water supply contains less than 0.6 ppm of fluoride, for children aged 6 months to 3 years where the water supply contains less than 0.3 pm fluoride, for infants who are exclusively breast-fed, and for

infants who are receiving only ready-to-feed formulas. Fluoride requirement is not related to exposure to sunlight. *(Rudolph CD:1290; MMWR 50:8, 2001)*

54. **(A)** Long-term sequelae of chemotherapy received in childhood is becoming more clearly defined as the survival rates improve. Pulmonary fibrosis most commonly is an adverse effect related to the administration of bleomycin. Pulmonary toxicity is dose related and can be exacerbated by other chemotherapeutic agents. Periodic monitoring of pulmonary function tests is recommended during such therapy. *(Rudolph CD:1609)*

55. **(E)** Neurotoxicity in the form of a peripheral neuropathy can occur with the use of vincristine. This most commonly presents as a peripheral mixed neuropathy involving both the sensory and motor nerves. Sensory loss involves a glove/stocking distribution while foot/ankle drop are the most common motor manifestations. *(Rudolph CD:2229)*

56. **(D)** The most likely diagnosis is acute pancreatitis given this clinical picture. You should also consider gastritis or ulcer. However, the epigastric pain with radiation into the back is more characteristic of pancreatitis. The most likely etiologies of pancreatitis in the pediatric age range include trauma, viral infections, gall bladder disease, drugs and toxins. The latter groups include corticosteroids, alcohol, valproic acid, tetracycline, and furosemide. Diagnostic evaluation should include a serum amylase and lipase. In children, the high GFR may result in rapid clearance of amylase resulting in false negative results. Lipase is cleared more slowly and may aid in the diagnosis. *(Tobias:452–453)*

57. **(C)** This patient with SVT was described with pallor and lethargy, thus indicating an unstable hemodynamic status. For patients with an unstable hemodynamic status, appropriate treatment of supraventricular tachycardia includes immediate electrical synchronized cardioversion (0.5 J/kg). With stable hemodynamics, adenosine is generally considered the drug of choice. Bretylium has no efficacy in the treatment of

atrial arrhythmias and is considered a second line drug for ventricular arrhythmias. *(Tobias: 172–173; Rudolph CD:1854–1855)*

58. **(D)** The goal of therapy in patients with "tet spells" is to increase systemic vascular resistance and relieve infundibular spasm to restore effective pulmonary circulation. Reduction of infundibular spasm includes the use of beta-adrenergic antagonists such as propranolol or esmolol, or opioids such as morphine. Agents to increase systemic vascular resistance and restore left-to-right flow of blood include phenylephrine. Sodium nitroprusside, by decreasing systemic vascular resistance, may increase right-to-left shunting and increase cyanosis. *(Tobias:162; Rudolph CD:1753, 1820–1822)*

59. **(E)** Treatment of gonococcal urethritis depends on achieving a high antimicrobial level in the serum for a short time; prolonged treatment is not required. Benzathine penicillin should never be used as it will not achieve sufficiently high blood levels. Ampicillin 3.0 g orally once, with 1 g of probenecid, or procaine penicillin 4.8 million units IM with 1 g of probenecid is effective against penicillin-sensitive strains. However, penicillin resistance is so common that a single dose of ceftriaxone, 250 mg IM, is generally the treatment of choice. This regimen should be followed with antimicrobial therapy such as doxycycline 100 mg PO bid for 7–10 days, or azithromycin 1 gm as a single oral dose, for possible chlamydial infection. *(Rudolph CD:969)*

60. **(A)** Liver injury is the major toxic effect of acetaminophen poisoning and generally is seen only with large overdoses or poisonings. The hepatic damage is not caused by the acetaminophen itself but rather by a toxic metabolic product. The metabolic pathway producing the hepatotoxic metabolite is less well developed in infants and young children, and therefore, the risks of liver injury are actually somewhat less in young children. Treatment involves oral administration of *N*-acetylcysteine, which minimizes metabolism of the acetaminophen to the toxic metabolite. Treatment is most effective if started within 24 h of ingestion. *(Rudolph CD:360–362)*

61. (D) Naloxone, an effective antagonist to opioids, will reverse the effects of drugs such as morphine and its derivatives. This includes methadone, codeine, pentazocine, and dextropropoxyphene. However, it is not effective against barbiturates such as phenobarbital. *(Rudolph CD:372)*

62. (A) Anecdotal case reports describe therapeutic responses to naloxone including increase in level of consciousness and respiratory function in patients that have ingested the alpha$_2$-adrenergic receptor agonist clonidine. Relatively larger doses of naloxone (up to 0.1 mg/kg) may be needed in distinction to lower doses (0.01 mg/kg) used to reverse opioid-induced respiratory depression. *(Rudolph CD:364)*

63. (C) The numerous side effects of corticosteroids include hyperglycemia, growth retardation, hypertension, osteoporosis, central obesity, moon facies, acne, hirsutism, myopathy, pseudotumor cerebri, cataracts, and glaucoma. *(Am J Dis Child 132:806–810, 1978)*

64. (E) Sotalol is classified as a class III antiarrhythmic based on its ability to alter the cardiac action potential. Although it has intrinsic beta-adrenergic antagonistic effects, these do not account for its therapeutic (antiarrhythmic) effects. All of the other agents are beta-adrenergic antagonists used to control blood pressure and heart rate. *(Rudolph CD:1849–1857)*

65. (B) Penicillin is the drug of choice to treat meningitis or infection related to group B *Streptococcus*. Ampicillin is also an appropriate choice. Treatment should be continued for 14–21 days. *(Rudolph CD:1000–1001)*

66. (E) The patient in question has obvious signs of increased intracranial pressure including Cushing triad and sixth nerve palsy. Ketamine increases ICP and is contraindicated in patients with intracranial hypertension. All of the other agents decrease the cerebral metabolic rate for oxygen and thereby decrease cerebral blood flow and intracranial pressure. *(Tobias:243–257; Pediatr Ann 25:317–328, 1996)*

67. (D) Although not commonly used except in extreme circumstances, the subcutaneous administration of beta agonists including albuterol and epinephrine works quickly in relieving bronchospasm. While inhaled albuterol and ipratropium (an anticholinergic agent) are valuable in the acute setting, cromolyn sodium requires 2—4 weeks of therapy before a beneficial effect is noted. *(Rudolph CD:1956–1960)*

68. (E) Malignant hyperthermia is an inherited metabolic disorder of muscle resulting from defective reuptake of calcium by the sarcoplasmic reticulum. As a result of this disorder, ongoing muscle contraction and metabolism occurs leading to rhabdomyolysis, myoglobinuria, hyperkalemia, acidosis, and hyperthermia. Halothane and succinylcholine are triggering agents and can precipitate an attack. Dantrolene is an effective agent for aborting an attack. Dantrolene blocks the release of calcium from the sarcoplasmic reticulum and prevents further muscle metabolism. *(Rudolph CD:2296)*

69. (B) Carnitine is the carrier involved in the transport of long chain fatty acids across the mitochondrial membrane. Carnitine deficiency can present as a myopathy limited to skeletal muscles, or as a more widespread form including cardiac muscles. *(Rudolph CD:2296–2298)*

70. (C) In newborns with tricuspid atresia, patency of the ductus arteriosus is ensured by the administration of PGE$_1$. This allows for blood to flow from the aorta through the ductus arteriosus, to the pulmonary artery and receive oxygen in the lungs. This blood is returned from the lungs by the pulmonary veins and then crosses over an atrial septal defect or a patent foramen ovale into the left atrium. Surgical palliation then is performed including a systemic-to-pulmonary shunt. *(Rudolph CD:1817)*

71. (D) Nitric oxide is also known as endothelial derived relaxing factor or EDRF. It functions as an autoregulatory compound in many vascular beds especially the lungs. Defects of nitric oxide production in patients with persistent fetal circulation lead to profound hypoxemia. Nitric oxide can now be delivered in a gaseous form as a therapeutic agent. *(Tobias:112–114; Rudolph CD:215–217, 1922)*

72. **(E)** Salicylates are weak acids that in an alkaline medium dissociate to the ionized form. The ionized form does not cross membranes and thus is not readily reabsorbed by the renal tubular cells. Severe cases of salicylate poisoning may require hemodialysis. *(Tobias:432)*

73. **(C)** Aztreonam is the first member of a class of antibiotics known as the monobactams. It is resistant to degradation by beta-lactamase. It has a wide spectrum of activity against gram-negative organisms with limited or no activity against gram-positive organisms. Unlike the aminoglycoside, it is not nephrotoxic. *(Rudolph CD:821–876)*

74. **(A)**, 75. **(B)** The tricyclic antidepressants act as sodium channel blockers in cardiac conduction tissue leading to prolongation of the QRS complex and the potential for the development of wide complex tachyarrhythmias. In addition to the usual supportive care, alkalinization can promptly reverse the cardiovascular changes. The mechanisms involved have not been fully elucidated, but may relate to alterations in the free fraction of the drug or changes in the ratio of ionized to nonionized drug. *(Tobias:436–437; Rudolph CD:364–365)*

76. **(C)** Methotrexate and other folic acid antagonists have been associated with midline facial defects including cleft lip and palate. *(Rudolph CD:775, 1530)*

77. **(C)** There is a significant risk of secondary cases of invasive *H. influenzae* (Hib) disease in susceptible children in the home. Therefore, chemoprophylaxis is recommended for all household contacts when one of the members is less than 48 months of age and is unimmunized or incompletely immunized against Hib. The suggested agent is rifampin and the prophylaxis should be initiated as soon as possible. *(2003 Red Book: 295–296)*

78. **(E)** Methadone has a plasma half-life of 12–24 h depending on the age of the patient. This effect

has been used to improve the quality of analgesia following surgical procedures by allowing a one-time dosing that provides a plasma level high enough to provide analgesia for up to 12 h. Fentanyl is the shortest-acting of the agents listed with a half-life of less than 30 min while the other three opioids have half-lives of 2–4 h. *(Pediatr Clin North Am 41:1269–1292, 1994)*

79. **(A)** Tularemia is a zoonotic infectious disease commonly associated with tick, rabbit, or deer exposure. Several clinical forms of tularemia have been described and are related to mode of infection and the portal of entry of the infecting organism, *Francisella tularensis*. Among children, ulceroglandular and glandular are the most common clinical forms. The recommended antibiotic is streptomycin. *(Rudolph CD:1009)*

80. **(C)** Cryoprecipitate contains factors I (fibrinogen), VIII (antihemophilia factor), and XIII (fibrin stabilizing factor). It also contains von Willebrand factor. It is used to treat deficiencies of fibrinogen which may occur due to disseminated intravascular coagulation or severe liver disease. Due to the relatively high infectious disease risks of cryoprecipitate, factor VIII concentrate is the recommended agent of choice for treatment of classic hemophilia. *(Tobias:341)*

81. **(B)** The patient's hemodynamic profile reveals findings consistent with cardiogenic shock including decreased cardiac output. The body's natural response to this process is to increase systemic vascular resistance in an attempt to maintain perfusion pressure. This is done through the activation of the renin-angiotensin system. Although the increase in SVR maintains blood pressure, the increase in afterload decreases cardiac output. Cardiac output equals stroke volume times heart rate. Stroke volume is controlled by preload, afterload (SVR), and contractility. The inotropic agent chosen should increase contractility and decrease SVR. Dopamine and norepinephrine increase SVR while dobutamine increases contractility and decreases SVR. *(Tobias:26–29)*

82. **(C)** Survival in hemolytic uremic syndrome has improved significantly with the institution of

early dialysis (peritoneal dialysis or hemodialysis). Anticoagulation or thrombolytic agents such as streptokinase have not been shown to improve survival nor has the use of plasmapheresis or the infusion of fresh frozen plasma. Antibiotic therapy is indicated only for documented infections. *(Rudolph CD:1698)*

83. **(A)** Clonidine and alpha-methyldopa (Aldomet) are centrally acting antihypertensive agents that act by decreasing the central sympathetic outflow. If these drugs are discontinued abruptly, rebound hypertension can occur. *(Rudolph CD: 1884)*

84. **(E)** Fluid administration to burn patients is based on estimates provided by various formulas such as the Parkland formula. These estimates are rough guidelines for starting rates for the administration of intravenous fluids. The rates should be adjusted to maintain urine output of 1–2 mL/kg/h. Inadequate urine output reflects depleted intravascular volume. Although it will temporarily increase urine output, the use of diuretics will only further decrease the intravascular volume. *(Tobias:284)*

85. **(B)** The penicillins are all administered as the sodium salt and can be problematic in patients susceptible to sodium or fluid overload. *(Rudolph CD:871–881)*

86. **(B)** Cyanosis due to congenital heart disease in the newborn is generally due to one of the five Ts including all of the above-mentioned answers. Tricuspid atresia is distinguished from the others because of the left-axis deviation on ECG due to the early origin of the left bundle from the common bundle. *(Tobias:161)*

87. **(D)** Antibiotic resistance patterns of *P. aeruginosa* vary from hospital to hospital, but many strains are sensitive to aminoglycosides, ciprofloxacin, aztreonam, and ticarcillin. Due to the rapid emergence of resistance, double therapy (usually a semisynthetic penicillin and aminoglycoside) is recommended. Ceftriaxone has very limited activity against this organism. *(Rudolph CD:924)*

88. **(B)** The anion gap is calculated by subtracting the serum bicarbonate and chloride from the serum sodium. Increased anion gap, suggesting the presence of an unmeasured acid, is seen with each of the aforementioned conditions except proximal renal tubular acidosis. In this condition, excessive loss of bicarbonate by the kidneys is compensated for by an increase in chloride reabsorption. This results in a normal anion gap. *(Rudolph CD:1710)*

89. **(C)** Nephrogenic diabetes insipidus may be caused by lithium. In this disorder, the plasma levels of ADH are normal; however, there is a defect in the response of the renal tubular cells to the ADH. As a result, the patient develops excessive loss of free water with an increase in the serum sodium. The diagnosis rests on the identification of a high serum osmolality with a low urine osmolality and no response to the administration of exogenous ADH. Treatment includes discontinuation of lithium and slow replacement of free water. *(Rudolph CD:1714)*

90. **(E)** As chemotherapy of leukemia has intensified, hyperuricemia as a complication of cell death (the *tumor-lysis syndrome*) has become more frequent. One of the major dangers of this complication is uric acid nephropathy with acute renal failure. Other problems include hyperphosphatemia (with secondary hypocalcemia) and hyperkalemia. Allopurinol inhibits the enzyme that accelerates the conversion of xanthine and hypoxanthine to uric acid and is used to prevent hyperuricemia in children at risk for the tumor-lysis syndrome when receiving chemotherapy. This primarily includes children with large tumor masses (lymphomas and leukemia with very high peripheral white blood cell counts) likely to respond to chemotherapy. *(Rudolph CD:1606)*

91. **(E)** Propranolol is a beta-adrenergic blocking agent that is useful in the management of chronic paroxysmal supraventricular tachycardias, especially when associated with the Wolff-Parkinson-White syndrome. The drug is contraindicated in conditions where beta-adrenergic blockade would be disadvantageous including asthma, abnormalities of cardiac

conduction, and myocardial dysfunction. *(Rudolph CD:1854–1857)*

92. (C) The child described most likely has viral croup (laryngotracheobronchitis). This common but potentially life-threatening seasonal condition is most often seen in children ages 3 months to 3 years. The administration of dexamethasone at a dose of at least 0.6 mg/kg has been shown to decrease the duration and severity of respiratory symptoms. Also important is the parental education and support. *(Rudolph CD:1275–1276)*

BIBLIOGRAPHY

American Academy of Pediatrics. *Report of the Committee on Infectious Diseases*, 26th ed. Elk Grove, IL: American Academy of Pediatrics, 2003.

American Academy of Pediatrics Committee on Quality Improvement, Subcommittee on Attention-Deficit/ Hyperactivity Disorder. Clinical practice guideline: diagnosis and evaluation of the child with attention-deficit/hyperactivity disorder. *Pediatrics* 2000;105: 1158–1170.

Bergeson PS, Singer SA, Kaplan AM. Intramuscular injections in children. *Pediatrics* 1982;70:944–948.

Cherington M, Lasater G. Prolonged paralysis in pseudo-cholinesterase deficiency. *Arch Neurol* 1973; 274–275.

Dorland's Illustrated Medical Dictionary, 29th ed. Philadelphia, PA: W.B. Saunders, 1999.

Hay WW, Hayward AR, Levin MJ, Sondheimer JM. *Current Pediatric Diagnosis & Treatment*, 16th ed. New York, NY: McGraw-Hill, 2003.

Kerns D, Shira JE. Ampicillin rash in children. Relationship to penicillin allergy and infectious mononucleosis. *Am J Dis Child* 1973;125:187–190.

Nichols DJ. Emergency management of status asthmaticus in children. *Pediatr Ann* 1996;25:394–400.

Rimsza ME. Complications of corticosteroid therapy. *Am J Dis Child* 1978;132:806–810.

Rudolph CD, Rudolph AM, Hostetter MK, et al. *Rudolph's Pediatrics*, 21st ed. New York, NY: McGraw-Hill, 2003.

Selden BS, Curry SC. Prolonged succinylcholine-induced paralysis in organophosphate insecticide poisoning. *Ann Emerg Med* 1987;215–217.

Tobias JD. Airway management for pediatric emergencies. *Pediatr Ann* 1996;25:317–328.

Tobias JD. Pain management and sedation in the pediatric intensive care unit. *Pediatr Clin North Am* 1994;41:1269–1292.

Tobias JD. *Pediatric Critical Care: The Essentials*. Armonk, NY: Futura Publishing Co., 1999.

Tobias JD. Postoperative pain management. *Pediatr Ann* 1997;26:490–500.

U.S. Department of Health and Human Services. Recommendations for using fluoride to prevent and control dental caries in the United States. *MMWR* 2001; 50:1–42.

CHAPTER 10

Case Diagnosis and Management

Mark A. Ward, MD

Joseph Y. Allen, MD

This chapter contains clinical scenarios followed by a set of questions. These "real life" scenarios and questions are designed to assess the examinee's clinical judgment and practical thinking ability as well as her or his fund of knowledge. Case-based questions are common on national examinations, so it is important to become comfortable with them. To maximize your learning experience, answer all of the questions about the case before looking at the answers. And, refrain from looking ahead at the next question about the case in hopes of obtaining additional information for the question at hand. Not only would this negate the learning-testing experience, it might actually lead to an incorrect answer! For example, diagnostic or therapeutic steps that might be correct later in the case might by considered incorrect earlier when certain information was not available.

Questions

Questions 1 through 3

An 18-month-old male toddler presents with pallor. He drinks 64 oz of cow milk per day. The examination is significant only for an obese and playful male with pallor. Stool is negative for blood.

1. Which lab test would most likely reveal the diagnosis?

    (A) chest x-ray
    (B) examination of stool for ova and parasites
    (C) complete blood count
    (D) serum haptoglobin
    (E) bone marrow aspirate

2. Testing reveals a mean corpuscular volume of 60 fL (nL 72–86 fL) and an elevated red cell distribution width. The most likely diagnosis is

    (A) B_{12} deficiency
    (B) B-cell leukemia
    (C) hemosiderosis
    (D) iron deficiency anemia
    (E) sickle cell disease

3. Appropriate therapy is started for this patient. When should reticulocytosis peak?

    (A) 12–24 h
    (B) 1–3 days
    (C) 5–10 days
    (D) 2–4 weeks
    (E) 1–2 months

Questions 4 through 6

A 10-month-old female presents in winter with 2 days of rhinorrhea, tachypnea, and wheezing. She has respirations of 60 breaths/min, heart rate of 160 bpm, and an oxygen saturation of 90% on room air. Examination reveals an alert infant in mild respiratory distress with mild intercostals retractions and coarse bilateral expiratory wheezing.

4. Appropriate therapy for this infant should begin with

    (A) intravenous access and a 20 cc/kg bolus of normal saline
    (B) oxygen by nasal canula
    (C) bag-valve mask followed by rapid sequence intubation
    (D) posterior-anterior and lateral chest radiographs
    (E) intravenous corticosteroids

5. Chest radiography reveals bilateral air trapping, chest hyperexpansion, and peribronchial thickening. The most likely diagnosis is

    (A) congestive heart failure
    (B) acute respiratory distress syndrome (ARDS)
    (C) pneumococcal pneumonia

(D) *Mycoplasma pneumoniae* pneumonia

(E) viral bronchiolitis

6. Additional therapeutic options for this patient include

(A) inhaled beta agonist therapy

(B) ribavirin

(C) RSV hyperimmune globulin (Respigam)

(D) palivizumab (Synagis)

(E) Heliox

Questions 7 through 9

A 6-year-old previously well male presents with 1 week of worsening elbow swelling and fever. He denies trauma. Examination reveals a male in mild distress with a temperature to 102°F. His left elbow is warm, erythematous, edematous, and tender around the joint. He is holding it in mid-flexion and strongly resists passive movement.

7. The most likely offending organism for his condition is

(A) *Neiserria gonorrhea*

(B) group B *Streptococcus*

(C) *Pseudomonas aeruginosa*

(D) *Mycobacteria tuberculosis*

(E) *Staphylococcus aureus*

8. Which of the following should be performed first?

(A) administration of oral antibiotics

(B) arthrocentesis of left elbow

(C) administration of nonsteroidal anti-inflammatory agents

(D) fasciotomy of the affected limb

(E) laboratory evaluation for immunologic deficiencies

9. Which of the following is a poor prognostic factor for this condition?

(A) age greater than 6 months

(B) gram-positive infection

(C) absence of physeal involvement

(D) positive Gram stain of joint fluid

(E) hip or shoulder involvement

Questions 10 and 11

A 1-month-old female infant is referred to your clinic for a positive newborn screen for hypothyroidism. On history, the mom reports she is "a good baby who sleeps all the time but is a slow eater." She was jaundiced for the first 2 weeks and stools twice a week. Examination reveals an awake infant with a large tongue, cool skin, a large umbilical hernia, edematous extremities, and hypotonia.

10. The most likely cause of this infant's condition is

(A) maternal ingestion of propylthiouracil

(B) thyroid dysgenesis

(C) iodide transport defects

(D) thyrotropin deficiency

(E) thyrotropin receptor–blocking antibodies

11. Which of the following management options should be initiated next?

(A) thyroxine therapy at a dose of 10–15 µg/kg per day

(B) thyroid scintiscan at the next available date

(C) neurodevelopmental consultation

(D) radiographs of the legs

(E) confirmation of the state screen findings with a TSH level

Questions 12 through 14

A 4-year-old previously healthy boy presents with 1 day of scrotal swelling. His mother noted his scrotum to be markedly swollen and thinks his eyes are puffy. Examination reveals an afebrile child with a blood pressure of 90/50 mmHg. He is alert with significant bilateral periorbital edema. His abdomen has ascites with no organomegaly. His scrotum and lower extremities have tense pitting edema.

12. The initial lab test most likely to point to the etiology of his illness is

(A) chest radiograph

(B) liver biopsy

(C) urinalysis

(D) hepatitis panel

(E) stool guaiac and pH

13. Subsequent testing reveals a serum albumin of 1 g/dL, a cholesterol level of 560 mg/dL (nL 109–189 mg/dL) and normal complement and liver enzyme levels. The most likely diagnosis for this patient is

   (A) membranous glomerulonephritis
   (B) focal segmental glomerulosclerosis
   (C) poststreptococcal glomerulonephritis
   (D) membranoproliferative glomeru-lonephritis
   (E) minimal-change disease

14. Which of the following statements regarding this patient's most likely condition is true?

   (A) It almost never responds to steroid therapy.
   (B) Spontaneous bacterial peritonitis is not a concern.
   (C) These patients have an increased tendency to hemorrhage.
   (D) A low salt diet is essential during flares of the illness.
   (E) Nonresponse to therapy for at least 1 year should prompt a nephrology referral for biopsy.

Questions 15 through 17
A 7-year-old well female presents to your emergency department with episodic headache and hypertension. During the episodes she is sleepy, complains of headaches, vomits, and becomes sweaty. Her current vital signs are: T 101°F, HR 150 bpm, BP 220/130 mmHg. She is diaphoretic, sleepy but arousable, and clutches her head. Pupils are reactive and papilledema is present. There is no organomegaly and femoral pulses are normal.

15. After determining that her airway is intact and breathing sufficient, the first course of action should be

   (A) immediate CT scan of the head to evaluate for a mass lesion
   (B) lumbar puncture to rule out meningitis
   (C) administration of an antihypertensive medication

   (D) administration of a benzodiazepine to relieve the patient's anxiety
   (E) placement of a large bore central catheter for dialysis

16. Her vital signs are stabilized on the appropriate therapy. Now happy and interactive, she is transferred to the ICU. The option most likely to lead to a diagnosis is

   (A) magnetic resonance imaging of the brain
   (B) urine for catecholamines
   (C) ECG and echocardiography
   (D) inquiry into a family history of essential hypertension
   (E) surgical consult for laparotomy

17. The urinary vanillyl mandelic acid level returns at 400 mg/g creatinine (nL < 8 mg/g creatinine). Treatment for this condition is

   (A) surgical removal of all tissue
   (B) radiologic injection of cyclophosphamide directly
   (C) watchful waiting as most regress spontaneously
   (D) oral mineralcorticoid therapy
   (E) oral propylthiouracil therapy

Questions 18 through 20
You are seeing a 7-day-old male infant for a well child check. The baby is breastfeeding well. He has had no fever or emesis. He passed his first stool at 3 days of age, and has not passed another stool. Examination reveals an afebrile, well-appearing and vigorous baby. The abdomen is firm and slightly distended with bowel sounds present. The perianal area is slightly erythematous and rectal examination reveals increased tone with no stool present in the rectal vault.

18. Of the following, which is the best initial diagnostic test?

   (A) stool culture for *Clostridium botulinum*
   (B) abdominal ultrasound
   (C) serum TSH
   (D) barium enema
   (E) diagnostic trial of mineral oil

19. The initial diagnostic approach is unsuccessful. The best test to perform next to diagnose this patient is

(A) serum TSH

(B) stool for esosinophils

(C) anal manometry

(D) upper gastrointestinal series with small bowel follow through

(E) rectal biopsy

20. Testing reveals an absence of the Meissner and Auerbach plexus. With proper treatment, the prognosis for this patient is that he will

(A) likely be continent

(B) need a colostomy for his entire childhood

(C) need a total colectomy and likely have serious incontinence problems

(D) need a small bowel transplant and require lifelong parenteral nutrition

(E) be at great risk for frequent life-threatening intraabdominal infections

Questions 21 and 22

A previously well 2-year-old girl is brought to you for evaluation of a "broken elbow." The father reports swinging her round and round by her left arm and leg. She now is crying and not moving her left arm as it is held in a flexed and slightly pronated position at her side. No effusions or point tenderness are discernible.

21. The most appropriate initial management is

(A) intravenous line placement for sedation and reduction

(B) hyperpronation or supination-flexion of the arm

(C) complete blood count and erythrocyte sedimentation rate

(D) social work evaluation for abuse

(E) radiographic evaluation of the left elbow

22. When counseling the father regarding his child's condition, you should tell him the following:

(A) recurrence is unlikely

(B) splinting at bedtime is desirable

(C) gymnastics should be avoided

(D) suspicion of abuse requires that you report this injury

(E) children outgrow predisposition for this condition

Questions 23 through 25

A 16-year-old female living in a shelter presents with 3 days of worsening lower abdominal pain. She reports multiple unprotected sexual encounters. She is febrile to 39°C and is ill appearing. She has bilateral lower quadrant tenderness without rebound. Her pelvic examination reveals purulent vaginal discharge with adnexal and cervical motion tenderness. Pregnancy test is negative.

23. The most appropriate management strategy at this time is

(A) inpatient admission with intravenous antibiotics for pelvic inflammatory disease

(B) social service referral for in loco parentis designation prior to initiation of therapy

(C) initiation of antibiotic therapy in the emergency department and discharge with close outpatient follow-up

(D) urinalyis and empiric intramuscular antibiotic therapy for cystitis

(E) nonsteroidal therapy and oral contraceptive pills for pregnancy prophylaxis

24. The patient remains febrile and has worsening abdominal pain despite 72 h of antibiotic therapy. At this time you decide to

(A) continue therapy at the scheduled doses

(B) add diphenhydramine for a potential drug reaction

(C) consult gynecology for imaging and drainage of a possible tubo-ovarian abscess

(D) repeat blood cultures and obtain a C-reactive protein to help monitor response to therapy

(E) consult infectious disease for evaluation of the possibility of methicillin-resistant *Staphylococcus aureus* infection

25. The patient improves and is ready for discharge. A true statement about this patient's condition is

    (A) recurrence is rare
    (B) recurrence is associated with an increased risk of infertility
    (C) douching and oral contraceptives may decrease the risk of recurrence
    (D) male partners with *Neiserria gonorrheae* are always symptomatic
    (E) ectopic pregnancies are not a concern after PID

Questions 26 and 27
An 11-year-old boy presents after cutting his ankle on a rusty piece of metal at the junkyard. His father reports he is positive his son's immunizations are current because the patient received booster doses just prior to kindergarten at 5 years of age. Examination reveals a healthy boy in no distress with a 4 cm bleeding laceration on the posterior aspect of the lower leg.

26. The first step in management of this wound is

    (A) radiography to evaluate for metallic particles
    (B) irrigation of the wound with normal saline
    (C) intravenous antibiotics directed against gram-positive organisms
    (D) surgery assistance for this complicated injury
    (E) direct pressure on the wound for hemostasis

27. The wound is treated. For tetanus prophylaxis, which of the following should this patient receive?

    (A) no prophylaxis
    (B) Td only
    (C) Td and tetanus immune globulin (TIG)
    (D) DTP
    (E) TIG only

Questions 28 and 29
A 6-month-old boy is brought in by his mother for crying. Your examination reveals a thin boy with tender swelling around the midshaft of his left femur. He cries when the leg is manipulated, but is comfortable when left alone. An x-ray reveals a transverse midshaft femur fracture. The father tells you the patient's 16-month-old brother lifted him off the bed and dropped him on the floor earlier that evening.

28. The next step in the management of this patient is

    (A) confrontation of the parents regarding the history of the injury
    (B) MRI of left lower extremity
    (C) skeletal survey
    (D) internal fixation of the fracture
    (E) fibroblast assay

29. During the evaluation the father asks that they be discharged immediately as he has to be at work early. The best response to this is to

    (A) let them go home and follow up with their pediatrician the next day
    (B) splint the child with follow-up by an orthopedist
    (C) call security to forcibly incarcerate the father
    (D) directly confront the parents of their complicity in allowing this to happen
    (E) inform the family that the safety of the child may be at risk as the history given does not match with her pattern of injuries

Questions 30 and 31
A 3-month-old female presents with 2 days of crying and decreased oral intake. She is afebrile, HR is 280 bpm, and BP is 85/40 mmHg. Her saturations are 99% on room air. She is alert and easily consolable, her lungs are clear, and she is tachycardic with no murmurs audible. There is no organomegaly and the peripheral pulses are normal in strength.

30. The first test to order to confirm the diagnosis is

   (A) complete blood count and differential
   (B) echocardiogram
   (C) blood glucose
   (D) thyroxine and TSH levels
   (E) electrocardiogram

31. Her heart rate and blood pressure remain unchanged after testing. The initial treatment for the most likely cause of her condition is

   (A) adenosine
   (B) defibrillation
   (C) verapamil
   (D) digoxin
   (E) ibuprofen

Questions 32 and 33

A 15-year-old previously well female presents with 1 week of hair loss. She denies fever, weight loss, or medications. On examination, she is pleasant but nervous about her hair loss. Her scalp reveals patches of complete hair loss with small broken hair that easily pull out at the edges. The scalp is smooth and no inflammation is seen. Microscopic examination of the shafts reveals the stubs to resemble exclamation points.

32. The most likely illness this patient has is

   (A) tinea capitis
   (B) alopecia areata
   (C) trichotillomania
   (D) hair traction alopecia
   (E) chemical exposure

33. You tell the patient the likely course of this illness is

   (A) spontaneous resolution
   (B) resolution after chemotherapy
   (C) difficult to predict
   (D) progression to total hair loss and then resolution
   (E) improvement with dietary change

Questions 34 through 36

A 6-month-old female develops a persistent cough with progressively worsening paroxysms and cyanosis. There is occasional posttussive emesis. The child is afebrile. Between coughing spells, the physical examination is normal.

34. At this time it would be most important to ask the family regarding

   (A) birth weight
   (B) immunizations
   (C) consanguinity
   (D) early infant deaths in relatives
   (E) family history of reactive airways disease

35. The white blood cell count on the patient is 32,000/mm^3, with 80% lymphocytes and 2% mononuclear cells. At this time it would be appropriate to

   (A) order a bone marrow examination
   (B) prescribe intravenous gammaglobulin
   (C) prescribe oral erythromycin
   (D) perform a lumbar puncture
   (E) repeat the blood count in 24 h

36. The most appropriate method to identify the responsible organism is via

   (A) throat swab
   (B) nasopharyngeal swab
   (C) blood culture
   (D) sputum culture
   (E) bronchoscopy

Questions 37 through 39

A 17-year-old female presents to your clinic with complaints of recurrent headaches for 6 months. They are described as circumferential; onset is not associated with time of day. There has been no emesis and the headaches have not interfered with activities. Her weight is 140 kg and her blood pressure is 140/90 mmHg. Her examination reveals bilateral papilledema, and an otherwise normal neurologic examination.

37.   The next step in management of this patient is

(A)   oral administration of nifedipine
(B)   determination of renin levels
(C)   intravenous nitroprusside drip
(D)   computerized tomography of the head
(E)   intravenous mannitol and furosemide

38.   The imaging study is normal, reveals no mass and normal sized ventricles. At this point you should

(A)   perform lumbar puncture
(B)   treat with dexamethasone
(C)   treat with acetazolamide
(D)   refer her for opthalmalogic evaluation
(E)   refer her for psychiatric evaluation

39.   You proceed and she has relief from her symptoms. Despite appropriate care she begins to develop visual loss and optic nerve atrophy is suspected. Your best course of action is now

(A)   increasing the dose of dexamethasone
(B)   increasing the frequency of lumbar punctures
(C)   increasing the dose of acetozolamide
(D)   referral her to a surgeon for gastric banding to speed up weight loss
(E)   referral to an ophthalmologist for evaluation for optic nerve fenestration

Questions 40 through 42
A 10-month-old female presents to the ED with a 2-day history of runny nose and fever to 102°F. On examination, her temperature is 103°F, HR 140 bpm, and a RR 30 times/min. She is alert and playful with copious rhinorrhea. After the examination is complete she becomes stiff and displays tonic-clonic movements of all four extremities.

40.   The most important first task is to

(A)   obtain whole blood glucose
(B)   administer intravenous lorazepam (Ativan)
(C)   perform lumbar puncture
(D)   establish airway patency
(E)   administer intramuscular fosphenytoin (Cerebyx)

41.   After 5 min, the seizure ceases and the respiratory rate is 30 breaths/min. The patient is sleepy but arousable. Fundoscopic examination is normal as is the remainder of the physical examination. Rectal acetaminophen is given. Which of the following tests should be performed at this time?

(A)   electroencephalogram
(B)   skull radiographs
(C)   arterial blood gas
(D)   computerized tomography scan of the head
(E)   lumbar puncture

42.   The patient quickly becomes alert, happy, and playful. She is afebrile and has a normal examination. All ordered tests are normal. Which of the following management plans is most appropriate at this time?

(A)   discharge home after instructions regarding home management of fever and seizures
(B)   discharge home on phenytoin
(C)   discharge home on phenobarbital
(D)   discharge home with alternating doses of ibuprofen and acetaminophen every 3 h for the next 3 days
(E)   admission for observation and MRI

Questions 43 through 45
A 6-year-old female presents with short stature. Her family reports she has been well and has had no other medical problems. Her diet and review of systems is unremarkable.

43.   Which of the following would be most important to know at this time?

(A)   maternal age at menarche
(B)   parental growth rate and height
(C)   paternal age at conception
(D)   maternal age at conception
(E)   sibling growth rate and height

44. The physical examination reveals a pleasant girl at less than the 5th percentile for height and 10th percentile for weight. In addition to her short stature, she has a broad chest, cubitum valgum, and 2/6 systolic ejection murmur at the right upper sternal border. The test most likely to confirm the etiology of her short stature at this time is

  (A) serum LH/FSH levels

  (B) abdominal ultrasound

  (C) growth hormone levels

  (D) karyotype

  (E) bone age analysis of the nondominant hand

45. Of the following management options, which is indicated for this patient?

  (A) transthoracic echocardiogram

  (B) halo bracing for cervical laxity

  (C) counseling regarding the likelihood of severe mental deficiency

  (D) hysterectomy to prevent the development of endometrial carcinoma

  (E) initiation of thyroid hormone replacement therapy

Questions 46 through 48

A 13-month-old boy presents with 5 days of fever to 103°F. His temperature is 102.8°F, HR 160 bpm, and RR 36 times/min. On examination, he is found to be irritable with markedly injected conjunctiva, a strawberry tongue, and red cracked lips. A 2 cm lymph node is present in the left anterior cervical chain. There is no meningismus. His lungs are clear and he is tachycardic. A diffuse erythematous blanching rash is present on his chest and extremities. No desquamation of the fingertips is noted.

46. The disease most likely to be causing this constellation of symptoms is diagnosed by

  (A) complete blood count

  (B) erythrocyte sedimentation rate

  (C) viral culture

  (D) clinical judgment

  (E) presence of antinuclear antibody

47. After the diagnosis is confirmed, therapy is initiated with improvement in symptoms within 24 h. Which of the following complications is most likely to occur in this illness?

  (A) thrombocytopenia

  (B) sterility

  (C) hydrops of the gallbladder

  (D) ulcerative colitis

  (E) transverse myelitis

48. Prior to discharge the parents state that their child needs his immunizations updated. You should counsel the parents that their son should

  (A) stay on schedule for his vaccinations

  (B) have measles and varicella immunizations deferred for several months after IVIG

  (C) not be given diphtheria-tetanus-acellular pertussis vaccine because it may potentiate a relapse of his illness

  (D) not receive influenza vaccine because he will be on chronic aspirin therapy

  (E) have his primary series of vaccines repeated

Questions 49 and 50

A 2-year-old is brought to your emergency department for refusal to walk after he tripped and fell while running. Examination reveals a well-appearing afebrile child in no distress. His left leg has full range of motion and some point tenderness in the distal tibia.

49. The most appropriate first step in your evaluation is to obtain

  (A) a C-reactive protein

  (B) a blood culture

  (C) radiographs of the tibia

  (D) a social work consultation

  (E) a serum alkaline phosphatase

50. Your initial evaluation confirms your suspicion. At this point you should

    (A) make a referral to child protective services for abuse

    (B) place a long-term intravenous catheter for intravenous antibiotics

    (C) arrange an immediate orthopedic referral

    (D) perform a needle aspirate of the affected area

    (E) immobilize the affected limb in a splint with outpatient follow-up

Questions 51 through 53

You are called to the nursery to evaluate a 3-day-old full-term male infant with lethargy. The nurse reports the infant was feeding well on standard formula until 4 h previously. He has had no emesis. There is no maternal history of fever or rash. The infant currently is afebrile with a HR 110 bpm, RR of 50 times/min, and a BP of 80/45 mmHg. He is lethargic but the examination is otherwise unremarkable. There are no dysmorphic features. Whole blood glucose is normal. Serum calcium and electrolyte results are pending.

51. The next step in the evaluation should be to

    (A) obtain emergent abdominal ultrasound

    (B) obtain complete blood count, urinalysis and lumbar puncture as well as cultures of blood, urine, and CSF

    (C) urine drug screen

    (D) obtain emergent upper gastrointestinal series with small bowel follow through

    (E) obtain emergent magnetic resonance imaging of the head to evaluate for an intracranial hemorrhage

52. The neonatal evaluation for sepsis is complete and the neonate is placed on antibiotics. The next day there is no evidence of infection and the infant has not improved. Additional studies are obtained, including a serum ammonia which is 1150 µmol/L (nL 64–107) and a blood pH of 7.36. Medical therapy is initiated. The urinary orotic acid level returns and is markedly elevated as well. At this point the most likely diagnosis is

    (A) ornithine transcarbamylase deficiency

    (B) carbamoyl synthetase deficiency

    (C) methylmalonic academia

    (D) carnitine palmitoyl transferase deficiency

    (E) glycogen synthetase deficiency

53. Six hours after institution of treatment with appropriate intravenous doses of arginine the serum ammonia is 1200 µmol/L. The best course of action at this time is

    (A) increase the rate of IV arginine to clear ammonia faster

    (B) begin a double volume exchange transfusion

    (C) transfer the patient to a center where hemodialysis can be performed

    (D) discuss DNR status with the family

    (E) allow another 6 h of therapy as ammonia in tissue needs to be metabolized first and therapy can be toxic as well

Questions 54 through 56

A 3-year-old girl is seen in the emergency department for bruising. Her family denies fever or weight loss but state she had a "cold" 3 weeks ago. She is afebrile and the remaining vital signs are normal. She is happy and playful and has generalized ecchymoses and petechiae.

54. The first test to obtain is a

    (A) bone marrow aspirate

    (B) *Neiserria meningitidis* latex assay of the cerebrospinal fluid

    (C) *Rickettsia rickettsiae* serology

    (D) skeletal survey looking for healing fractures

    (E) complete blood count and differential

55. The labs return and the platelets are 10,000/mm³. A bone marrow aspirate demonstrates increased megakaryocytes but is otherwise normal. Which of the following is an indication for WinRho (anti-RhoD antibodies)?

    (A) platelet count less than 100,000/mm³

    (B) fever greater than 39°C

    (C) splenomegaly

(D) epistaxis

(E) bone marrow with megakaryocyte hypoplasia

56. Which of the following would be an indication for splenectomy in this patient?

   (A) platelet count below 10,000/mm^3

   (B) gingival bleeding

   (C) persistence of thrombocytopenia for more than 1 month

   (D) persistence of thrombocytopenia for more than 1–2 years

   (E) presence of splenomegaly and anemia

Questions 57 and 58
A 4-year-old boy presents to the emergency department with a chief complaint of pallor. He was well until 1 week previously when he developed bloody diarrhea that resolved with oral antibiotics. He is afebrile with a BP of 150/100 mmHg and a HR of 130 bpm. He is alert and fundoscopic examination is normal. His examination is significant for pallor.

57. The test most likely test to reveal the diagnosis is

   (A) complete blood count and smear

   (B) stool culture

   (C) computerized tomography of the head

   (D) renal ultrasound

   (E) urine myoglobin levels

58. The laboratory results reveal a hemoglobin of 8 g/dL, a BUN and creatinine of 40 and 1.8, respectively. The urine output is normal. Regarding the treatment of this disease you tell the family that

   (A) aggressive medical management and dialysis result in the majority of the patients doing well

   (B) high dose steroids are essential in the treatment of this illness

   (C) most patients eventually require renal transplantation

   (D) antibiotics need to be continued for 21 days

   (E) recurrence of this illness is frequent

Questions 59 and 60
An 18-month-old female presents to the emergency department with fever to 102°F, a barky cough, and stridor. The examination shows a RR of 60 breaths/min with an oxygen saturation of 95% while breathing room air, marked stridor, moderate substernal retractions, and equal aeration without wheezes or rhonchi.

59. As the patient is being evaluated, initial therapy for this patient should begin with

   (A) acetaminophen per rectum

   (B) nebulized dexamethasone

   (C) nebulized racemic epinephrine

   (D) humidified air only in a position of comfort

   (E) stat portable AP and lateral neck films

60. Despite therapy the patient becomes more toxic appearing and is drooling. The parents subsequently report the child has received no immunizations. Her respiratory rate is now 70 times/min and she appears sleepy. At this point the best intervention is

   (A) blind intubation with a laryngeal mask airway

   (B) humidified oxygen and observation with the patient in a position of comfort

   (C) rapid sequence intubation in the emergency department

   (D) anesthesia assistance for intubation in the operating room with surgical availability

   (E) prompt administration of intravenous cefotaxime (Claforan)

Questions 61 and 62
A 12-year-old male presents to the office with wheezing and increased work of breathing for the fifth time in the past year. On examination, his RR is 30 breaths/min and oxygen saturation is 98% while breathing room air. He is talking in complete sentences and there is expiratory wheezing with a prolonged expiratory phase.

61. The first treatment he should receive is

    (A) nebulized beta agonist therapy
    (B) intravenous beta agonist therapy
    (C) subcutaneous epinephrine
    (D) oxygen via 15 L nonrebreather
    (E) intramuscular steroids

62. The patient improves after receiving the treatment selected. Further history reveals that the patient has been using inhaled albuterol three times per week to control wheezing. In addition to albuterol and a short course of oral steroids the best additional medicine he should receive is

    (A) epinephrine auto injector (Epi-Pen) to used as needed
    (B) salmeterol (Serevent) to be used in divided doses daily
    (C) fluticasone (Flovent) to be used in divided doses daily
    (D) theophylline to be used in divided doses daily
    (E) cetirizine (Zyrtec) to be used in divided doses daily

Questions 63 through 65
A previously well 9-year-old Hispanic male presents with 2 days of yellow eyes and abdominal pain. He visited Mexico 1 month previously. On examination he is febrile to 101°F, has scleral icterus, and moderate right upper quadrant tenderness. The liver is moderately enlarged.

63. What would be the most helpful additional history?

    (A) sickle cell disease in the family
    (B) excessive carrot intake
    (C) history of malar rash
    (D) acetaminophen usage
    (E) vaccination status prior to travel

64. The test most likely to confirm his diagnosis is

    (A) hepatitis A serology
    (B) hepatitis B serology
    (C) 24-h copper excretion

    (D) abdominal ultrasound
    (E) acetaminophen level

65. Diagnostic testing confirms the diagnosis and the family has questions about the disease. You tell them

    (A) an effective vaccine is not routinely available
    (B) the recurrence risk is approximately 25%
    (C) if he were to contract hepatitis D simultaneously he would likely need a liver transplant
    (D) fulminant hepatitis is uncommon in children with hepatitis A infection
    (E) intimate sexual contact is the most common route of transmission

Questions 66 through 68
You are called to see a 2-h-old male with cyanosis and tachypnea. Oxygen saturation is 80% while breathing room air and the RR is 60 breaths/min with a BP of 80/50 mmHg. The baby is cyanotic and there are no murmurs. The rest of the examination is unremarkable. The baby is placed in on an FiO_2 of 1.0 by head hood and arterial blood gases reveal the PaO_2 to be 30 mmHg.

66. The most likely etiology of the hypoxemia is

    (A) methemoglobinemia
    (B) cyanotic congenital heart disease
    (C) sepsis
    (D) pneumonia
    (E) arteriovenous fistula

67. A chest x-ray shows normal lung fields, slightly generous cardiothymic silhouette, and a narrow upper mediastinum. An electrocardiogram is normal. The most likely diagnosis based on this information would be

    (A) transposition of the great arteries
    (B) tetralogy of Fallot
    (C) ventricular septal defect
    (D) endocardial fibroelastosis
    (E) total anomalous pulmonary venous return

68. The airway is stabilized and prostaglandin E$_1$ therapy is initiated. Echocardiography confirms the diagnosis. At this point the best intervention is

(A) emergent cardiac catheterization and atrial septostomy

(B) nothing until the patient's hypoxemia improves

(C) empiric antibiotics for sepsis

(D) emergent cardiovascular surgery consultation for immediate arterial switch

(E) dobutamine and milrinone to enhance cardiac function

Questions 69 through 71
A 6-year-old previously well African American child presents with new onset jaundice, dark urine, and pallor. There is a history of a recent mild upper respiratory tract infection. Vital signs are normal. Physical examination is remarkable for icterus and pallor. Laboratory examination reveals a hemoglobin of 7 g/dL with a normal platelet and white blood cell count. The total bilirubin is 4 mg/dL.

69. Which of the following historical findings is most likely to indicate the diagnosis?

(A) His father has sickle cell trait.

(B) Baby aspirin given to him last year was associated with dark urine.

(C) His grandmother was diagnosed with leukemia last year.

(D) He was diagnosed as being iron deficient 4 years ago.

(E) His healthy cousin returned from a trip to Mexico 1 month ago.

70. The bilirubin is predominantly unconjugated and the reticulocyte count is 12%. Further history reveals that for the past 2 days he has been given an antibiotic that his grandfather was taking for a urinary tract infection. What is the most likely diagnosis?

(A) sickle cell disease

(B) preleukemia

(C) infectious hepatitis

(D) spherocytosis

(E) glucose-6-phophate-dehydrogenase deficiency

71. The most appropriate management at this time is

(A) immediate transfusion to bring the hemoglobin to 14 g/dL

(B) immediate transfusion to bring the hemoglobin to 10 g/dL

(C) withhold transfusion and follow vital signs and hemoglobin level

(D) initiate prednisone at 2 mg/kg per day

(E) transfusion to bring the hemoglobin to 10 g/dL and prednisone at a dose of 2 mg/kg per day

Questions 72 and 73
A 16-year-old female presents with leg weakness after recovering from an upper respiratory illness. On examination her vital signs are normal. She is unable to stand alone. Motor strength is 5/5 in the arms and 2/5 in the legs. Deep tendon reflexes are absent in the legs.

72. A finding classically associated with this illness is

(A) hydrocephalus

(B) elevated serum C-reactive protein

(C) myoglobulinuria

(D) elevated cerebrospinal fluid protein

(E) presence of *Clostridium* species on stool culture

73. Testing demonstrates marked slowing of nerve conduction velocity. At this point the most appropriate intervention would be

(A) administration of intravenous immune globulin

(B) discharge and reassurance about the overall benign nature of this disease.

(C) administration of intravenous fresh frozen plasma

(D) supplemental oxygen via nasal canula

(E) administration of intravenous interferon-beta

Questions 74 and 75

A 5-year-old male presents with a 5-lb weight loss over the previous 2 weeks and nighttime enuresis. On examination, he is alert and talkative with a BP of 90/60 mmHg and a HR of 130 bpm. Mucous membranes are sticky and respirations are rapid and deep. The bedside whole blood glucose is 750 mg/dL. Intravenous access is obtained.

74. The first step in the management should be

   (A) regular insulin 0.1 U/kg IV push
   (B) bicarbonate 1 meq/kg IV over 1 h
   (C) endotracheal intubation
   (D) 20 cc/kg isotonic crystalloid solution over 1 h
   (E) a diet soda

75. After your intervention, the whole blood glucose is 485 mg/dL. Intravenous fluids and insulin are given, and the patient is admitted for further care. Which of the following metabolic abnormalities is most likely to occur during insulin therapy?

   (A) hypokalemia
   (B) hyperkalemia
   (C) hyperphosphatemia
   (D) hypercalcemia
   (E) hypermagnesemia

Questions 76 through 78

A 13-month-old female in day care presents to the outpatient clinic with 3 days of rhinorrhea, cough and fever to 101°F. Her examination is significant for clear nasal congestion and red tympanic membranes that are mobile with insufflation. The mother asks for antibiotics.

76. The most appropriate therapy at this time is

   (A) amoxicillin 80–90 mg/kg per day for 10 days
   (B) amoxicillin 40–50 mg/kg per day for 5 days
   (C) ceftriaxone 50 mg/kg IM in one dose
   (D) otorhinolaryngology consult for tympanocentesis
   (E) acetaminophen and fluids

77. The mother brings her child in 6 days later for persistent fever (up to 103°F) and pulling at the left ear. On examination, the left tympanic membrane is bulging and immobile. The bony landmarks are not visible. The mother states the day care won't let her back in without antibiotics. The most appropriate therapy is

   (A) amoxicillin 80–90 mg/kg per day for 10 days
   (B) erythromycin 40–50 mg/kg per day for 10 days
   (C) ceftriaxone 50 mg/kg IM in one dose
   (D) otorhinolaryngology consult for drainage
   (E) acetaminophen and fluids

78. The patient returns again in 2 days with continued fevers to 104°F. The child is still fussy. There is redness, swelling, and tenderness posterior to the left ear and the pinna is displaced forward. The most appropriate therapy at this time is

   (A) amoxicillin 80–90 mg/kg per day for 10 days
   (B) amoxicillin 40–50 mg/kg per day for 5 days
   (C) ceftriaxone 50 mg/kg IM in one dose
   (D) otorhinolaryngology consult for drainage
   (E) acetaminophen and fluids

Questions 79 through 81

A mother brings her 17-year-old daughter to your clinic for evaluation of 6 weeks of fatigue, 10-lb weight loss, and listlessness. The vital signs include a HR of 70 bpm and BP of 90/50 mmHg. Examination reveals a thin girl with a flat affect, but no other abnormalities.

79. The best next step in this patient's management would be

   (A) obtain a serum beta-human chorionic gonadotrophin (β-HCG)
   (B) a referral to an oncologist for a bone marrow aspirate
   (C) obtain stat urine drug screen

(D) reassure the mother that this is normal behavior

(E) interview the patient alone

80. Further discussion with the patient reveals signs of depression. However, she is interactive and denies any drug use or suicidal ideation. She has friends and makes As and Bs in school. The results of screening laboratory work are normal. Appropriate initial management would be

(A) immediate psychiatry consultation due to the medicolegal risk posed by the patient

(B) immediate inpatient admission with 24 h suicide watch

(C) urine collection for illicit substances against the patient's will

(D) initiation of a selective serotonin reuptake inhibitor (SSRI) and scheduling of outpatient counseling with a therapist

(E) reassurance to the patient that it is a sign of puberty and the feelings will pass

81. You are called 3 weeks later as the patient is brought to an outside ED because of increasing hyperactivity, loquaciousness, and 3 days of insomnia. The patient's parents state that she purchased a large amount of goods. Urine toxicology is negative. This patient most likely has

(A) a drug reaction

(B) bipolar disorder

(C) schizophrenia

(D) reaction to sexual abuse

(E) normal adolescent behavior

Questions 82 through 84

A 7-year-old girl presents with a 3-week history of fatigue, 5-lb weight loss, and listlessness. Examination is significant for a thin girl who appears tired. Petechiae and ecchymoses are present over her trunk and extremities. The complete blood count reveals a white blood cell count of $85,000/mm^3$, hemoglobin of $7 g/dL$, and platelets of $15,000/mm^3$. The differential reveals 80% blasts and 20% lymphocytes. She is febrile to 103°F and has a BP of 90/50 mmHg.

82. Appropriate empiric antibiotic therapy would begin with

(A) intramuscular ceftriaxone (Rocephin)

(B) intravenous clindamycin and cefuroxime (Zinacef)

(C) intravenous ceftazidime (Fortaz)

(D) intravenous amphotericin (Fungizone) and voriconazole (Vfend)

(E) oral ciprofloxacin (Cipro)

83. Bone marrow examination confirms the diagnosis of acute lymphocytic leukemia. Which of the following would indicate a poor prognosis?

(A) patient's age (7 years)

(B) patient's initial white blood count ($85,000/mm^3$)

(C) hyperdiploidy

(D) absence of the Philadelphia chromosome (9:22)

(E) absence of blasts in the cerebrospinal fluid

84. Induction chemotherapy is begun. Which of the following patterns of metabolic abnormalities might be expected to occur?

(A) hypokalemia, hypouricemia, hypophosphatemia

(B) hypokalemia, hypouricemia, hyperphosphatemia

(C) hyperkalemia, hyperuricemia, hyperphosphatemia

(D) hyperkalemia, hypouricemia, hypophosphatemia

(E) hypokalemia, hyperuricemia, hypophosphatemia

Questions 85 through 87

A first time mother brings her 6-week-old full-term male infant in because of excessive crying. She states he is feeding well and has had no fever but seems to cry "all the time" for the last 3 weeks. Examination reveals an alert and vigorous infant who has gained weight very well since the 2-week check-up and is currently cooing with no abnormalities noted on examination.

85. The initial approach to management should be

    (A) a full sepsis evaluation
    (B) a skeletal survey
    (C) a radioisotope milk scan
    (D) a urinalysis and urine culture
    (E) counseling, reassurance, and close follow-up

86. The most appropriate management option at this time would be

    (A) suggesting that a single individual, preferably the mother, act as the sole caregiver
    (B) swaddling of the infant
    (C) warm water feedings three times a day to decrease gastric upset
    (D) vigorous shaking of the baby back and forth to simulate uterine movements
    (E) oral paregoric to calm the infant's immature nervous system

87. Potential causes of prolonged crying include

    (A) hair tourniquet around a digit
    (B) milk protein intolerance
    (C) occult fracture
    (D) corneal abrasion
    (E) all of the above

Questions 88 and 89
A 10-month-old female is brought to the emergency department for evaluation of streaks of blood on the surface of the stools. The parents deny any history of travel, diarrhea, or fever.

88. What additional history would be most likely to point to a specific diagnosis in this patient?

    (A) family history of hemophilia
    (B) dietary iron intake
    (C) history of constipation
    (D) presence of rotavirus in day care contacts
    (E) family history of Crohn's disease

89. Examination reveals a small fissure without erythema in the posterior area of the anus. Appropriate treatment at this time would include

    (A) prescribing milk of magnesia
    (B) encouraging the use of a rectal dilator to stretch the internal anal sphincter
    (C) prescribing a stool softener and titrating the dose to desired stool consistency
    (D) prescribing an oral antibiotic to prevent secondary infection of the fissure
    (E) referral to a naturopathic practitioner for colonic irrigation

Questions 90 and 91
An 8-year-old girl presents with a 3-month history of intermittent joint swelling and stiffness and is subsequently diagnosed with juvenile rheumatoid arthritis.

90. The type of JRA most associated with development of severe arthritis is

    (A) systemic onset JRA
    (B) pauciarticular type 1 JRA
    (C) pauciarticular type 2 JRA
    (D) polyarticular RF positive JRA
    (E) polyarticular RF negative JRA

91. Vision loss associated with JRA is most commonly due to

    (A) optic neuritis
    (B) retinal artery thrombosis
    (C) retinal detachment
    (D) beta carotene malabsorption
    (E) chronic iridocyclitis/uveitis

Questions 92 through 94
A 4-month-old male infant presents with 3 days of profuse watery nonbloody diarrhea and nonbilious emesis. He was being fed milk, orange juice, and rice water. Vital signs are T 99°F, HR 170 bpm, and BP 80/40 mmHg. His eyes and fontanelle are sunken and he has poor skin turgor with a capillary refill time of 3–4 s; pulses are normal.

92. This description is most consistent with

    (A) hypovolemic shock, compensated
    (B) hypovolemic shock, uncompensated
    (C) cardiogenic shock, compensated
    (D) septic shock, uncompensated
    (E) normal cardiovascular state

93. His weight just prior to intravenous fluid therapy is 6.3 kg. His fluid deficit is approximately

    (A) 50 cc
    (B) 250 cc
    (C) 650 cc
    (D) 850 cc
    (E) 1100 cc

94. Assuming normal kidney function, the initial hydrating fluid bolus in this patient should contain

    (A) sodium 140 meq/L
    (B) sodium 100 meq/L
    (C) sodium 80 meq/L
    (D) sodium 40 meq/L
    (E) glucose 10 mg%

Questions 95 through 97

An 8-day-old full-term neonate presents with 1 day of vesicular lesions of the skin and mouth. She is afebrile and is alert. There are multiple 3–5 mm vesicles on an erythematous base present on her trunk and mouth. The pregnancy was uncomplicated and the parents have no history of genital lesions.

95. At this point the best course of action is to

    (A) discharge home and follow up in 72 h
    (B) culture the lesions and begin treatment with oral clindamycin (Cleocin)
    (C) check a complete blood count and urinalysis and, if normal, discharge patient after intramuscular ceftriaxone (Rocephin)

    (D) perform bacterial cultures of blood, urine, cerebrospinal fluid, bacterial and viral cultures of the lesions and initiate broad spectrum antibacterial therapy
    (E) perform bacterial cultures of blood, urine, cerebrospinal fluid, bacterial and viral cultures of the lesions and initiate broad spectrum antibacterial therapy and acyclovir

96. Viral shedding due to maternal HSV reactivation is associated with transmission to the fetus in approximately what proportion of cases?

    (A) 2%
    (B) 10%
    (C) 35%
    (D) 70%
    (E) 90%

97. Risk factors for vertical transmission of HSV type 2 include

    (A) maternal coinfection with HSV type 1
    (B) physician rupture of membranes just prior to delivery
    (C) scalp electrode usage
    (D) coinfection with the human immunodeficiency virus
    (E) delayed administration of acyclovir to the mother in labor

Questions 98 and 99

A 15-day-old full-term large for gestational age infant is brought to your clinic for evaluation of a chest mass. Examination reveals an afebrile vigorous baby with a firm, nontender mass palpable over the middle third of the right clavicle.

98. What is the most appropriate course of action for this patient?

    (A) reassurance to the family about the condition
    (B) weight bearing and comparison views of the clavicles
    (C) skeletal survey to rule out abuse
    (D) fibroblast assay for osteopetrosis
    (E) report to child protective services for failure to seek care in a timely fashion

99. Risk factors for this condition include

(A) congenital syphilis
(B) breech presentation
(C) maternal drug use
(D) female gender
(E) thanatophoric dysplasia

Questions 100 through 102

You are called to evaluate the cause of hypotonia in a 1-day-old full-term female infant born to a 28-year-old mother. The baby is alert and moves all extremities well but is hypotonic. She has upward slanting palpebral fissures, speckled irides, a large tongue, short 5th digits, and bilateral transverse palmar creases. Karyotype is 46,XX.

100. The most likely reason for this result is

(A) the number of chromosomes was miscounted
(B) she has a partial translocation involving chromosome 21
(C) there is no chromosomal abnormality
(D) interference of the test by maternal-fetal blood transfusion
(E) she has Turner syndrome

101. The frequency of Down syndrome is closest to

(A) 1/12 live births
(B) 1/600 live births
(C) 1/4000 live births
(D) 1/8000 live births
(E) 1/20,000 live births

102. Patients with Down syndrome are at increased risk for

(A) hyperthyroidism
(B) arthritis of the cervical spine
(C) streak gonads
(D) cardiac malformations
(E) rhabdomyosarcoma

103. You are seeing a previously well 22-month-old male with fever to 102°F, rhinorrhea, and cough for 3 days. His parents report that he remains playful with no alteration in his activity. Your examination reveals rhinorrhea and is otherwise unremarkable. The complete blood count reveals a white cell count (WBC) of 6000/mm^3, normal hemoglobin and platelet count; WBC differential is 8% neutrophils, 40% lymphocytes, 50% monocytes, 2% basophils. At this point the best course of action is

(A) hospitalization and treatment with intravenous ceftazidime and tobramycin
(B) intramuscular dosages of ceftriaxone for a 7-day period
(C) bone marrow aspirate to rule out leukemia
(D) initiation of treatment with granulocyte colony stimulating factor
(E) close outpatient follow-up and repetition of the complete blood count in 1–2 days

Questions 104 through 106

A 10-year-old boy with sickle cell disease (hemoglobin SS) presents with a 1-h history of right-sided weakness. Examination reveals right hemiparesis. A CT scan of the brain is normal.

104. Acute treatment for this patient's condition is

(A) observation
(B) anticoagulation with heparin
(C) exchange transfusion
(D) intravenous tissue plasminogen activator
(E) hydroxyurea

105. The patient recovers completely, but prior to discharge develops a fever to 102°F. He appears otherwise well. Infection with which of the following organisms would be of most concern in this patient?

(A) *Mycobacterium tuberculosis*
(B) *Clostridium botulinum*
(C) group A beta-hemolytic *Streptococcus*
(D) *Streptococcus pneumoniae*
(E) influenza A

106. The patient's father inquires about the possibility that his son's children will have sickle cell disease. You should inform him that the risk

(A) is negligible

(B) is approximately 25%

(C) is approximately 50%

(D) approaches 100%

(E) cannot be determined at this time

Questions 107 through 109

During a well child examination, the mother of a previously healthy 5-year boy inquires whether you think her child is unusually clumsy. The mother thinks her son is going to be strong as he has "big calves," but her family tells her he seems to trip a lot. Your examination reveals a pleasant male with a slightly waddling gait and mildly enlarged calves.

107. Which of the following physical examination findings would suggest the diagnosis of Duchenne muscular dystrophy?

(A) Rovsing's sign

(B) opisthotonus

(C) Gower sign

(D) Chovstek's sign

(E) Grey Turner sign

108. Complications of Duchenne muscular dystrophy include

(A) renal failure from myoglobinuria

(B) ophthalmoplegia

(C) seizures

(D) immunosuppression

(E) aspiration pneumonia

109. The mother is devastated to learn the diagnosis and that she carries the affected gene. A true statement about Duchenne muscular dystrophy inheritance is

(A) 50% of her daughters will be affected with the disease

(B) about 25% of the cases are from new mutations

(C) women are never affected with the disease

(D) the risk of recurrence is minimal

(E) an affected male will pass the illness on to all his sons

Questions 110 and 111

An 8-year-old girl is seen in the emergency department with a complaint of 1-week worsening shortness of breath. She denies fever or cough. Vital signs include HR 140 bpm and BP 78/40 mmHg. She is alert with mild tachypnea and is most comfortable leaning forward. Cardiac examination reveals tachycardia and muffled heart tones.

110. The finding that would be most suggestive of pericardial tamponade is

(A) pulsus paradoxus of greater than 10–20 mmHg

(B) electrocardiogram with low voltages in all leads

(C) chest radiograph demonstrating an enlarged cardiothymic silhouette

(D) egophany over the left anterior chest

(E) bounding carotid pulses

111. Echocardiography confirms a large pericardial effusion compromising left ventricle function. After insuring that the airway is stable, the next intervention should be

(A) intravenous solumedrol 30 mg/kg rapid infusion

(B) continuous intravenous milrinone infusion

(C) thoracotomy and placement of a pericardial window

(D) pericardiocentesis under ultrasound guidance

(E) intravenous albumin and furosemide

Questions 112 through 114

A previously healthy 7-day-old full-term infant presents to your clinic with jaundice which began on the first day of age. He is afebrile with normal vital signs and growth indices. He is breastfeeding well and has five gray stools and six wet diapers per day. Examination reveals a vigorous infant with marked scleral icterus and jaundice to the level of the umbilicus. The liver is palpable 3 cm below the right costal margin. Your nurse was only able to obtain a limited sample of blood.

112. The most important tests to direct further evaluation at this time are

    (A) complete blood count and culture
    (B) total and direct bilirubin
    (C) blood type and Coomb's test
    (D) aspartate aminotransferase and alanine aminotransferase
    (E) alpha$_1$-antrypsin levels

113. The child is sent to the emergency department, and testing reveals the total bilirubin to be 16 mg/dL with a conjugated fraction of 14 mg/dL. Which of the following tests would be most likely to reveal the cause of this infant's conjugated hyperbilirubinemia?

    (A) urinalysis and culture
    (B) urine succinylacetone
    (C) sweat chloride test
    (D) abdominal ultrasound
    (E) thoracolumbar films

114. The above test is ordered and is abnormal. A subsequent liver biopsy to confirm the diagnosis reveals a paucity of biliary channels and plugging with the channel diameter of greater than 150 μm. The treatment for this condition is

    (A) phenobarbital to promote bile flow
    (B) immediate liver transplant using a parental split liver graft
    (C) hepatocyte infusion directly into the residual portal vein
    (D) Kasai hepatoportoenterostomy after 6 months of life to make it technically easier
    (E) Kasai hepatoportoenterostomy as soon as possible after diagnosis

Questions 115 and 116
A 4-year-old boy is brought in for evaluation because of perianal irritation and itching and parental concern that this might be a manifestation of sexual abuse. Examination reveals a playful boy; inspection of the perianal region demonstrates several superficial excoriations and several thread-like worms.

115. The next step in management is

    (A) antiparasitic treatment and reassurance about the benign nature of the condition
    (B) stool for ova and parasite examination
    (C) social work evaluation and child protective services referral
    (D) instructions to the family regarding improved hygiene
    (E) antiparasitic treatment of household pets, the most likely reservoir for this parasite

116. Treatment of this condition is with

    (A) mebendazole
    (B) metronidazole
    (C) diethylcarbamazine
    (D) praziquantel
    (E) thiabendazole

Questions 117 through 119
A 2-year-old 13-kg female is brought to the emergency department by her parents after they found her with an empty bottle of cherry-flavored acetaminophen drops about 2 h prior. You note that the bottle contained 1 oz at a concentration of 80 mg/0.8 cc. The parents report they just purchased it earlier in the day for her 2-month-old brother. No treatment was given prior to arrival at the emergency department. The patient's vital signs are normal, and her physical examination is unremarkable.

117. The next step in this patient's management is

    (A) intubate to secure the airway
    (B) do nothing until 4 h have elapsed since the purported time of ingestion
    (C) give activated charcoal with sorbitol at a dose of 1 g/kg orally or via nasogastric tube
    (D) induce emesis with syrup of ipecac
    (E) proceed with gastric lavage using a 12-french orogastric tube

118. You proceed with management. The 4-h acetaminophen level is 200 μg/kg. You should now

    (A) continue observation in the emergency department for 6 h and discharge if the patient remains asymptomatic
    (B) start the antidote, N-acetylcysteine

(C) continue activated charcoal every 4 h in addition to the antidote, *N*-acetylcysteine

(D) begin preparations for liver transplant

(E) place a hemodialysis catheter for initiation of hemodialysis

119. The toxicity of acetaminophen comes from

(A) its renal metabolite

(B) acetaminophen directly

(C) its glucoronidate metabolite

(D) its sulfated metabolite

(E) its cytochrome p450 metabolite

Questions 120 and 121

A previously healthy 3-year-old male is brought in by his parents with a chief complaint of increased sleepiness which began during a visit to his grandmother's house earlier that day. The patient's vital signs are HR of 50 bpm, temperature of 97°F, RR of 8 times/min, and a BP of 98/65 mmHg. Examination reveals an obtunded male toddler who is unresponsive to sternal rub and lacks a gag reflex. He also has miosis.

120. The first step in managing this patient is

(A) bedside whole blood glucose

(B) urinary catherization to obtain urine drug screen

(C) intravenous flumazenil

(D) securing an airway and insuring adequate breathing

(E) intravenous epinephrine for bradycardia

121. The grandmother reports that she has multiple medications in her house and is concerned that the patient's problems may be due to an ingestion. Which one of her medicines would most likely cause the symptoms reported?

(A) clonidine

(B) nifedipine

(C) meperidine

(D) labetalol

(E) diazepam

Answers and Explanations

1. **(C)** Given the history of excessive intake of milk, a food known to be low in iron, and the presentation of pallor, initial testing should focus on the hemoglobin and iron status. The reticulocyte count and the mean corpuscular volume (MCV) generally are low in iron deficiency. Chest radiography and stool smears for ova and parasites are not indicated. Serum haptoglobin is low in state of hemolysis, but that is not the most likely cause of anemia in this case. A bone marrow biopsy is not indicated at this time. *(Behrman:1469–1471)*

2. **(D)** In iron deficiency anemia, the red blood cells are smaller than normal and are variable in size; therefore a decreased MCV and elevated red cell distribution width (RDW) are classic with this history. B_{12} deficiency from a poor diet or intrinsic factor deficiency presents with an elevated MCV. No blasts indicating leukemia or stippling suggesting hemosiderosis were noted on the smear. Additionally, there is no evidence of sickled cells. *(Behrman: 1469–1471)*

3. **(C)** When iron deficiency anemia is suspected, elemental iron at a dose of 6 mg/kg per day divided into two or three doses should be initiated. Appetite will return to normal in 12–24 h. Bone marrow response will begin in 36–48 h. Reticulocytosis will peak around 5–7 days. Repletion of stores will occur in 1–3 months depending on the severity of the anemia. Contrary to common belief, iron does not constipate patients. Increasing vitamin C intake via diet or supplementation can increase iron absorption. Parents should be counseled regarding the importance of a diverse diet.

Milk intake should be limited to 16–24 oz per day. *(Behrman:1469–1471)*

4. **(B)** The initial step in the management of patients presenting in respiratory distress is assessment of the "ABCs" (airway, breathing, and circulation). The presence of hypoxemia is an indication for administration of supplemental oxygen. There is no indication of a compromised airway (e.g., stridor) in this patient. While there is mild distress, there is no indication at this time of respiratory failure necessitating emergent intubation. Chest radiographs and administration of corticosteroids may be necessary, but are not the first priority in this patient's management. *(Behrman:991–993, 1285–1287)*

5. **(E)** The age, physical findings, and season all point to bronchiolitis, most likely due to respiratory syncytial virus (RSV), as the most likely cause of this patient's problem. RSV is the etiologic agent in about 70% of patients with bronchiolitis and results in approximately 70,000 inpatient admissions yearly in the United States. Congestive heart failure likely would be associated with other physical findings such as hepatomegaly, or have demonstrable cardiomegaly on the chest radiograph. Respiratory distress syndrome typically has a ground-glass appearance on chest radiography and presents with more severe clinical symptoms. Pneumococcal pneumonia classically presents with a more focal infiltrate with consolidation, is unilateral, and is not associated with wheezing. Mycoplasmal infections are not common at this age. *(Behrman:991–993, 1285–1287)*

6. **(A)** A trial of beta agonist therapy, such as albuterol or racemic epinephrine should be offered to all patients with bronchiolitis with symptoms of distress; however, not all patients will respond. Guidelines as delineated by the American Academy of Pediatrics recommend the use of ribavirin in patients with congenital heart lesions, immunodeficiencies, and chronic lung disease; its use can also be considered in the very young or very ill, intubated patient in the early course of the illness. Ribavirin can present some technical challenges in its administration. And, while teratogenicity has been demonstrated only in rodents, it is a category X drug. Respigam and Synagis are both anti-RSV immune globulin products. However, the polyclonal antibodies in Respigam are pooled from donors with high titers of anti-RSV and the humanized mouse monoclonal antibodies in Synagis are recombinantly produced. Both have been shown to reduce the incidence of infection with RSV but have no role in treatment of confirmed infections. Heliox (70/30 mixture of helium/oxygen) has been used for upper airway obstructions and severe bronchiolitics but is not indicated here. *(Behrman: 991–993, 1285–1287)*

7. **(E)** Gram-positive organisms, in particular *Staphylococcus aureus*, are a significant source of soft tissue infections in the immunocompetent child. Spread to deep tissues can occur directly or hematogenously. Arthritis due to infection with *Neisseria* typically presents as a monoarticular septic joint in sexually active individuals. Group B streptococcal arthritis is most commonly seen in neonates. *Pseudomonas aeruginosa* or other gram negatives should be considered in drug users or immunodeficient individuals. Arthritis due to *Mycobacteria tuberculosis* is uncommon and would have a more indolent course. *(Behrman:777–780)*

8. **(B)** The examination is very concerning for a septic arthritis of the left elbow. Erosion and permanent damage of the joint can occur quickly. Obtaining fluid for cultures by arthrocentesis prior to antibiotic therapy is preferred, particularly in light of the increasing frequency of antibiotic resistant organisms.

Oral antibiotics are inappropriate for initial treatment of septic arthritis. Nonsteroidal anti-inflammatory agents provide symptomatic relief only and are not a primary treatment modality in septic arthritis. *(Behrman:777–780)*

9. **(E)** Young infants, patients with hip and shoulder involvement, and those whose antibiotic therapy is delayed are at increased risk of a poor outcome following bacterial arthritis. Additionally, septic arthritis due to gram-negative and fungal organisms is more difficult to eradicate. The Gram stain is only positive in approximately 50% of cases, and the presence or absence of organisms on Gram stain is of no prognostic value in septic arthritis. *(Behrman: 777–780)*

10. **(B)** Thyroid dysgenesis accounts for 90% of the cases of congenital hypothyroidism. Maternal ingestion of propylthiouracil causes a transitory hypothyroidism, but history should reveal maternal use of this drug. The other causes of congenital hypothyroidism are uncommonly seen. *(Behrman: 1698–1703)*

11. **(A)** When a patient presents with a state screen that is positive and has obvious clinical symptoms of hypothyroidism, initiating thyroxine prior to confirmation is essential. Therapy initiated prior to 2–4 weeks of life can ensure near normal intelligence. Dosing for infants starts at 10–15 μg/kg per day. Older children require about 4 μg/kg per day and adults require only 2 μg/kg per day. A scintiscan to look for ectopic thyroid tissue is helpful. Close neurodevelopmental follow-up is necessary. Radiography of the distal femur of patients with congenital hypothyroidism frequently reveals absent distal epiphysis. This finding is occasionally used as a quick indirect screen for hypothyroidism. *(Behrman:1698–1703)*

12. **(C)** Edema results from two pathophysiologic conditions: increased venous hydrostatic pressure or decreased oncotic pressure. Increased hydrostatic pressure, resulting in extravasation of fluid into the interstitial space, results from conditions such as venous thrombosis and congestive heart failure. Reduced oncotic pressure

most commonly results from hypoalbumine-mia due to decreased production of albumin (e.g., liver failure) or increased loss of albumin (e.g., via the gastrointestinal tract or kidneys); reduction in oncotic pressure in turn results in fluid extravasation into the interstitial tissues. Of the choices given, a urinalysis for protein is the quickest, cheapest, least invasive, and most helpful initial test to direct further evaluation. *(Behrman:1592–1595)*

13. **(E)** In conjunction with proteinuria, elevated serum cholesterol, hypoalbuminemia, and edema constitute the nephrotic syndrome. Membranous glomerulonephritis, focal segmental glomerulosclerosis, membranoproliferative disease, and acute poststreptococcal glomerulonephritis all may be associated with the nephrotic syndrome. However, minimal-change disease is much more common in children, accounting for 85% of protein-losing nephropathies. *(Behrman:1592–1595)*

14. **(D)** Fortunately, 90% of patients with minimal-change disease respond rapidly to steroids. Loss of properdin factor B that opsonizes bacteria can occur, leading to an increased risk of spontaneous bacterial peritonitis. Antithrombin III is also lost in the urine, so children are at increased risk of thrombosis, not hemorrhage. During flares low sodium diets, combined with diuretics and albumin infusions may be necessary to decrease edema. A referral and renal biopsy should be performed after 1 month (not 1 year) of nonresponse to steroid therapy to determine the etiology of the illness. *(Behrman: 1592–1595)*

15. **(C)** Hypertension presenting with symptoms (headache, altered mental status, papilledema) requires immediate antihypertensive therapy. Causes of severe hypertension (>95th percentile) include renal artery stenosis, malignant hyperthyroidism, aldosteronism, pheochromocytoma, and a coarctation of the aorta. An intracranial mass with Cushing's triad causing hypertension should present with bradycardia

but this can be a late presenting sign. An LP should be deferred in a patient with papilledema until imaging demonstrates the absence of an intracranial mass. *(Behrman:1184, 1741–1742)*

16. **(B)** Determination of urine level of vanillyl mandelic acid (VMA, a metabolite of epinephrine), thyroid function analysis, and CT imaging of the abdomen for a mass as well as renal artery caliber delineation are all essential in looking for the etiology of her hypertension. Laparotomy may be needed for eventual therapy but is not a part of the initial evaluation. *(Behrman:1184, 1741–1742)*

17. **(A)** An elevated VMA level with this patient's symptoms point to a pheochromocytoma as the cause of her hypertension. Pheochromocytomas arise from the chromaffin cells of the sympathetic nervous system; they can arise in the adrenal medulla or anywhere along the sympathetic chain. They can be inherited sporadically or as a component of types IIA and IIB multiple endocrine neoplasia syndromes from a mutation in the RET proto-oncogene. The definitive treatment is surgical with exquisite detail to peri- and postoperative hypertension. *(Behrman:1184, 1741–1742)*

18. **(D)** Ninety-nine percent of healthy neonates pass their first stool (meconium) within 48 h after birth. Delayed passage of the meconium raises concern for Hirschsprung disease. Barium enema may demonstrate a "transition zone" at the junction of the dilated normal bowel proximally and the narrowed aganglionic segment distally. As frequent rectal stimulation and digital examination may alter the radiographic appearance, the barium enema should be delayed until 2–3 days after these procedures if feasible. Botulism and hypothyroidism may present with constipation, but this neonate's vigorous appearance and history of feeding make these unlikely. Mineral oil should not be given to infants because of the risk of aspiration and subsequent lipoid pneumonia. *(Behrman: 1139–1141)*

19. **(E)** The diagnostic ability of the barium enema depends on demonstration of a transition zone of narrow distal bowel expanding into more normal caliber proximal bowel. However, false negative studies occur, especially if performed after previous rectal stimulation (e.g., digital examination). Biopsy above the dentate line remains the gold standard for diagnosis; in Hirschsprung disease, it reveals a lack of the neuronal plexus (Meissner and Auerbach), hypertrophied nerve bundles, and increased acetylcholinesterase levels. Stool examination for eosinophils may be useful in cases of milk protein allergy, but is not indicated in this breast-fed baby. Anal manometry to measure pressure changes of the rectum is technically challenging in young infants but can be performed in older patients. Upper GI series with small bowel follow through is useful in the diagnosis of intestinal malrotation, but is not indicated in the patient described. *(Behrman: 1139–1141)*

20. **(A)** The prognosis for surgically treated HD generally is satisfactory with a majority of patients achieving fecal continence. In 75% of patients the aganglionic segment is limited to the distal rectosigmoid area. Colostomy placement is rare and is only temporary until the proximal segment recovers from its dilated state. A total colectomy is necessary in fewer than 10% of patients. A small bowel transplant is needed only if a large proportion of the small bowel is aganglionic (total intestinal Hirschsprung disease). Enterocolitis can occur in untreated Hirschsprung disease but is uncommon following surgical correction. *(Behrman:1139–1141)*

21. **(B)** The history of longitudinal traction in a child less than 4 years old, the lack of tenderness or effusion on examination, and the characteristic posture (arm flexed at elbow and slightly pronated) point to nursemaid's elbow (radial head subluxation) as the most likely diagnosis. This occurs when the radial head is subject to longitudinal traction causing the developing annular ligament to remain partially entrapped in the radiohumeral joint. In patients with a typical history and physical examination, maneuvers to reduce the subluxation are both diagnostic and therapeutic. Hyperpronation or supination/flexion of the forearm are two maneuvers that can reduce the subluxation. Although causing brief pain, reduction does not require sedation. On successful reduction a "clunk" can be felt over the lateral portion of the elbow, and the patient will generally begin using the arm normally within a short period. Radiographs are not indicated as they will be normal. While nonaccidental trauma may result in a nursemaid's elbow, the history given is compatible with the injury and, in the absence of other suspicious findings, is not an indication for social service evaluation. *(Behrman:2092)*

22. **(E)** Recurrence of nursemaid's elbow has been reported in as many as 30% of children. Therefore, counseling the parents on the mechanism of this injury is important. No splints are necessary and physical activity as tolerated should be permitted. A radial head subluxation by itself typically is not indicative of abuse. The annular ligament and radial head strengthen with age and radial head subluxation is rare after 4 years of age. *(Behrman:2092)*

23. **(A)** This adolescent has several risk factors that make her a candidate for admission. The fever and toxic appearance she has indicate an illness beyond a cystitis or simple cervicitis caused by *N. gonorrhea* or *C. trachomatis*. Residence in a shelter also suggests increased difficulty with outpatient follow-up. Treatment for an emergent condition as well as for sexually transmitted diseases does not require legal proceedings. Appropriate pain control will be necessary, but admission and intravenous antibiotic therapy are the first critical step in this patient with pelvic inflammatory disease (PID). Prior to discharge from the hospital and hopefully after this patient has developed a trusting professional relationship with her

physician, counseling regarding contraception and further protection as well as life's choices are indicated. *(Red Book:470–472)*

24. **(C)** Complications of PID include chronic pelvic pain, perihepatitis, ectopic pregnancies, infertility and tubo-ovarian abscess should be worsening signs and symptoms despite appropriate antimicrobial therapy are suggestive of tubo-ovarian abscess. Consultation with a gynecologist and diagnostic imaging (usually ultrasound) is appropriate at this time. A C-reactive protein to monitor therapy is not needed when the clinical picture clearly suggests lack of response to therapy. Methicillin-resistant *S. aureus* is an uncommon cause of PID. *(Red Book:470–472)*

25. **(B)** PID causes scarring of the reproductive tract and can lead to many complications later in life. There is a 10% risk of tubal infertility after a single episode of PID, with a 50% risk after 3 or more episodes. Patients who have had PID are at increased risk for repeat infections, and douching or oral contraceptives do not prevent them. Male carriers are not always symptomatic. PID is a risk factor for future ectopic pregnancies. *(Red Book:468–472)*

26. **(E)** The first step in management of any laceration is hemostasis. Once this is achieved, irrigation, evaluation of the wound for foreign bodies, and antimicrobial therapy can begin. If the wound injury is found to involve tendons, ligaments, vessels, or may be associated with severe cosmetic imperfection, surgical assistance for repair is appropriate. *(Red Book:613)*

27. **(B)** Two questions to ask when confronted with tetanus prophylaxis are (1) has the patient received three or more doses of tetanus toxoid and (2) is the wound clean. The following table from the 26th edition of the AAP Red Book (used by permission) is a guide to this frequently encountered issue. *(Red Book:614)*

GUIDE TO TETANUS PROPHYLAXIS IN ROUTINE WOUND MANAGEMENT

History of absorbed tetanus toxoid (doses)	Clean, minor wounds		All other wounds[a]	
	Td^b	TIG^c	Td^b	TIG^c
Unknown or <3	Yes	No	Yes	Yes
≥3[d]	No[e]	No	No[f]	No

Td indicates adult-type diphtheria and tetanus toxoids vaccine; TIG, tetanus immune globulin (human).

[a] Such as, but not limited to, wounds contaminated with dirt, feces, soil, and saliva; puncture wounds; avulsions; and wounds resulting from missiles, crushing, burns, and frostbite.

[b] For children younger than 7 years of age, diphtheria and tetanus toxoids and acellular pertussis (DTaP) vaccine is recommended; if pertussis vaccine is contraindicated, diphtheria and tetanus toxoids (DT) vaccine is given. For persons 7 years of age or older, Td vaccine is recommended.

[c] Equine tetanus antitoxin should be used, if available, when TIG is not available.

[d] If only three doses of fluid toxoid have been received, a fourth dose of toxoid, preferably an adsorbed toxoid, should be given. Although licensed, fluid tetanus toxoid rarely is used.

[e] Yes, if more than 10 years since last dose.

[f] Yes, if more than 5 years since last dose. More frequent boosters are not needed and can accentuate adverse effects.

28. **(C)** The injury this child suffered is not consistent with the story that is presented. Other "red flags" suggesting nonaccidental trauma include stories that are developmentally impossible or change over time, reticence on the part of one caregiver to speak, and delay in seeking medical care. This child clearly is at risk and needs an evaluation with a skeletal survey. Findings suggestive of abuse are multiple healing injuries, rib fractures, bucket handle fractures, or healing long bone fractures. A hip spica is the treatment for a femur fracture in infants; internal fixation is not indicated. Although osteogenesis imperfecta may present with long bone fractures, it is rare and evaluation for more common conditions such as abuse takes precedence. Eighty percent of inflicted skeletal trauma occurs in children under 18 months of age. Among fractures resulting from abuse, skull fractures are most common followed by fractures of the extremities. *(Rudolph CD:463–469, 561)*

29. **(E)** When confronted with possible nonaccidental trauma, the safety of the affected child as well as other members of the household is of primary importance. Evaluation for factors that may contribute to the potential for abuse should be undertaken. The assistance of a social

worker is often valuable in this regard. All states mandate that physicians report any case of suspected abuse. Mandated reporters are immune from prosecution, even if abuse is not proven, as long as the report is made in good faith. Direct confrontation and accusation are not productive and may hinder further efforts in the investigative process. Incarcerating the father is not appropriate as he has made no threats nor is there sufficient evidence to implicate him as the perpetrator of the injury. However, this child should not be discharged until there is sufficient investigation of the social situation to permit safe placement. (Rudolph CD:463–469, 561)

30. **(E)** A patient with this degree of tachycardia needs immediate assessment of her cardiorespiratory status. As her airway, breathing and circulation are intact with no evidence of impending failure, a brief evaluation can be performed to evaluate her tachycardia. Obtaining an electrocardiogram during the episode likely will be valuable for analysis of the rhythm and determining the best treatment modality. The other tests are helpful in evaluating sinus tachycardia, which usually peaks around 220–230. A tachycardia over 230 is more suggestive of a supraventricular tachycardia (SVT), which is the most common dysrhythmia requiring medical intervention in children. (Rudolph CD:1854–1856)

31. **(A)** Once the diagnosis of supraventricular tachycardia is made, adenosine 0.1 mg/kg (maximum 6 mg) rapid intravenous push is the treatment of choice. If the initial attempt is unsuccessful, the dose can be doubled and repeated (to a maximum of 12 mg). Side effects include transient headache, flushing, and chest pain. Serious side effects of adenosine include atrial fibrillation, apnea, bronchospasm, brief asystole, accelerated ventricular rhythms, and wide complex tachycardia. Cardioversion (not defibrillation) at a dose of 0.5–1 J/kg is indicated if the patient is unstable. Digoxin is also used for recalcitrant SVT. Calcium channel blockers are contraindicated for children under 1 year of

age as they may precipitate cardiovascular collapse. Ibuprofen would be useful for sinus tachycardia due to fever, but this patient had no fever and the heart rate is above that seen with sinus tachycardia. (Rudolph CD:1854–1856)

32. **(B)** All of the listed answers may cause hair loss. Tinea capitis generally has more patchy hair loss and may have "black dots," representing broken hair. Trichotillomania will have bizarre patterns of hair loss in linear bands that has stubs of varying length. Hair traction alopecia occurs in areas of stress where the hair is pulled into braids or ponytails. It may become permanent if scarring occurs. Chemical exposure should be elicited from history. Alopecia areata is the most likely cause in this patient, given the complete hair loss and the characteristic exclamation point appearance of the hair. (Rudolph CD:1210–1212)

33. **(C)** Alopecia areata occurs when hair that is in a growing phase (anagen) abruptly stops growing, causing the hair shafts to taper and lose adhesion to the follicle. Round patches of hair anywhere on the body can be affected, but are most noticeable when on the scalp. Clues to diagnosis include lack of inflammation, easily removed hair at the borders and the exclamation point appearance of the hair under the microscope. Unfortunately the course is difficult to predict, a fact that should be stressed to the patient. Treatments with steroids, minoxidil, and immunomodulators such as cyclosporine have shown some success, but their use should be undertaken in consultation with a dermatologist. (Rudolph CD:1210–1212)

34. **(B)** This history is highly suggestive of pertussis. The clinical course is divided into three stages: (1) the catarrhal stage, 2–10 days in duration, characterized by rhinorrhea, lacrimation, and sometimes low-grade fever; (2) the paroxysmal stage, lasting 1–6 weeks, during which there are intermittent episodes of coughing that may terminate with a forced inspiration against a partially closed glottis resulting in a "whoop" or may terminate with

vomiting; (3) the convalescent stage, lasting up to 6 months, during which the coughing episodes gradually resolve. Infants with pertussis often do not whoop because of their inability to generate sufficient inspiratory forces. Between episodes of cough, the examination is often normal. Of the choices given, the immunization status is of most importance. (McMillan:990–993)

35. **(C)** A high white blood count with a marked lymphocytosis is characteristic of pertussis. Therefore, prescribing erythromycin is the most appropriate choice. A repeat CBC is not needed to follow the treatment. In fact, antibiotics do not hasten the resolution of the illness, but will decrease spread to other household members, who should also be treated. (McMillan: 990–993)

36. **(B)** *Bordetella pertussis* is most likely to be recovered from the nasopharynx and more likely to be positive early in the illness. Throat swabs are less likely to be positive and sputum is almost never obtainable from infants. Bronchoscopy is not necessary to make the diagnosis and bacteremia does not occur. Special media are needed for cultivation of the organism. (McMillan:990–993)

37. **(D)** This history and the finding of papilledema is strongly suggestive of pseudotumor cerebri, a condition marked by overproduction of cerebrospinal fluid leading to increased intracranial pressure. However, imaging to rule out a mass or a sinus thrombosis should be performed. A history of ingestion of vitamin A, tetracycline, or steroids, or a history of pregnancy would further support the diagnosis of pseudotumor cerebri. Her blood pressure is mildly elevated, but does not warrant treatment at this time with oral or intravenous antihypertensive agents. Mannitol and furosemide would be used in the emergent management of suspected herniation, but the patient currently has no signs to suggest that problem. (Rudolph CD:2398; Behrman:1862)

38. **(A)** The next step would be lumbar puncture with determination of opening and closing pressures. Removal of sufficient fluid to reduce the CSF pressure is therapeutic. At times a nonsteroidal drug or even a narcotic may be necessary to temporarily relieve the headaches associated with pseudotumor cerebri. Serial lumbar punctures may be needed for continued symptomatic relief. Medications to reduce CSF production include acetazolamide and steroids. (Rudolph CD:2398; Behrman:1862)

39. **(E)** Indications for surgical interventions include vision loss despite adequate therapy or inability to tolerate treatment. Surgical options include optic nerve fenestrations or placement of a lumboperitoneal shunt; repeat or additional (MRI) imaging should also be performed in case a small tumor was missed initially. (Rudolph CD:2398; Behrman:1862)

40. **(D)** The first priority in managing this patient is insuring that the airway is patent and ventilation/oxygenation is adequate. Suction of vomitus may be needed as well. (McMillan:579, 1949–1952; Pediatrics 97:769–772, 1996)

41. **(E)** Given the patient's age, fever, and paucity of abnormal physical findings, the most likely diagnosis is febrile seizure. The most pressing need is to rule out meningitis. The American Academy of Pediatrics strongly recommends consideration of a lumbar puncture in all patients less than 12 months of age who present with a simple febrile seizure. In the absence of signs of increased intracranial pressure, a head CT is not indicated prior to lumbar puncture. Skull x-rays, arterial blood gas, and electroencephalograms have very low yield in this clinical situation and are not routinely warranted. (McMillan:579, 1949–1952; Pediatrics 97:769–772, 1996)

42. **(A)** It is reassuring that this patient's physical examination has returned to normal, compatible with the diagnosis of a simple febrile seizure. The parents should be counseled that about one-third of children experiencing a febrile seizure will have at least one recurrence.

The risk is higher in children experiencing the first seizure before the age of 1 year. Chronic anticonvulsant prophylaxis is not indicated for simple febrile seizures. While attempts to control fever are certainly warranted in patients with a history of febrile seizures, the use of antipyretics alone has not proven effective in the prevention of recurrence. In particular, there is no evidence that the use of alternating doses of acetaminophen and ibuprofen is necessary or effective in seizure prevention. Hospital admission and neuroimaging are not necessary in patients whose examination returns to normal prior to discharge from the emergency department. (McMillan:579, 1949–1952; Pediatrics 97:769–772, 1996)

43. **(B)** Before a lengthy and expensive diagnostic evaluation is undertaken the growth patterns of the biological parents should be evaluated, as they are predictive of the child's growth pattern. Sibling height may be helpful, but is not predictive. Parental age doesn't affect offspring height per se, but may be indirectly associated in cases of age-related disorders such as Down syndrome. Social factors may influence growth rate as psychosocial dwarfism is seen in institutionalized and maltreated children. (Behrman: 1753–1754)

44. **(D)** The physical findings described suggest the diagnosis of Turner syndrome. As patients with Turner syndrome have dysgenic ovaries, their estrogen levels are low resulting in a lack of negative feedback on the pituitary gland. Consequently, luteinizing and follicle stimulating hormone levels are high. An abdominal ultrasound will reveal the streak ovaries. Growth hormone levels are low and the bone age is delayed. Although all of the tests listed will likely reveal abnormalities, it is the karyotype that will ultimately confirm the diagnosis. (Behrman:1753–1754)

45. **(A)** Echocardiograph is indicated in patients with Turner syndrome because of the association with various cardiac anomalies, including bicuspid aortic valve, aortic stenosis, and anomalous pulmonary venous return. While

characteristic of Down syndrome, cervical laxity is not a feature of Turner syndrome. Growth hormone may increase adult height, and estrogen replacement therapy can improve bone density, growth, and sexual maturation. However, thyroid hormone replacement is not routinely indicated. The risk of endometrial carcinoma is not increased in these patients. Although Turner syndrome is associated with increased risk for some learning problems, mental retardation is not a feature of the disorder. Psychosocial support is important as well; the Turner Syndrome Society has chapters in the United States that can provide a support network for patients and their families. (Behrman:1753–1754)

46. **(D)** The constellation of these symptoms is strongly suggestive of Kawasaki disease. The disease is most commonly seen in children under 5 years of age. Diagnostic criteria include fever of at least 5 days' duration together with at least four of the following features: (1) conjunctival injection; (2) oral changes, including erythema of the oral mucosa and pharynx, strawberry tongue, and red cracked lips; (3) an erythematous, generalized rash; (4) changes in the peripheral extremities consisting of swelling of the hands or feet, erythematous palms or soles, or desquamation of the fingertips; and (5) a unilateral lymph node at least 1.5 cm in diameter. In addition, other potential causes of the illness (e.g., measles, scarlet fever, and Stevens-Johnson syndrome) must be excluded. (Red Book:382–395)

47. **(C)** Kawaski manifestations and complications include arthralgias, irritability, vomiting, sterile pyuria, mild hepatic dysfunction, aseptic meningitis, pericardial effusion, myocarditis, and coronary artery ectasia and aneurysms. In addition to these problems, hydrops of the gallbladder is a well-described complication. Although thrombocytopenia has rarely been described in association with this disease, thrombocytosis is the more characteristic finding. Sterility, ulcerative colitis, and transverse myelitis are not associated with this disease. (Red Book:382–395)

48. **(B)** Receipt of IVIG may interfere with the immune response to some live viral vaccinations. Therefore, measles and varicella immunization should be deferred for 11 months following IVIG administration. Other routine vaccines should be given as scheduled. Influenza vaccine should be encouraged, as the disease (and not the vaccine) is associated with Reye syndrome when aspirin is given. No repetition of previously administered vaccines is necessary. *(Red Book:423)*

49. **(C)** The history of trauma with the presence of localized tenderness on examination and the lack of systemic symptoms such as fever make infection unlikely. Therefore, C-reactive protein and blood culture are not indicated. At this point there is no indication of underlying metabolic bone disease and alkaline phosphatase is not warranted. Although a high index of suspicion for nonaccidental trauma is appropriate, the history given is consistent with the physical findings described, and social service consultation is not warranted at this time. Given the possibility of fracture, performance of radiographs would be the most appropriate choice. *(Behrman:2097)*

50. **(E)** The history and physical findings described are suggestive of a "toddler's fracture," also termed childhood accidental spiral tibial (CAST) fracture. These fractures occur most commonly in the distal tibia, often following relatively minor trauma. They are not suggestive of abuse. The diagnosis is confirmed by radiographs; occasionally, the fracture may be radiographically occult or demonstrable only on oblique films. Immobilization of the limb in a posterior short leg splint will provide support and reduce the pain that occurs with movement of the limb. Casting can occur later when swelling has subsided. Healing typically occurs in 4–6 weeks. *(Behrman:2097)*

51. **(B)** The differential diagnosis of the lethargic neonate is extensive and includes infection, effect of maternal medications, electrolyte disturbances, metabolic abnormalities, congenital abnormalities, and trauma. The delay in onset of symptoms until day of life three make maternal medications an unlikely cause of lethargy in this neonate. There is no history of abdominal distention or bilious emesis to suggest an intraabdominal emergency such as midgut volvulus and diagnostic imaging is therefore not indicated. If there were reason to suspect head trauma or intracranial bleeding, CT would be the imaging modality of choice. Of the options presented, performance of an evaluation for infection is the most appropriate first step. *(Rudolph CD:106–107)*

52. **(A)** Inborn errors of metabolism are likely in this patient. While rare individually, these disorders in aggregation approximate the incidence of sepsis. Therefore, consideration of one of these disorders, particularly when the evaluation for infection does not yield any definite evidence of infection, should not be delayed. In a male with an elevated ammonia level, especially without acidosis, a urea cycle defect is the most likely possibility. Elevation of urine orotic acid, a by-product produced in increased amounts due to a lack of ornithine transcarbamylase, is consistent with ornithine transcarbamylase deficiency. Inheritance is X-linked dominant, and there are over 20 variants. Females with the defective gene typically have milder forms of the illness. *(Behrman: 368–369)*

53. **(C)** Therapy for suspected urea cycle defects involves parenteral nutrition with glucose, lipids, and essential amino acids to promote anabolism. Arginine hydrochloride intravenously is essential to supply the urea cycle with ornithine, which now becomes an essential amino acid. Additional emergent medications to lower the ammonia include sodium benzoate, that combines with glycine to form hippuric acid, and sodium phenylacetate, that combines with glutamine to from phenylacetylglutamine, both of which are more easily excreted by the kidney than ammonia. Citrulline is necessary as 1 mol of citrulline will remove 1 mol of ammonia. Frequent monitoring of ammonia levels is necessary. If no appreciable change in ammonia is noted within a few hours, the only therapeutic option left is dialysis, which may be

technically difficult or impossible if access cannot be obtained. Increasing arginine infusion rates or prolonging an ineffective therapy will provide no benefit to this child. Exchange transfusion has little effect on lowering total body ammonia. While many children do suffer permanent debilitating effects of the initial hyperammonemia, consideration of DNR status at this time is inappropriate. (*Behrman: 367–370*)

54. **(E)** In a well-appearing child with a recent viral illness and without fever, toxicity, or systemic signs of illness who presents with unexplained petechiae and ecchymoses, idiopathic thrombocytopenic purpura (ITP) is the most likely diagnosis. A complete blood count is indicated to establish the presence of thrombocytopenia and assess the other cell lines. If other cell lines are affected, a bone marrow may be needed to rule out leukemia and other hematologic disorders. Trauma presenting only with generalized petechiae would be rare. Rickettsial or Neisserial infections can cause petechiae but most affected patients have other symptoms. (*Rudolph CD 1556–1557*)

55. **(D)** The presence of isolated thrombocytopenia and increased megakaryocytes on bone marrow examination establishes the diagnosis of idiopathic thrombocytopenic purpura. If examination of the bone marrow reveals a lack of megakaryocytes, the diagnosis is not ITP and other causes of thrombocytopenia should be pursued. Several treatment options for ITP exist, including simple observation. Corticosteroids, intravenous immunoglobulin, and anti-Rho antibodies have all been used with success. Indications for treatment include evidence of bleeding, thrombocytopenia less than 50,000, or prolonged thrombocytopenia. The presence of fever is not relevant to the treatment decision. The mechanism of action of anti-Rho antibodies is uncertain. However, it is thought that reticuloendothelial Fc receptor blockade is involved. This type of therapy will only be effective in patients that are Rh-positive. (*Rudolph CD:1556–1557*)

56. **(D)** ITP resolves completely within 6 months in 80–90% of cases. Splenectomy is seldom necessary, and usually is reserved for chronic cases lasting greater than 6–9 months. Splenectomy may also be required for control of severe recalcitrant bleeding. Low platelet counts, bleeding, splenomegaly, and anemia are not in themselves indications for splenectomy. (*Rudolph CD:1556–1557*)

57. **(A)** In a patient presenting with hypertension and pallor following a history of hemorrhagic enteritis, the presence of hemolytic-uremic syndrome (HUS) should be considered. The most frequent cause is infection with *E. coli* O157:H7. The primary event in this condition is endothelial injury from verotoxin release, resulting in a microangiopathic hemolytic anemia. Renal vascular involvement results in hypertension. The CBC and smear will show anemia, thrombocytopenia, and schistocytes. The other tests may be abnormal but will not establish the diagnosis. (*Behrman :367–370*)

58. **(A)** Additional evidence for HUS is manifested by the elevated BUN and creatinine. Care for HUS is primarily careful medical management in conjunction with early and frequent dialysis to control fluid overload, manage electrolyte abnormalities, and remove plasminogen activator inhibitor-1 so that endogenous fibrinolytic mechanisms can dissolve vascular thrombi. Plasmapheresis and fresh frozen plasma have been used with some success as well. Steroids and antibiotics have no ameliorative effect, and the illness rarely recurs. Ninety percent of patients survive the acute phase and the majority of patients regain normal renal function. (*Behrman:367–370*)

59. **(C)** This patient has typical signs and symptoms of croup which is caused primarily by parainfluenza viruses. Infection results in tracheal airway inflammation and edema. In mild cases, positive intrathoracic airway pressure generated by coughing generates a high-pitched, seal-like barky cough. As narrowing continues, the negative thoracic pressure generated by the diaphragm will cause the airway to collapse,

requiring more accessory muscle effort to generate airflow. Nebulized epinephrine provides immediate effect in relief of edema, primarily through its alpha agonist effect. Steroids are effective in relieving the edema of croup, but typically take several hours for effects to be seen. The hypoxia and degree of respiratory distress this child is manifesting requires more than just humidified air. While the other options presented may all be useful in the management of croup, racemic epinephrine will provide the fastest relief. *(Behrman 836:1275–1278)*

60. **(D)** If a patient is not responsive to initial therapies, other etiologies of upper airway obstruction must be considered. Of those (a foreign body, retropharyngeal abscess, epiglottitis, peritonsillar abscess, or Ludwig's angina), epiglottitis is most likely in this patient. Compared to patients with viral croup, patients with bacterial epiglottitis typically are more toxic appearing. They present with lethargy, drooling, and a rapid onset of respiratory failure. When the diagnosis of bacterial epiglottitis is highly suspected, intervention (intubation) should not be delayed to await radiographic confirmation (*thumb print sign*), antibiotic administration, or observation. Because of the

risk of the development of complete airway obstruction, establishment of an artificial airway is the first priority. Controlled endotracheal intubation, performed in the operating suite if possible, should be undertaken with immediate surgical backup. Rapid sequence intubation in the emergency department may become necessary, but is not preferred to the more controlled environment of the operation suite. *(Behrman:836, 1275–1278)*

61. **(A)** The patient described is not in severe distress as indicated by the ability to talk in complete sentences and the lack of hypoxia. The recurrent episodes of wheezing suggest asthma as the most likely etiology. An initial trial of an inhaled beta agonist is the most appropriate choice. These agents' primary mode of action is relaxation of airway smooth muscle. The other therapies listed are sometimes used, but not as the initial management for acute exacerbations of mild-to-moderate asthma. *(Rudolph CD:1950–1963; Behrman:674–679)*

62. **(C)** The National Asthma Education and Prevention Program classification of asthma divides asthma into four groups based on severity (see table).

Asthma severity	Symptoms	Nighttime Symptoms	Lung Function
Severe persistent	Continual symptoms Limited physical activity Frequent exacerbations	Frequent	FEV_1 or PEF $\leq$ 60% predicted PEF variability >30%
Moderate persistent	Daily symptoms Daily use of inhaled short-acting beta$_2$ agonist Exacerbations affect activity Exacerbations >2 times per week; may last days	>1 time a week	FEV_1 or PEF > 60– <80% predicted PEF variability >30%
Mild persistent	Symptoms >2 times a week but <1 time a day Exacerbations may affect activity	>2 times a month	FEV_1 or PEF >80% predicted PEF variability 20–30%
Mild intermittent	Symptoms <2 times a week Asymptomatic and normal PEF between exacerbations Exacerbations brief; intensity may vary	≤2 times a month	FEV_1 or PEF >80% predicted PEF variability >20%

Source: Adapted from National Asthma Education and Prevention Program: Clinical Practice Guidelines. Expert Panel Report 2. Guidelines for the diagnosis and management of asthma. NIH Publication No. 97–4051, July 1997.

The panel also provides guidelines for management based on the severity of the disease. The patient described has mild, persistent asthma. Recommended management includes the daily use of an anti-inflammatory agent. Therefore, inhaled fluticasone is the most appropriate choice given. Autoinjectable epinephrine should be used for anaphylaxis and is not indicated in the routine management of asthma. Salmeterol, a long-acting beta$_2$-adrenergic agonist, is indicated for patients with more severe asthma. Because of its narrow therapeutic index and need for frequent monitoring, theophylline's use has declined and currently is considered only a second line agent for patients with mild persistent asthma. Antihistamines do not decrease bronchoconstriction and are not routinely part of chronic asthma management. *(Rudolph CD: 1950–1963; Behrman:674–679)*

63. **(E)** The history of recent travel to a country with high rates of contagious illness makes an infectious etiology more likely in this previously healthy child. His icterus and hepatomegaly point to an infectious hepatitis. Whether he had received the hepatitis A vaccine would be most useful to know. Sickle cell may be associated with jaundice, but is most common in individuals of African descent. Consumption of large amounts of carotene-containing vegetables such as carrots may result in carotenemia. This may cause cutaneous discoloration resembling jaundice, but would not cause scleral icterus or systemic symptoms. Malar rash might suggest the possibility of systemic lupus erythematosis which might be associated with hepatitis, but the constellation of findings presented is more suggestive of an infectious illness. Acetaminophen can result in hepatic dysfunction but generally in the context of overdose. *(Behrman:769–771)*

64. **(A)** Given the history of travel to Mexico, hepatits A is the most likely etiology of this illness, and may be diagnosed by serology. The aspartate aminotransferase will be elevated but does not establish the etiology of the hepatitis. Twenty-four hour urinary copper excretion is useful in the diagnosis of Wilson's disease which can present with hepatic dysfunction, but is not indicated in the clinical context presented here. Unless there is a suspicion of acetaminophen overdose, determination of serum level is not warranted. *(Behrman:769–771)*

65. **(D)** Hepatitis A is a picornavirus spread via the oral-fecal route that has a mean incubation period of approximately 4 weeks. Most infected children are asymptomatic. In certain developing countries, prevalence of infection with this agent approaches 100%. After infection, protective antibodies persist for life. An effective vaccine currently is available and in widespread use. Fortunately, most children completely recover from hepatitis A infection. Rarely, it will progress to fulminant hepatic failure. In patients with hepatitis B infection, coinfection with hepatitis D can lead to fulminant hepatic failure. Hepatitis B, C, and D are spread via exposure to blood products or via intimate sexual contact. Hepatitis A could theoretically be spread this way but that is not the most common manner. *(Behrman: 769–771)*

66. **(B)** Response to supplemental oxygen is helpful in the differential diagnosis of cyanosis in the neonate. The lack of response to increased oxygen suggests a right-to-left shunt, which in a newborn would most likely be due to cyanotic congenital heart disease. Hypoxemia associated with sepsis and pneumonia should respond to an increase in inspired oxygen. Because the PaO$_2$ is a measure of oxygen dissolved in plasma, it will be normal in patients with methemoglobinemia and will increase with administration of oxygen. However, cyanosis will persist as oxygen saturation of hemoglobin will remain impaired. While an arteriovenous fistula might produce right-to-left shunting and would not respond to increased oxygen, this is a much less likely entity than cyanotic congenital heart disease. *(Rudolph CD:1824–1836)*

67. **(A)** Transposition of the great arteries (TGA) is the most likely cardiac malformation to present in the early newborn period with cyanosis and absence of heart murmur. TGA occurs in about

1/5000 live births and is more common in males and infants of diabetic mothers. The mediastinum often appears narrowed on chest radiographs. Tetralogy of Fallot usually presents slightly later in infancy with cyanosis and a systolic murmur from the associated ventricular septal defect. Total anomalous pulmonary venous return presents in a similar fashion but usually is associated with increased pulmonary vascular markings on chest radiography. (*Rudolph CD:1824–1836*)

68. **(A)** This infant is critically ill and immediate intervention is needed. The hypoxemia requires immediate cardiac catheterization for atrial septostomy to create a shunt and improve oxygenation. Antibiotics or pressors such as dobutamine may slightly improve the clinical state but do nothing to correct the underlying problem. An arterial switch generally is deferred until the patient's electrolytes and medical status have stabilized. (*Rudolph CD:1824–1836*)

69. **(B)** The presence of anemia, jaundice, and dark urine suggests hemolysis as the most likely cause of the anemia. Evaluation should inquire about previous illnesses, episodes of pallor, and a list of all medicines taken, such as aspirin, antibiotics, or antimalarials. A family history of leukemia or sickle cell trait alone in a previously healthy child is unlikely to be relevant. Hepatitis A may cause jaundice but not pallor; also the cousin is described as healthy. Initial labs to obtain include a smear to define red cell morphology, a reticulocyte count to determine marrow response and the type of bilirubin made. A bone marrow may need to be performed at a later time. (*Behrman:1474, 1489–1491*)

70. **(E)** The unconjugated bilirubinemia is compatible with increased bilirubin production resulting from hemolysis. Initial presentation of sickle cell disease at 6 years of life would be unusual. Absence of spherocytes on the peripheral smear weighs against the diagnosis of spherocytosis although they may be absent in the face of acute hemolysis. Glucose-6-phosphate-dehydrogenase deficiency is the most likely etiology of those presented. Hemolysis associated with this disorder may

be precipitated by sulfa-based antibiotics, antimalarials, aspirin, as well as organic solvents. Diagnosis depends on measurement of G6PD levels in older red cells. (*Behrman:1474, 1489–1491*)

71. **(C)** The patient described has no evidence of cardiovascular instability; therefore, transfusion is not necessary or indicated. Close observation and serial hemoglobin determinations to monitor for continued hemolysis are sufficient. Removal of the offending agent usually results in cessation of hemolysis. Prednisone and other steroids have not been shown to change the course of the illness. (*Behrman:1474, 1489–1491*)

72. **(D)** This is a classic presentation of Guillan-Barré syndrome (GBS), a postinfectious polyneuropathy. Illness is frequently preceded by a nonspecific viral illness. The patient experiences ascending paralysis with the bulbar muscles affected last if at all. Deep tendon reflexes are lost, usually early in the course of the illness. Sensory function usually is spared. Nerve conduction velocity is decreased in Guillan-Barré syndrome. While there is no specific diagnostic test, the clinical picture combined with a cerebrospinal fluid showing an elevated protein and normal cell count is highly suggestive. Occasional cases of GBS can be associated with infection due to *Mycoplasma pneumonia* or *Campylobacter* species. The other lab abnormalities listed are not associated with Guillan-Barré syndrome. (*Behrman :1335–1336, 1892–1893*)

73. **(A)** Patients in the early phase of the illness should be admitted for monitoring of their respiratory status as the muscles of respiration may become affected. Administration of IVIG has been shown to decrease the length of illness and lessen the associated long-term disability. Most patients will recover fully within 2–3 weeks and supportive care is all that is routinely needed. Other therapies that have been used for rapidly progressive courses include plasmapheresis, high dose steroids, and immunosuppressive agents. Intravenous interferon-beta is a therapeutic agent that has shown promise in the treatment of multiple sclerosis but not GBS. (*Behrman:1335–1336, 1892– 1893*)

74. **(D)** The most likely cause of this patient's illness is diabetes mellitus with diabetic ketoacidosis (DKA). After assessing mental status and insuring airway and breathing are intact, restoration of circulating volume using isotonic fluids is the first priority in the treatment of DKA. Diabetic ketoacidosis usually has an insidious onset as the body tries to compensate for the hyperglycemia and acidosis. The deficiency of insulin increases production of fatty acids and ketone bodies resulting in metabolic acidosis. Breathing becomes deep and rapid (Kussmaul respirations) as the respiratory centers increase ventilation to compensate for the metabolic acidosis. Additional lactic acidosis when the osmotic diuresis associated with hyperglycemia results in increased urinary output (polyuria) and volume depletion. Dehydration and the caloric loss from glucosuria lead to weight loss. As thirst increases patients will increase volume intake (polydipsia), but the acidosis and other metabolic derangements may lead to nausea, vomiting, and abdominal pain. Once these compensatory mechanisms are overwhelmed, DKA will become manifest as in this patient. Bicarbonate boluses have been associated with the development of cerebral edema. Although oral intake is not necessarily contraindicated in DKA, it is not the initial step in management. *(Berhman:1772–1777)*

75. **(A)** A variety of metabolic derangements may result from the treatment of DKA. One of the more common is hypokalemia. Although serum potassium may be elevated in the untreated state, total body potassium is actually low. With insulin replacement and resolution of acidosis, hypokalemia may become manifest. Hypophosphatemia may also occur, as phosphate is transported intracellularly to restore adenosine triphosphate stores. Likewise, depletion of total body stores of magnesium and calcium occurs during DKA. *(Berhman: 1772–1777)*

76. **(E)** Parental requests for antibiotic therapy are frequent. A red eardrum alone is not diagnostic of otitis media. Diagnosis should be made only in the presence of a bulging tympanic membrane, opaque middle ear fluid, and abnormal membrane mobility on pneumatic otoscopy. For this child's likely viral illness, antipyretic therapy and fluids are all that is indicated at this time. The physician should take the time to discuss the development of a bacterial ear infection so the parents understand why antibiotics are not necessary at this time, but may become necessary over the course of the illness. *(Rudolph CD:1249–1255)*

77. **(A)** The child now has developed acute otitis media with effusion. Viral upper respiratory infections are the most frequent antecedent of otitis media in young children. They result in eustachian tube dysfunction that predisposes to middle ear bacterial superinfection, most commonly by *Streptococcus pneumoniae,* nontypeable *Haemophilus influenzae,* or *Moraxella catarrhalis.* Amoxicillin is considered by many authorities to be first-line therapy for otitis media. Because of increasing pneumococcal penicillin resistance, high doses (i.e., 80–90 mg/kg per day) are appropriate. This is especially true in the context of day care attendance because of the increased risk for resistant pneumococci among children in this setting. Ceftriaxone has been demonstrated to be effective in the management of otitis media, but should generally be reserved for cases not responsive to initial antibiotic management. Erythromycin is not appropriate in the treatment of this infection because many of the offending organisms are resistant. An otorhinolaryngology consult is not routinely necessary in the management of acute otorrhea. *(Rudolph CD:1249–1255)*

78. **(D)** The physical findings described indicate that mastoiditis has developed as a complication of the otitis media. The organisms causing mastoiditis are the same as for otitis media. Computerized tomography of the mastoids permits delineation of the area of involvement. Intravenous antibiotic therapy including a third generation cephalosporin and possibly additional gram-positive coverage are also indicated. Consultation with an otolaryngologist for drainage is appropriate. The other choices are inappropriate at this stage. *(Rudolph CD:1249–1255)*

79. **(E)** Diagnostic options for evaluating the etiology of this patient's problems are numerous.

However, the first step is to interview the patient alone. Her symptoms and flat affect warrant a frank, private discussion with the patient regarding issues such as depression, suicidal ideation, abuse (physical, mental, and sexual), eating disorders, and drug abuse. It should be stressed that theses discussions will be kept in confidence. Although both organic and psychiatric conditions may cause the constellation of findings seen in this patient, the initial step in the evaluation of either is a careful history. The behavior described is not typical for a healthy adolescent and should not be ignored. *(Behrman:80, 92)*

80. **(D)** Psychiatric illness needs to be aggressively addressed. The healthcare professional needs to assess whether the patient poses a threat to herself or others; the rate of suicide in the 15–19-year-old age group is around 9/100,000. If there is any indication of suicidal ideation, the patient should be evaluated emergently by a psychiatrist. Inpatient admission with close monitoring may be warranted in such cases. Collection of urine for drug screening against this patient's will increases barriers to establishing a therapeutic alliance. Although comorbidity with drug use is often seen in patients with psychiatric disorders, screening for drug use should only proceed with the patient's consent. Variation in mood is characteristic of adolescents, but the severity indicated here is outside the norm. Selective serotonin reuptake inhibitors are safe and possess minimal side effects. Initiation of this class of therapeutic agent along with counseling and close follow-up is appropriate in the case described. *(Behrman:80, 92)*

81. **(B)** Bipolar disorder usually presents in the third decade of life but can present in late adolescence. Patients with this disorder vacillate from depression to mania or may present with mania alone. During manic spells the patient's behavior is characterized by high levels of activity, loquaciousness, insomnia, feelings of grandiosity, a tendency toward overspending, and an expansive mood that may persist for weeks. SSRIs can heighten energy but not to this extent. The lack of delusions and the ability

to function well enough to purchase items make schizophrenia less likely. Sexual abuse can present in a variety of fashions but given her history, a bipolar disorder is more likely. Lithium carbonate, valproic acid, and/or carbamazepine along with intense psychiatric therapy may be necessary to control the symptoms of this illness. *(Behrman:80, 92)*

82. **(C)** The findings indicate that this patient has leukemia and is presently neutropenic. Most infections in neutropenic patients arise from endogenous flora, primarily the gastrointestinal tract. Bacteria intermittently seed the blood stream by translocating across the mucosal surface due to impaired immune surveillance. Empiric antibiotics should be directed against gram-negative organisms, including *Pseudomonas aeruginosa*. Of the options presented, ceftazidime (Fortaz) is the most appropriate, offering coverage of gram-negative organisms including *P. aeruginosa*. Despite broad activity against gram-negative bacteria, including *P. aeruginosa*, ciprofloxacin given orally is not appropriate in the situation described. *(Behrman: 785–787, 1543–1546)*

83. **(B)** Indicators of a more favorable prognosis in acute lymphocytic leukemia include age 1–10 years, hyperdiploidy over 50 chromosomes, absence of blasts in the CSF, initial white blood cell count of less than 50,000, absence of the 9:22 translocation (Philadelphia chromosome), and a TEL/AML-1 translocation. Poor prognostic factors include 11q23 or 4:11 translocations or lack of the previously described favorable conditions. *(Behrman:785–787, 1543–1546)*

84. **(C)** Induction chemotherapy may produce the tumor lysis syndrome, a constellation of metabolic abnormalities resulting from destruction of large numbers of tumor cells with release of intracellular constituents. In particular, potassium, calcium, and phosphorus levels can rise precipitously. Hyperkalemia can lead to dangerous arrhythmias. Simultaneous development of hyperphosphatemia and hypercalcemia can lead to heterotopic calcifications in various organ systems; kidney involvement

may result in renal failure. The release of uric acid can lead to nephrolithiasis. Preventative measures for these complications include aggressive hydration, alkalinization of the urine, and allopurinol administration. Dialysis may be needed if these preventative efforts fail. *(Behrman:785–787, 1543–1546)*

85. **(E)** Colic typically begins prior to 3 months of age, and is characterized by 3 or more hours of unexplained crying at least three times a week. The cry is spontaneous and continuous, with the face appearing flushed, the legs drawn up and the hands clenched. Bouts of crying associated with colic may resolve when the patient becomes exhausted or with the passage of flatus or belching. Without fever, ill appearance, vomiting, weight loss, or other abnormal signs or symptoms, reassurance and follow-up are the most appropriate initial steps. *(Rudolph CD:414–417)*

86. **(B)** A wide variety of colic treatment modalities have been suggested. The most effective one remains time, as colic rarely persists over 3 months of age. Swaddling has been shown to calm some infants. Stress is a precipitant of colic, and subjecting a single caregiver to the unremitting crying associated with colic is likely to worsen the stress (of both caretaker and baby). Water has not been demonstrated to be effective in this condition and excessive amounts given to young infants may precipitate hyponatremia. Likewise, vigorous shaking obviously is very harmful to infants. Paregoric (morphine, alcohol, and anise oil) is ineffective and potentially harmful. *(Rudolph CD:414–417)*

87. **(E)** A preverbal child cries to express him- or herself, and this needs to be stressed to parents. A search for causes of discomfort needs to be performed by the physician. Potential causes include hair tourniquets, occult fractures or infection, corneal abrasions, and severe diaper rashes. Irritability can also be due to sepsis, intussusception, hernia, or feeding intolerance. Given this patient's well appearance, it is unlikely that one of these more serious causes of crying is present. *(Rudolph CD:414–417)*

88. **(C)** A history of constipation and the potential for an associated anal fissure would be useful given the history of streaks of blood on the surface of the stools. Hemophilia rarely presents with gastrointestinal bleeding. Iron intake is irrelevant as iron (except in overdose) does not cause gastrointestinal bleeding. Rotavirus is unlikely in the absence of diarrhea and typically does not result in the presence of gross blood in the stools. Crohn's disease would be rare in a patient of this age. *(Behrman: 1181)*

89. **(C)** Anal fissures are the most common cause of bloody stools in the pediatric population. Continued passage of hard stool may prevent healing, a fact that should be stressed to the parents. Initial treatment should be aimed at softening the stool. Increasing fiber intake is very useful but hard to do as it may require drastically altering the diet of the child (and the parents as well). A stool softener (such as lactulose or mineral oil) titrated to the desired consistency is usually needed as well. Infections of anal fissures are rare; parents should be taught what to look for, but routine antibiotics are not warranted. The use of rectal dilators, frequent rectal temperatures, or colonic manipulation should not be performed. *(Behrman:1181)*

90. **(D)** Juvenile rheumatoid arthritis (JRA) affects about 250,000 children in the United States with a yearly incidence of approximately 14/100,000 children under 16 years of age. Joint symptoms are typically more severe in the morning and improve through the day. Large joints are usually affected. Progression of disease may result in persistent joint effusion, arthritis, and fusion of wrist joints with loss of movement. JRA is classically divided into three types: polyarticular, pauciarticular (with two subtypes), and systemic onset. Of these, polyarticular, rheumatoid factor positive JRA tends to have the worst prognosis with respect to joint involvement. *(Behrman:704–709)*

91. **(E)** Eye involvement can be seen in either polyarticular or pauciarticular type of JRA but is more commonly seen in the pauciarticular type. Affected children complain of redness, pain, photophobia, and decreased visual acuity.

Early detection by serial ophthamologic examinations is essential for prevention of blindness in these children. *(Behrman:704–709)*

92. **(A)** The patient described is in shock which is characterized by inadequate end organ perfusion. Evidence of inadequate perfusion in this patient includes tachycardia and delayed capillary refill time. Shock is considered to be compensated in the presence of a normal blood pressure. Hypotension is defined by a blood pressure less than the 5th percentile for age. For children aged 1–10 years, the lower limits of normal systolic blood pressure (in mmHg) can be estimated using the following formula: 70 + (age in years × 2). Other causes of shock include cardiogenic (e.g., due to myocarditis) and sepsis. However, the presence of sunken eyes and fontanelle, along with poor skin turgor and the history of fluid loss from vomiting and diarrhea implicate hypovolemia as the most likely etiology of this patient's shock. *(McMillan: 68–72, 2192–2198)*

93. **(C)** Mild dehydration (3–6%) loss of body weight is manifested by increased thirst and tachycardia but normal skin turgor and capillary refill time. Moderate dehydration in young infants such as this patient occurs when there is a fluid loss approximating 10% body weight, whereas older children have moderate dehydration with fluid losses of about 6–9% body weight. Moderate dehydration is characterized by the signs and symptoms of mild dehydration together with weak peripheral pulses. Patients with severe dehydration (fluid loss >10% body weight) frequently have associated hypotension, not present in the patient under discussion. Therefore, this child has an estimated fluid loss of 10% body weight (approximately 600–700 cc). *(McMillan:68–72, 2192–2198)*

94. **(A)** The initial hydrating solution should have close to 130–155 meq/L of sodium so that it can expand the intravascular volume quickly. If the patient is hypernatremic, it will not decrease the serum sodium too quickly, and will also correct any hyponatremia slowly as well. Appropriate resuscitation fluid could be normal saline (154 meq/L) or lactated Ringer's (130 meq/L). *(McMillan:68–72, 2192–2198)*

95. **(E)** Onset of a vesicular exanthem and enanthem in the early neonatal period should suggest the possibility of herpes simplex infection. Most women giving birth to infected babies have no known history of herpes infection. Evaluation of babies with suspected herpes infection should include cultures of the lesions for virus. Examination of the CSF is also important to evaluate for concomitant central nervous system infection. Prompt initiation of acyclovir is important in reducing morbidity and mortality. Institution of antiviral therapy in patients with compatible signs and symptoms should not await culture confirmation. *(Red Book:347)*

96. **(A)** The overall incidence of HSV infection is from 1/3000 to 1/20,000 of all live births. The risk of vertical transmission in cases of primary maternal infection is 33–50%. The risk of transmission is substantially lower (approximately 2%) in the setting of reactivated disease. *(Red Book:345–346)*

97. **(C)** Risk factors for vertical transmission include prolonged rupture of membranes greater than 4–6 h, primary maternal infection, presence of active lesions on the vaginal mucosal surface, and the use of scalp electrodes. Maternal coinfection with HSV type 1 or human immunodeficiency virus is not known to increase risk of transmission of HSV type 2. Peripartum administration of acyclovir has not been demonstrated effective in reducing the risk of transmission. *(Red Book: 350–351)*

98. **(A)** This child has a healing clavicle fracture that likely occurred during childbirth. Large babies have an increased risk of this problem. Associated symptoms may be minimal or absent. Callus formation does not become apparent until about 2 weeks of age, so it is not surprising that this is when the parents brought the infant in for evaluation. Some infants will not display irritability despite this obvious fracture. Comparison views are not necessary in the evaluation. A fibroblast assay is not warranted as

this fracture is most commonly seen in otherwise normal neonates. *(Behrman:492–493)*

99. **(B)** Factors that increase the difficulty of delivery may increase the risk of clavicular fracture. These include maternal diabetes (because of the association with fetal macrosomia), cephalopelvic disproportion, shoulder dystocia, or extension of the arms in breech position. Congenital syphilis may be associated with skeletal abnormalities, but there is no increase in risk for clavicle fractures. Likewise, maternal drug use has not been implicated as a cause of this problem. Thanatophoric dysplasia is a rare, lethal form of chondrodysplasia with associated defects in bone growth. These infants have short limbs, narrow chests, and large heads, but do not have an increased risk of clavicle fractures. *(Behrman:492–493, 2096, 2120–2122)*

100. **(B)** The patient described has features typical of Down syndrome. Ninety-five percent of patients with Down syndrome have trisomy of chromosome 21, usually due to mitotic nondisjunction of maternal gonadal cells. About 4% of affected patients have a centromeric translocation of chromosome 21 onto another chromosome, usually 13, 14, 15, or 21. Translocations account for 9% of Down syndrome patients born to mothers under 30. *(Behrman:324–328)*

101. **(B)** Down syndrome is the most common trisomy, occurring in about 1/600–1/800 births. For comparison, sickle trait occurs in approximately 1/12 of African Americans, trisomy 18 (Edwards syndrome) occurs in about 1/8000 births, and trisomy 13 (Patau syndrome) occurs in about 1/20,000 births. *(Behrman:324–328)*

102. **(D)** Individuals with Down syndrome are at increased risk for a variety of disorders. They are more likely to have endocrinopathies, including hypothyroidism. Congenital heart disease (most commonly endocardial cushion defects) occurs in almost half of these children. They also have an increased likelihood of leukemia, but not solid tumors. Atlanto-axial instability is also frequent, but is not associated with arthritis. Streak gonads are a finding seen in Turner syndrome. *(Behrman:324–328, 1864, 2091)*

103. **(E)** Neutropenia generally is defined as an absolute neutrophil count less than 1500/mm^3. Neutropenia is one of the major risk factors for infection in patients undergoing chemotherapy for malignancy. Conversely, the previously healthy child with an acute undifferentiated febrile illness and a nontoxic appearance has a very low risk of serious infection. The fact that the other blood cell lines are normal is reassuring. The most likely cause of the neutropenia is transient bone marrow suppression from a viral infection. Antibiotic therapy is not routinely necessary. Observation and follow-up of the WBC count to document resolution of the neutropenia would be the most appropriate management. *(Behrman:621–626)*

104. **(C)** The onset of hemiparesis most likely is due to a thrombotic stroke, a known complication of sickle cell disease. Rapid intervention is essential in order to minimize morbidity. Computerized tomography may not show evidence of ischemia for several hours after onset of symptoms. Exchange transfusion, which acts by decreasing the proportion of hemoglobin S, is the therapeutic intervention of choice. Unlike the situation in adults where strokes are primarily due to atherosclerosis and activation of the clotting cascade, heparinization or infusion of plasminogen activator provides no benefit in stroke associated with sickle cell. Hydroxyurea may be helpful in long-term treatment to increase hemoglobin F but is not useful in the acute management of stroke. *(Behrman: 1479–1483)*

105. **(D)** Patients with sickle cell disease have functional asplenia by 1–2 years of age and are particularly susceptible to infection by polysaccharide-encapsulated bacteria, including *Streptococcus pneumoniae, Haemophilus influenzae,* and *Neisseria meningitidis.* Of these, the pneumococcus is the most frequent cause of bacteremia. *(Behrman:1479–1483)*

106. **(E)** Sickle cell disease is an autosomal recessive disorder. Approximately 12% of African Americans are heterozygous for the abnormal gene. However, this risk varies in other ethnic/racial groups and the risk of this patient's children cannot be determined without knowing

the risk of his future mate carrying the abnormal gene. However, the risk for future children of couples *with an affected child* is approximately 25%. *(Behrman:1479–1483)*

107. **(C)** This boy has stigmata of Duchenne muscular dystrophy (DMD) including pseudohypertrophy of the calves and a waddling gait. Because of muscle weakness, patients with DMD may use their hands to "walk" up their legs when arising from a sitting position (Gower sign). Rovsing sign occurs in appendicitis when palpation of the left lower quadrant elicits pain in the right lower quadrant. Opisthotonus (hyperextension of the head, neck, and trunk) occurs in tetanus and kernicterus. Chvostek's sign is present when tapping over the course of the facial nerve causes contraction of the muscles of the eye, mouth, or nose and occurs with hypocalcemia. Grey Turner sign (bruising of the flanks) is associated with hemorrhagic pancreatitis. *(Behrman: 1873–1877)*

108. **(E)** As weakness progresses and difficulty handling oral secretions ensues, aspiration pneumonia becomes a problem for patients with Duchenne muscular dystrophy. Other complications seen include osteopenia and scoliosis due to the weakness and immobility. Scoliosis may become severe enough to contribute to impaired ventilation. Cardiomyopathy progressing to congestive heart failure may also occur. The myoglobinuria associated with this condition does not cause renal failure and the bulbar muscles are rarely affected. *(Behrman: 1432, 1797, 1873–1877)*

109. **(B)** DMD is primarily an X-linked recessive disorder, occurring in about 1/3600 male infants. As with other X-linked recessive diseases, approximately 50% of male offspring will be affected while 50% of female offspring will be carriers. Affected males will not pass the disease to their sons, but all of their daughters will be carriers. Although female carriers are generally not severely affected, Barr body inactivation can result in the expression of some stigmata of disease. Approximately 30% of cases result from new mutations. *(Behrman:1432, 1797, 1873–1877)*

110. **(A)** Of the findings listed, pulsus parodoxus (decline in systolic blood pressure >10 mmHg during inspiration) is the most suggestive of cardiac tamponade. This results from impeded left ventricular outflow and restricted left atrial filling during inspiration caused in part by the decent of the diaphragm exerting traction on the taut pericardium. Enlargement of the cardiac silhouette is neither sensitive nor specific for the diagnosis of tamponade. Neither bounding pulses nor egophany result from cardiac tamponade. Although the electrocardiogram may demonstrate low voltage, this finding can also be seen with myocarditis. *(Rudolph CD:1865–1866)*

111. **(D)** In the presence of symptoms, particularly hypotension, prompt intervention to remove the fluid can be lifesaving. Steroids, inotropes, diuretics, and/or pericardial window may be needed as part of further management, but immediate pericardiocentesis is needed to permit patient stabilization. *(McMillan:2271–2272; Rudolph CD:1865–1866)*

112. **(B)** Fractionation of the bilirubin will guide further workup of the jaundice. The history of acholic stools suggests the presence of an obstructive jaundice. The other tests listed may all be indicated, but it is the bilirubin determination that will provide the most immediately useful data. *(Behrman:1205–1206)*

113. **(D)** The presence of an elevated conjugated bilirubin in a thriving infant makes an obstructive lesion such as bile duct paucity or a choledochal cyst within the liver most likely. The initial diagnostic study in the evaluation of this condition is ultrasound. Tyrosinemia, which is characterized by elevated urinary succinylacetone levels might present with conjugated hyperbilirubinemia but not acholic stools. Cystic fibrosis is less likely to present with jaundice alone, especially at this age. Finally, plain film radiography will not add specific information. *(Behrman:1205–1206)*

114. **(E)** Biliary atresia affects about 1/10,000–1/15,000 infants and varies in severity. An exploratory laparotomy and cholangiography should be done to determine if a surgically

correctable lesion is present. For those in whom none is seen, the Kasai hepatoportoenterostomy should be performed as soon as possible to prevent worsening of cholestasis and hepatic damage. The rationale is that minute channels may be present in the porta hepatis and permit reestablishment of some bile flow, particularly if the channels are greater than 150 μm in diameter. The rate of success with this procedure is greatest if performed prior to 8 weeks of age. Some patients can survive indefinitely with this procedure; for others it is palliative, permitting increased time for growth and location of a suitable liver for transplantation. Hepatocyte infusion has been performed on an experimental basis, but is not currently part of standard care for this condition. *(Behrman: 1205–1206)*

115. **(A)** The signs and symptoms presented are typical of pinworm infestation. Treatment includes antiparasitic agents and reassurance regarding the benign nature of the condition. Visualization of the worms establishes the diagnosis and obviates the need to perform stool ova and parasite examination. Pinworms are easily transmitted and lack of personal hygiene is not thought to be of primary importance in spread. Household pets do not harbor pinworms and are therefore not involved in perpetuation of transmission. Finally, the pruritis and perianal excoriations noted are common with pinworm infestation and are not suggestive of sexual abuse in this setting. *(Rudolph CD:1105–1106)*

116. **(A)** Appropriate choices for treatment of pinworms include mebendazole, albendazole, and pyrantel pamoate. An antipruritic agent such as hydroxyzine or diphenhydramine may be given for symptomatic relief. No special local hygiene is necessary. The other drugs listed are useful in a variety of other parasitic infections but not for pinworm infections. *(Rudolph CD:1105–1106)*

117. **(C)** The initial history in cases of accidental ingestion should include specific substance ingested, amount and concentration of ingested substance, potential for coingestants, and interventions (e.g., induction of emesis) prior to emergency department evaluation. For this

patient, it would be prudent to assume she drank the entire bottle of acetaminophen. This would be about 3000 mg (100 mg/cc × 30 cc = 3000 mg). If so, the ingested dose would be approximately 230 mg/kg, a potentially toxic dose. Administration of activated charcoal with sorbitol to bind acetaminophen still within the gastrointestinal tract is the best option of those presented. There is no evidence of airway compromise, and acetaminophen is not associated with rapid loss of airway reflexes; therefore, intubation is not indicated. Gastric emptying by lavage or induced emesis is not recommended more than 1–2 h following ingestion, unless the ingested substance is known to delay gastric emptying. Although an acetaminophen level should be obtained at 4 h ingestion, administration of charcoal should not delay until the results are available. *(Rudolph CD:356–362)*

118. **(B)** The Rumack-Matthew nomogram is used to assess the risk of acetaminophen toxicity after an acute overdose. The initial serum level should be determined 4 h after ingestion. At that time, levels over 150 μg/mL fall into the possible hepatic toxicity range, while levels over 200 μg/mL fall into the probable hepatic toxicity range.

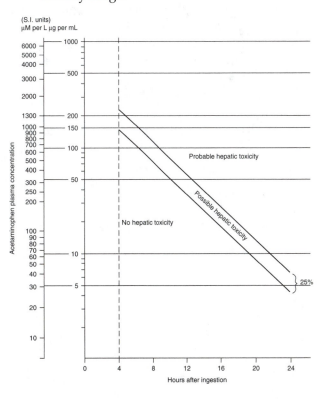

For patients with levels in the possible or probable toxic range, institution of *N*-acetyl-cysteine is indicated. Prompt initiation may be lifesaving, and long-term follow-up indicates that most patients receiving prompt treatment recover completely. *(Rudolph CD:356–362)*

119. **(E)** Acetaminophen is metabolized primarily (94%) to the sulfate or glucoronide form within the liver. About 4% is metabolized via the cytochrome p450 system and glutathione reductase to the mercapturic acid conjugate; the rest is secreted unchanged by the liver and, to a small amount, the kidney. When the load of acetaminophen depletes the glutathione to less than 70% of normal, the highly reactive p450 metabolite generates significant amounts of free radicals, leading to hepatocyte destruction. NAC serves as a precursor for glutathione synthesis and prevents the free radical formation. *(Rudolph CD:356–362)*

120. **(D)** The first priority in this patient's management is to secure the airway. The deep depression of consciousness, reflected by lack of response to painful stimuli and absence of gag reflex, place the patient at risk for aspiration. In addition, ventilation is likely inadequate. Drug screen and determination of blood glucose will likely be indicated, but should not delay establishment of a secure airway. Flumazenil may be useful in benzodiazepine overdose, but is not the next step in this patient's management. *(Gunn:19–20, 39–40, 748, 752, 894)*

121. **(C)** The toxidrome of bradycardia, hypopnea, marked lethargy, and miosis is most suggestive of a narcotic overdose. Clonidine ingestion can have bradycardia, hypotension, and respiratory depression but usually not miosis. Labetalol would cause bradycardia and hypotension but usually not the mental status changes. Diazepam can cause sleepiness but not usually miosis. *(Gunn:19–20, 39–40, 748, 752, 894)*

BIBLIOGRAPHY

American Academy of Pediatrics. *2003 Red Book, Report of the Committee on Infectious Diseases*, 26th ed. Elk Grove, IL: American Academy of Pediatrics, 2003.

American Academy of Pediatrics Policy Statement. Practice parameter: the neurodiagnostic evaluation of a child with a first simple febrile seizure. *Pediatrics* 1996; 97(5):769–772.

Berhman RE, Kleigman RM, Arvin AM. *Nelson's Textbook of Pediatrics*, 16th ed. Philadelphia, PA: W.B. Saunders, 1998.

Gunn VL, Nechyba C. *The Harriet Lane Handbook*, 16th ed. Philadelphia, PA: Mosby, 2002.

McMillan JA, DeAngelis CD, Feigin RD, Warshaw JB. *Oski's Pediatrics: Principles and Practice*, 3rd ed. Philadelphia, PA: JB Lippincott, 1999.

National Asthma Education and Prevention Program, National Heart, Lung, and Blood Institute. Expert panel report 2, guidelines for the diagnosis and management of asthma. NIH publication no. 97-4051, July 1997.

Ruddy S, Harris ED, Sledge CB, et al. *Kelley's Textbook of Rheumatology*, 6th ed. Philadelphia, PA: W.B. Saunders, 2001.

Rudolph CD, Rudolph AM, Hostetter MK, et al. *Rudolph's Pediatrics*, 21st ed. New York, NY: McGraw-Hill, 2003.

Dorland's Illustrated Medical Dictionary, 29th ed. Philadelphia, PA: W.B. Saunders, 1999.

──────────── CHAPTER 11 ────────────

Practice Test

Sara S. Viessman, MD

This chapter, a 162-question sample examination, provides a final opportunity to review, evaluate, and improve your clinical knowledge in general pediatrics. You should be able to complete the sample examination within 3 hours Good luck!

Questions

1. Among children, short stature and infertility are most commonly associated with

    (A) Klinefelter syndrome
    (B) Beckwith-Wiedemann syndrome
    (C) Turner syndrome
    (D) Marfan syndrome
    (E) Pierre Robin sequence

2. Unilateral multicystic dysplastic kidney in an infant usually presents with

    (A) an abdominal mass
    (B) hematuria
    (C) hypertension
    (D) nephrotic syndrome
    (E) oliguria

3. The Fanconi syndrome is characterized by

    (A) azotemia, edema, and hypertension
    (B) glycosuria, amino-aciduria, and phosphaturia
    (C) hematuria, glycosuria, and proteinuria
    (D) hypoglycemia, glycosuria, hypoglycinemia, and glycinuria
    (E) uremia, phosphaturia, and albuminuria

4. Which of the following sets of values is most suggestive of proximal renal tubular acidosis?

	Urine (pH)	Serum bicarbonate (meq/L)	Serum chloride (meq/L)
(A)	8	22	98
(B)	8	15	115
(C)	7	22	115
(D)	6	22	98
(E)	6	15	115

5. The presence of bilateral renal masses and a midline suprapubic mass in a newborn male infant is most suggestive of

    (A) bilateral Wilms tumor
    (B) congenital neuroblastoma
    (C) congenital rubella infection
    (D) rhabdomyosarcoma of the bladder
    (E) congenital urethral or bladder neck obstruction

6. Wilms tumor (nephroblastoma) is the most frequent malignant tumor of the genitourinary tract in childhood. The most common presenting sign of this neoplasm is

    (A) abdominal mass
    (B) abdominal pain
    (C) edema
    (D) hematuria
    (E) hypertension

7. A newborn with abdominal distension is found to have a meconium ileus. Which of the following conditions is most likely present in this neonate?

    (A) trisomy 13
    (B) trisomy 21
    (C) Tay-Sachs disease
    (D) cystic fibrosis
    (E) maple syrup urine disease

8. A 5-year-old male presents with a 48-h history of headache, and meningismus. Evaluation of the CSF reveals clear fluid with normal protein and glucose content. The CSF cell count reveals 300 WBC/hpf, 90% lymphocytes. Which of the following is the most likely etiologic agent?

    (A) *Streptococcus pneumoniae*
    (B) *Haemophilus influenzae*
    (C) *Neisseria meningitidis*
    (D) adenovirus
    (E) enterovirus

9. Compared to other methods of dialysis, peritoneal dialysis offers many advantages for children and their families including increased autonomy and flexibility, with resultant enhanced school attendance and peer interactions. Peritoneal dialysis is less costly than hemodialysis and can be used to treat even small infants. The major complication of peritoneal dialysis, either continuous ambulatory (CAPD) or continuous cycling (CCPD), is

    (A) a high incidence of disequilibrium syndrome
    (B) a high incidence of peritonitis
    (C) a need for severe dietary restriction
    (D) frequent electrolyte problems
    (E) poor growth

10. Which of the following represents the occurrence of significant bilateral hearing loss in infants in well newborn nurseries in the United States?

    (A) 1/100
    (B) 1/1000
    (C) 1/5000

    (D) 1/10,000
    (E) 1/100,000

11. The peak age of onset of childhood nephrotic syndrome associated with minimal-change morphology is

    (A) under 6 months of age
    (B) between 12 and 18 months of age
    (C) between 2 and 5 years of age
    (D) between 5 and 10 years of age
    (E) between 10 and 15 years of age

12. The finding of a low serum concentration of C3 component of complement in a child with nephrotic syndrome

    (A) indicates a high likelihood of spontaneous remission
    (B) indicates a high likelihood of good response to steroid therapy
    (C) suggests the presence of focal segmental sclerosis
    (D) suggests the presence of membranous glomerular nephritis
    (E) suggests the presence of membranoproliferative glomerular nephritis

13. A 4-year-old presents for a well-child visit. The parents state their family has practiced a strict vegan diet since the child was 2 years of age. Of the following, which is most likely to be deficient now or in the near future?

    (A) vitamin C
    (B) folic acid
    (C) thiamine
    (D) vitamin B_6
    (E) vitamin B_{12}

14. The most common roentgenographic abnormality in a child with asthma is

    (A) bronchiectasis
    (B) generalized hyperinflation
    (C) lower lobe infiltrates
    (D) pneumomediastinum
    (E) right middle lobe atelectasis

15. The pattern of inheritance of achondroplasia is

(A) autosomal recessive
(B) autosomal dominant
(C) X-linked recessive
(D) X-linked dominant
(E) polygenetic

16. The bacterial pathogens most commonly encountered in the lungs of patients with cystic fibrosis are

(A) *Escherichia coli* and alpha *Streptococcus*
(B) *Escherichia coli* and *Pseudomonas*
(C) *Staphylococcus aureus* and *Proteus*
(D) *Staphylococcus aureus* and *Pseudomonas*
(E) *Haemophilus influenzae* and *Streptococcus pneumoniae*

17. A 16-year-old male presents for a sports physical. Examination reveals hypermobile joints, pes planus, and a high-arched palate. Which of the following would be most appropriate at this time?

(A) chromosomal analysis
(B) cardiac ultrasound
(C) urine for organic acids
(D) cerebrospinal fluid for amino acids
(E) urine for calcium to creatinine ratio

18. A 2-month-old infant presents with irritability and congestive heart failure. An ECG is interpreted as characteristic of myocardial infarction. Which of the following is the most likely explanation for these findings?

(A) viral myocarditis
(B) ventricular septal defect
(C) endocardial fibroelastosis
(D) anomalous origin of the left coronary artery
(E) atherosclerotic heart disease secondary to a congenital lipid disorder

19. A 6-month-old infant is found to be lethargic and cyanotic. Blood obtained by venipuncture appears chocolate brown and does not become bright red when shaken in the presence of air. It is especially important to seek a history of exposure to

(A) automobile exhaust
(B) fava beans
(C) paint fumes
(D) undercooked meat
(E) well water

20. Peak height velocity for girls most often occurs around sexual maturity rating

(A) zero
(B) one
(C) three
(D) five
(E) seven

21. Which of the following is characteristic of a night terror?

(A) most often occur during the first one-third of the night
(B) onset usually is during the elementary school years
(C) rarely persists until adolescence
(D) occurs during REM sleep
(E) the event is vividly recalled by the child

22. The primary lesion in acne is

(A) hyperplasia of the sweat gland
(B) sterile inflammation of the sweat gland
(C) plugging of the sebaceous gland
(D) infection of the sebaceous gland
(E) increased cornification of the epidermis

23. A 7-year-old child is brought to the office because of chronic nasal obstruction. Examination reveals bilateral clear, serous discharge from the nose, but is otherwise unremarkable. The most likely diagnosis is

(A) a defect in the cribriform plate
(B) allergic rhinitis
(C) choanal atresia
(D) cystic fibrosis
(E) immunodeficiency

24. Atopic dermatitis in children

    (A) tends to spare the face and arms
    (B) is frequently associated with uveitis
    (C) rarely begins during the first 2 years of life
    (D) is characterized by pruritus and lichenification
    (E) is associated with elevated serum levels of IgA and IgM and decreased levels of IgE

25. A 15-year-old boy is bitten on the hand by a snake, which he then kills and brings to the emergency room. The snake is identified as a copperhead measuring 14 in in length. The most likely complication to be expected in this child would be

    (A) fever
    (B) local tissue necrosis
    (C) paralysis
    (D) renal failure
    (E) shock

26. The major concern regarding chronic otitis media with effusion is the development of

    (A) meningitis
    (B) mastoiditis
    (C) permanent nerve deafness
    (D) perforation of the tympanic membrane
    (E) impaired speech and language development

27. Which of the following is the most common indication for surgical repair of pectus excavatum?

    (A) thoracic scoliosis
    (B) cardiac dysfunction
    (C) pulmonary compromise
    (D) cosmetic appearance
    (E) cervical pain

28. Most nasal polyps in children are due to either

    (A) allergy or immunodeficiency
    (B) allergy or infection
    (C) allergy or cancer
    (D) cystic fibrosis or cancer
    (E) cystic fibrosis or allergy

29. The most common manifestation of alpha$_1$-antitrypsin deficiency in infancy is

    (A) pulmonary cysts
    (B) myocarditis
    (C) hepatic cirrhosis
    (D) pancreatic insufficiency
    (E) obstructive lung disease

30. The earliest indicators of Cushing syndrome (glucocorticoid excess) in children are

    (A) weight gain and growth arrest
    (B) growth arrest and acne
    (C) acne and hypertension
    (D) hypertension and striae
    (E) acne and striae

31. A 12-year-old girl presents with headache, visual changes, and papilledema. A CT scan reveals a mass lesion in the region of the anterior pituitary gland. The most likely diagnosis is a

    (A) chromophobe adenoma
    (B) craniopharyngioma
    (C) ganglioneuroma
    (D) medulloblastoma
    (E) neuroblastoma

32. An 8-year-old male with sickle cell disease presents with 2–3 days of runny nose and mild-to-moderate anterior chest pain. On chest x-ray a new infiltrate is noted in the right middle lobe. Of the following diagnoses, which is most likely?

    (A) acute chest syndrome
    (B) right middle lobe syndrome
    (C) aspiration pneumonia
    (D) foreign body
    (E) RSV bronchiolitis

33. Which of the following is frequently seen in sickle cell patients with splenic sequestration?

    (A) hyposplenism
    (B) pneumonia
    (C) polycythemia
    (D) eosinophilia
    (E) thrombocytopenia

34. Which of the following is the most common cause of infant (from 1 to 12 months of age) deaths each year in the United States?

    (A) sudden infant death syndrome (SIDS)
    (B) RSV bronchiolitis
    (C) child abuse
    (D) infantile leukemia
    (E) congenital heart disease

35. Of the following, which is a significant risk factor for SIDS?

    (A) firm mattress
    (B) breastfeeding
    (C) early introduction of solid foods
    (D) pacifier use
    (E) maternal smoking during pregnancy

36. Which of the following in an 8-year-old child is most likely to indicate an underlying psychologic or behavioral problem?

    (A) enuresis
    (B) encopresis
    (C) motion illness
    (D) migraine headache
    (E) recurrent pharyngitis

37. A 5-year-old girl presents with a 1 year history of monthly episodes of fever and aphthous stomatitis. A CBC about 6 months prior was reportedly normal, but a CBC now reveals a total neutrophil count of less than 200/mm³. The remainder of the CBC is normal. Physical examination reveals an inflamed pharynx and oral mucosa with several aphthous lesions on the gingival and buccal mucosa. There are bilateral, tender anterior cervical lymph nodes, the largest of which is about 4 cm in diameter.

The remainder of the physical examination is normal. The most likely diagnosis is

    (A) Chediak-Higashi syndrome
    (B) cyclic neutropenia
    (C) HIV infection
    (D) leukemia
    (E) Schwachman-Diamond syndrome

38. A 3-year-old male presents with random eye movements, ataxia, and developmental delay. Of the following, which is most likely the diagnosis?

    (A) acute cerebellar ataxia
    (B) migraine variant
    (C) neuroblastoma
    (D) retinoblastoma
    (E) rhabdomyosarcoma

39. An 11-month-old male presents with a 1 week history of poor feeding and constipation. On examination, you note poor head control and a weak cry. Though the infant's face is expressionless, he displays a paradoxical alertness and has normal features. The most likely condition of this infant is

    (A) bacterial meningitis
    (B) infantile botulism
    (C) hypothyroidism
    (D) Hirschsprung disease
    (E) iron poisoning

40. Chronic upper airway obstruction from enlarged tonsils and adenoids in a child may cause

    (A) convulsions
    (B) cor pulmonale
    (C) a pneumothorax
    (D) thymic hyperplasia
    (E) reactive airway disease

41. Febrile seizures occur most frequently

    (A) in the first month of life
    (B) in the first 6 months of life
    (C) between 6 months and 5 years of age

(D) between 5 and 10 years of age

(E) around the time of puberty

42. A mother calls to inform you that her previously well 4-year-old child has been complaining of headaches for about a month. For the past 2 weeks he has been keeping his head in a tilted position, and for the past few days he has been vomiting in the morning. The most likely diagnosis is

(A) acute torticollis

(B) brain abscess

(C) brain tumor

(D) degenerative brain disease

(E) meningitis

43. Episodes of cerebellar ataxia may be seen in

(A) cystinuria

(B) Gaucher disease

(C) Hartnup disease

(D) oxalosis

(E) tyrosinosis

44. An 8-year-old child develops an intensely pruritic rash on the legs only. There are patches of erythematous papules and vesicles and several streaks of erythematous vesiculation. The child is afebrile and otherwise well. The most likely diagnosis is

(A) eczema

(B) Henoch-Schönlein purpura

(C) poison ivy dermatitis

(D) scabies

(E) varicella

45. A 2-day-old male presents with upper abdominal distension and bilious vomiting. He passed a normal meconium stool shortly after birth. Abdominal x-rays suggest duodenal obstruction. An upper gastrointestinal contrast study reveals a "bird's beak" appearance of the distal portion of the duodenum. Which of the following is most likely?

(A) malrotation with midgut volvulus

(B) infantile hypertrophic pyloric stenosis

(C) duodenal atresia

(D) intussusception

(E) Hirschsprung disease

46. The usual presentation of an annular pancreas in childhood is

(A) hypoglycemia

(B) hyperglycemic acidosis

(C) jaundice

(D) vomiting

(E) steatorrhea

47. The classic radiologic finding in duodenal atresia is

(A) a totally gasless abdomen

(B) free air below the diaphragm

(C) the double bubble sign

(D) the anchor sign

(E) the string sign

48. During the first year of life, birth length increases by about

(A) 25%

(B) 50%

(C) 75%

(D) 100%

(E) 125%

49. Infants typically double their birth weight by age

(A) 2 weeks

(B) 2 months

(C) 4 months

(D) 8 months

(E) 12 months

50. A female-appearing infant is operated on for bilateral inguinal hernias only to have the surgeon discover that the masses are undescended testes. Chromosomal analysis reveals XY constitution. The patient's adolescent sister has primary amenorrhea. Chromosomal analysis of the sister also reveals XY constitution. The most likely cause of this syndrome in the patient and sister is

   (A) 20, 22-desmolase deficiency complex
   (B) end-organ insensitivity to androgens
   (C) congenital adrenal hyperplasia
   (D) true hermaphrodism
   (E) Turner syndrome

51. The normal, or average, hemoglobin concentration in a 12-month-old infant is about

   (A) 8 g/dL
   (B) 10 g/dL
   (C) 12 g/dL
   (D) 15 g/dL
   (E) 17 g/dL

52. Breath-holding spells

   (A) are most common between 4 and 6 years of age
   (B) are a common cause of sudden infant death
   (C) are a manifestation of infantile colic
   (D) represent a type of epilepsy
   (E) may terminate in cyanosis and loss of consciousness

53. The most common presentation of *Enterobius vermicularis* infection is

   (A) appendicitis
   (B) diarrhea
   (C) intussusception
   (D) perianal pruritus
   (E) vaginitis

54. A 10-day-old infant is evaluated for recurrent blisters and sores, mostly on the extremities at areas of friction or trauma. The child has been afebrile and well except for irritability. Examination is unremarkable except for blisters,

varying in stage from fresh to ruptured and crusted, mostly on the extremities, especially the dorsal surfaces of the hands and feet. Which of the following would be highest on your differential diagnosis?

   (A) bullous impetigo
   (B) congenital syphilis
   (C) drug-induced toxic epidermal necrolysis
   (D) epidermolysis bullosa
   (E) staphylococcal-scalded skin syndrome

55. Juvenile gastrointestinal polyps

   (A) occur most commonly in the ileum
   (B) rarely present in the first 5 years of life
   (C) usually present as blood-streaked stools
   (D) often already have malignant elements when first discovered
   (E) have a significant risk of malignant transformation after puberty

56. A 2-week-old male presents with irritability, decreased feeding, and fever. Cerebrospinal fluid examination reveals cloudy fluid with 5500 WBC/mm^3 and a low glucose. Gram stain revealed no bacteria. Which of the following is the most likely causative agent?

   (A) *Treponema pallidum*
   (B) cytomegalovirus
   (C) *Mycobacterium tuberculosis*
   (D) group B *Streptococcus*
   (E) *Staphylococcus epidermidis*

57. In comparison to cow milk, human milk contains more

   (A) protein
   (B) sodium
   (C) casein
   (D) calcium
   (E) calories

58. On routine examination, a 2-month-old Black male infant is noted to have a moderate size umbilical hernia. The contents of the hernia are easily reduced, and it is noted that the abdominal wall defect easily admits one examining finger but not quite two. The remainder of the

examination is normal and the infant is asymptomatic. The appropriate next step in management would be to

(A) order thyroid function tests

(B) refer the infant to a surgeon

(C) instruct the parent in how to tape the defect

(D) obtain an abdominal roentgenogram or ultrasound

(E) advise the parent that the defect will probably close spontaneously

59. Which of the following statements regarding chylous ascites in infancy is true?

(A) Congenital nephrosis is the most common cause.

(B) Hypoalbuminemia and lymphopenia are common.

(C) The condition usually is benign and transient.

(D) Hypergammaglobulinemia is common.

(E) Hepatic involvement is common.

60. A 12-year-old child presents with severe abdominal pain, nausea and vomiting, abdominal distension, and epigastric tenderness. Chest roentgenogram reveals a small pleural effusion. The child is afebrile but blood count reveals a marked leukocytosis. Of the following, the most likely cause for this condition is

(A) blunt abdominal trauma

(B) systemic lupus erythematosis

(C) hemolytic uremic syndrome

(D) alcohol ingestion

(E) Kawasaki disease

61. Idiopathic scoliosis is

(A) more common in boys than in girls

(B) diagnosed by x-ray

(C) generally associated with mental retardation

(D) most commonly noted during preadolescence or adolescence

(E) usually associated with considerable pain on motion of the back

62. A 6-month-old male presents with failure to thrive, eczema, and a history of recurrent bacterial infections. On evaluation, a thrombocyte count of $20,000/mm^3$ is noted. The peripheral smear reveals microthrombocytes. The most likely condition causing these signs and symptoms is

(A) Wiskott-Aldrich syndrome

(B) DiGeorge syndrome

(C) celiac disease

(D) idiopathic thrombocytopenic purpura

(E) leukemia

63. A 10-year-old male presents with an acute episode of nausea, vomiting, and severe testicular pain. On examination, scrotal edema and erythema with lack of cremasteric relex are noted. Color-flow Doppler ultrasonography confirms the suspected diagnosis. The initial treatment of choice is

(A) observation for 24 h

(B) immediate surgical exploration

(C) chemotherapy

(D) intravenous antibiotics

(E) intramuscular ceftriaxone

64. You examine a school-age child because of itchy scalp and note minute white-gray structures firmly attached to the hair shafts. You recommend

(A) a selenium containing shampoo

(B) a 1% permethrin cream rinse

(C) oral tetracycline

(D) oral and topical tetracycline

(E) oral griseofulvin

65. A 2-year-old child drinks kerosene that had been left in a glass. After the first swallow, she cries and drops the glass. She is most likely to develop

(A) aplastic anemia

(B) chemical pneumonitis

(C) coma and/or convulsions

(D) hepatitis

(E) peripheral neuritis

66. Congenital hypothyroidism should be included in the differential diagnosis of a newborn with

    (A) coma
    (B) prolonged jaundice
    (C) pulmonary edema
    (D) renal failure
    (E) severe anemia

67. A 2-month-old infant has had inspiratory stridor since the first month of life, but has been otherwise well. Physical examination is unremarkable except for moderate inspiratory stridor and retractions which are worse when the infant is supine or agitated and better when he is prone and quiet. The most likely cause of these findings is

    (A) reactive airway disease
    (B) laryngomalacia
    (C) viral croup
    (D) an aspirated foreign body
    (E) a tracheoesophageal fistula

68. A significant number of children with recurrent gross or microscopic hematuria, normal renal ultrasound, and normal tests of renal function have

    (A) hyperkaliuria
    (B) hypercalciuria
    (C) hypercalcemia
    (D) hyperphosphatemia
    (E) hemorrhagic urethritis

69. A 4-year-old child, previously well, presents with the rather sudden onset of wheezing which does not respond to treatment with aerosolized albuterol. An x-ray examination of the chest (see figure) is obtained. The most likely diagnosis is

    (A) asthma
    (B) foreign body
    (C) infantile lobar emphysema
    (D) pulmonary hypoplasia
    (E) right middle lobe syndrome

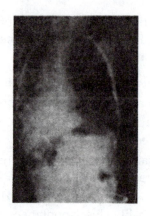

70. Physical examination of a 1-year-old child who does not walk reveals the findings shown below. The most likely diagnosis is

    (A) arthrogryposis congenita
    (B) congenital hip dislocation
    (C) equinovarus deformity
    (D) rickets
    (E) tibial torsion

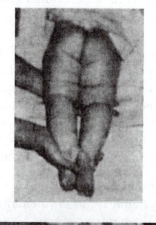

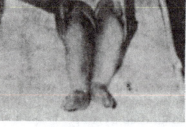

71. A 12-year-old girl complains of decreasing visual acuity and a slight feeling of discomfort in both eyes. Examination by an ophthalmologist reveals anterior uveitis. You suspect that the child may have

    (A) leukemia
    (B) toxoplasmosis
    (C) toxocara infection
    (D) hypoparathyroidism
    (E) juvenile rheumatoid arthritis

72. A 5-year-old female presents with intoeing. Her mother states the child is very limber and has no complaints of pain. On examination, with the child in prone position and knees flexed 90 degrees the child can easily place her lateral malleoli on the table. The most likely condition described here is

    (A) Perthes disease
    (B) acute slipped femoral epiphysis
    (C) metatarsus adductus
    (D) tibial torsion
    (E) femoral anteversion

73. For which of the following would laboratory testing for group A *Streptococcus* (GAS) be recommended in the United States?

    (A) an 18-month-old with pharyngitis
    (B) a 5-year-old with pharyngitis and anterior stomatitis with discrete ulcerative lesions
    (C) a 10-year-old with pharyngitis, conjunctivitis, and cough
    (D) all household contacts of a child with documented GAS pharyngitis
    (E) all household contacts of a child with documented poststreptococcal glomerulonephritis

74. The most consistent finding in lymphocytic thyroiditis (Hashimoto thyroiditis) is

    (A) enlargement of the thyroid gland
    (B) hyperthyroidism
    (C) hypothyroidism
    (D) eosinophilia
    (E) associated disturbances of the parathyroids

75. A 6-month-old male presents with diaper rash that is resistant to therapy. He has intermittent diarrhea. He is breastfeeding, and rarely seems interested in solid foods. Mom is a vegetarian. On examination, he is thin and listless. He has dry plaque-like sharply demarcated lesions around his mouth and eyes. His hair is coarse and scanty. A deficiency of which of the following could explain this condition?

    (A) iron
    (B) zinc
    (C) vitamin A
    (D) vitamin B_6
    (E) vitamin D

76. A 2-year-old child has had recurrent episodes of fever, cough, and pulmonary infiltrates on chest roentgenograms. Diagnostic evaluation reveals a normal sweat test, barium swallow, and serum immunoglobulins, but a severe microcytic, hypochromic anemia. The child's diet is normal for age. Which of the following would be highest on your list of differential diagnoses?

    (A) cystic fibrosis
    (B) diffuse pulmonary hemangiomatosis
    (C) extramedullary pulmonary erythropoiesis
    (D) gastroesophageal reflux and hemorrhagic esophagitis
    (E) primary pulmonary hemosiderosis

77. A 13-year-old female athlete presents with anterior knee pain of 2–3 weeks' duration. She has no history of trauma. On examination, she has good flexibility of lower extremities. There are no effussions. There is no tenderness over the tibial tubercle, or at the inferior pole of the patella. She has a positive patella glide test. Of the following causes of anterior knee pain, which is most likely in this patient?

   (A) Osgood-Schlatter disease
   (B) chondromalacia patellae
   (C) Sinding-Larsen-Johansson disease
   (D) osteochondritis dissecans
   (E) slipped capital femoral epiphysis

78. On a 6-month well-child visit, you note a healthy well-grown male with a normal physical examination except for a closed anterior fontanelle. Which of the following should you consider?

   (A) hypothyroidism
   (B) trisomy 18
   (C) hydrocephalus
   (D) craniosynostosis
   (E) hypophosphatasia

79. A previously well 9-year-old boy develops an intensely pruritic rash consisting of raised hive-like lesions with pink edges and pale centers. Lesions are well circumscribed and range in size from 2 to 6 cm in diameter. The history is unremarkable and physical examination is unrevealing except for the rash. Careful diagnostic workup probably will disclose

   (A) a food allergy
   (B) an occult malignancy
   (C) a collagen vascular disease
   (D) C1-esterase inhibitor deficiency
   (E) no specific cause for the rash

80. Most patients with XYY constitution are

   (A) short
   (B) homosexual
   (C) behaviorally normal
   (D) impulsive and antisocial
   (E) severely mentally retarded

81. A petechial rash is noted in a 10-hour-old newborn who is otherwise appearing normal and vigorous. There is no hepatosplenomegaly and radii are present. There are no risk factors for sepsis. A complete blood count reveals a normal WBC count with differential hemoglobin 17 g/dL; and platelet count 11,000/mm^3 with large platelets present. Which of the following would be the most appropriate next step?

   (A) maternal platelet count
   (B) abdominal ultrasound
   (C) bone marrow aspiration
   (D) Chest x-ray
   (E) PT and PTT

82. A 2-month-old male presents with a cough that has persisted for over 2 weeks. Mom has noted he coughs in spells and at the end of these spells, he vomits. She feels he has lost weight. On examination, you note a thin male infant who otherwise appears normal. Complete blood count reveals 30,000 white blood cells with 95% lymphocytes. Which of the following is the most likely diagnosis?

   (A) respiratory syncitial virus bronchiolitis
   (B) pneumococcal pneumonia
   (C) pertussis
   (D) laryngomalacia
   (E) vascular ring

83. Pseudohypoparathyroidism is associated with

   (A) short stature
   (B) renal failure
   (C) long, spindly fingers
   (D) generalized increased mineralization of bone
   (E) decreased serum levels of parathyroid hormone

84. The most consistent abnormality in von Willebrand disease is a

   (A) decreased platelet count
   (B) prolonged bleeding time
   (C) prolonged prothrombin time

(D) prolonged partial thromboplastin time

(E) decreased plasma level of factor XII

85. The most common cause of congenital hypothyroidism is

(A) dysgenesis of the thyroid gland

(B) a defect in thyroid synthesis

(C) Hashimoto's thyroiditis

(D) maternal ingestion of iodides

(E) maternal iodine deficiency

86. A 6-year-old Latin American male presents with a first-time generalized seizure lasting less than 5 min. There is no history of trauma or illness. The family recently immigrated to the United States from Mexico. The child is afebrile, and his examination is completely normal. Of the following, which would be the most likely cause for the seizure?

(A) herpes encephalitis

(B) cysticercosis

(C) lead poisoning

(D) vitamin B_{12} deficiency

(E) hypocalcemia

87. A 17-year-old boy with cystic fibrosis complains of a 5–10 lb weight loss over the past month, unaccompanied by changes in his pulmonary or gastrointestinal symptoms. You suspect that he has developed

(A) a bronchogenic carcinoma

(B) an eating disorder

(C) biliary cirrhosis

(D) cor pulmonale

(E) diabetes mellitus

88. The diagnosis of cystic fibrosis is usually confirmed by the finding of

(A) elevated sweat chloride

(B) decreased sweat chloride

(C) elevated serum chloride

(D) decreased serum chloride

(E) elevated sweat and serum chloride

89. A 2-year-old male presents with upper respiratory symptoms for 3 days and 1 day of fever, irritability, and right ear pain. Examination reveals a temperature of 39°C, clear rhinorrhea, an immobile right tympanic membrane with diffuse light reflex. The most appropriate initial therapy is

(A) antihistamines and ibuprofen

(B) antihistamines and acetaminophen

(C) penicillin

(D) amoxicillin

(E) erythromycin

90. An inguinal hernia in a 2-month-old girl

(A) may contain an ovary

(B) is usually a direct hernia

(C) does not require surgical repair

(D) is a sign of pseudohermaphroditism

(E) is generally associated with an imperforate anus

91. Which of the following would be expected in a 6-month-old child with a large ventricular septal defect?

(A) cyanosis

(B) an enlarged heart

(C) a continuous cardiac murmur

(D) decreased pulmonary vasculature on roentgenogram

(E) evidence of predominantly right ventricular hypertrophy on ECG

92. The most common presentation of hypoparathyroidism beyond the neonatal period is

(A) syncope secondary to prolonged QT intervals

(B) tingling of extremities

(C) seizure

(D) bronchospasm

(E) laryngospasm

93. The most common cause of school absenteeism among adolescent females is

    (A) depression
    (B) asthma
    (C) headache
    (D) dysmenorrhea
    (E) drug overdose

94. An irritable 12-month-old male has a 1 week history of high fevers and macular truncal rash. Examination reveals bulbar conjuctivitis, bright red cracked lips, and cervical adenopathy. The most appropriate next step is

    (A) immediate isolation
    (B) intravenous antibiotics
    (C) intravenous antibiotics for the infant and oral antibiotics for all household members
    (D) intravenous gammaglobulin
    (E) intravenous corticosteroids

95. An 8-month-old female presents with failure to thrive, constipation, fevers, and polydipsia. On evaluation, you find hypokalemia and hyper-chloremic metabolic acidosis and suspect Fanconi syndrome. Which of the following would be the most likely inherited cause?

    (A) cystinosis
    (B) cystic fibrosis
    (C) glycogen storage disease
    (D) Tay-Sachs disease
    (E) tyrosinemia

96. A 13-year-old male presents with a 3 cm annular scaling lesion on his right posterior trunk unresponsive to 2 weeks of a topical antifungal. On follow-up visit he presents with dozens of elliptical scaling lesions on his trunk. He has no palmoplantar or mucous membrane lesions and no adenopathy. The most likely diagnosis is

    (A) pityriasis rosea
    (B) secondary syphilis
    (C) lichen planus
    (D) tinea versicolor
    (E) Munchausen syndrome by proxy

97. An 18-month-old female presents for a well-child visit. On examination, there is an asymmetric red reflex, with the left appearing normal and the right appearing cream colored. Of the following, which is the most likely diagnosis?

    (A) rhabdomyosarcoma
    (B) retinoblastoma
    (C) neuroblastoma
    (D) leukemia
    (E) lymphoma

98. Which of the following represents the ethnic group with the highest neonatal and infant mortality rates in the United States?

    (A) American Indian
    (B) Asian and Pacific Island
    (C) Black
    (D) Hispanic
    (E) White

99. Patients with constitutional growth delay

    (A) will begin puberty at the same time as their peers
    (B) have a bone age equal to their chronological age
    (C) are usually obese
    (D) will achieve normal adult height
    (E) demonstrate height that is inappropriate for bone age

100. A 4-year-old male presents with a 1-day history of abdominal pain and vomiting. He is afebrile and has no diarrhea. He complains of knee pain bilaterally, and there is some tenderness of the knee joints but no effusions. Within 24 h he develops a rash on his legs and buttocks which is petechial and purpuric, and his platelet count is normal. The most likely diagnosis is

    (A) hemolytic uremic syndrome
    (B) Henoch-Schönlein purpura
    (C) acute glomerulonephritis
    (D) Kawasaki disease
    (E) systemic lupus erythematosis

101. A 4-year-old female presents with a limp. The week prior she had an upper respiratory infection. There is no history of trauma. Examination reveals limitation of motion of the right hip joint, especially with internal rotation. She remains afebrile. X-ray reveals some swelling in soft tissues surrounding the hip joint. A complete blood count and sedimentation rate are normal. What would be the next most appropriate step?

(A) aspirate the hip joint
(B) order bed rest and nonsteroidal anti-inflammatory agents
(C) order a CT scan of the hip
(D) order an MRI of the hip
(E) begin intravenous antibiotics

102. A newborn is noted to have a large head and short limbs. On further examination, short broad fingers, a small face, and low-normal length are noted. The trunk appears long and narrow. To confirm the diagnosis you should

(A) order an ophthalmologic examination
(B) obtain skeletal radiographs
(C) order chromosome analysis
(D) examine the parents
(E) perform the routine newborn screen

103. Infants fed exclusively goat milk are susceptible to
(A) vitamin A deficiency
(B) vitamin B_6 deficiency
(C) vitamin E deficiency
(D) folate deficiency
(E) thiamine deficiency

104. A 5-month-old female presents in the winter with a 2-day history of vomiting, diarrhea, and fever. The diarrhea is without blood or mucus. On examination, she is moderately dehydrated and has a serum sodium of 152 meq/L. The most likely etiologic agent is

(A) *Giardia lamblia*
(B) *Salmonella*
(C) influenza

(D) enterovirus
(E) rotavirus

105. Among adolescents of 15–19 years of age, motor vehicle accidents cause the greatest number of deaths each year. Which of the following is the second leading cause of death in this age group?

(A) homicide and legal intervention
(B) suicide
(C) heart disease
(D) cancer
(E) cystic fibrosis

106. The most common congenital infection is infection with cytomegalovirus, affecting 3–4/1000 livebirths. Of those babies infected, approximately what percent are normal at birth and develop normally?

(A) 5%
(B) 15%
(C) 25%
(D) 75%
(E) 90%

DIRECTIONS (Questions 107 through 128): This part of the test consists of a series of cases followed by a group of related questions. For each question, study the case and select the ONE best answer to complete each statement that follows. [*Note*: Try to complete all questions about a case before looking at the answers.]

Questions 107 through 110
On the second day of treatment for pneumococcal meningitis, a 10-month-old child who had been alert is noted to be lethargic. Serum electrolytes reveal: Na 120 meq/L; Cl 82 meq/L; K 3.1 meq/L; BUN 2 mg/dL.

107. The most likely cause of the lethargy and hypo-electrolytemia in this patient is

(A) acute hepatic failure
(B) acute renal failure
(C) congestive heart failure
(D) inappropriate secretion of ADH
(E) subdural effusions

108. The appropriate test to confirm this diagnosis would be

    (A) chest roentgenogram

    (B) measurement of serum and urine osmolality

    (C) determination of serum creatinine

    (D) measurement of hepatic enzymes

    (E) CT scan of the head

109. One would also expect this patient to exhibit

    (A) polyuria

    (B) hypotension

    (C) metabolic alkalosis

    (D) high urine specific gravity

    (E) high serum alkaline phosphatase

110. The most appropriate management of this problem would be

    (A) administration of hypertonic (3%) saline

    (B) restriction of fluid intake to about 50–70% of maintenance requirements

    (C) restriction of sodium intake to about 10% of normal

    (D) administration of a diuretic such as furosemide

    (E) discontinue intravenous fluids and begin oral fluids as tolerated

Questions 111 through 113
A 12-year-old child is admitted because of the sudden onset of coma. The child had been well until about 6 h prior to admission, when he began to complain of a headache. The headache became more severe and the child lapsed into coma. Physical examination reveals a temperature of 38.2°C. The child is flaccid and comatose. The remainder of the physical examination is unremarkable. A lumbar puncture reveals grossly bloody spinal fluid. After centrifugation, the fluid appears xanthochromic. There are 3000 RBCs and 7 WBCs/mm³. The protein concentration is 400 mg/dL and the glucose is 62 mg/dL.

111. The most likely etiology of the coma is

    (A) intraventricular hemorrhage

    (B) subarachnoid hemorrhage

    (C) aqueductal stenosis

    (D) viral encephalitis

    (E) subdural effusion

112. Which of the following underlying structural abnormalities would most likely have led to the above event or condition?

    (A) absence of the corpus callosum

    (B) porencephalic cyst

    (C) cerebral arteriovenous malformation

    (D) cerebral aneurysm

    (E) Arnold-Chiari malformation

113. The most appropriate next step at this time would be to

    (A) obtain a CT of the head

    (B) repeat the lumbar puncture

    (C) administer fresh frozen plasma

    (D) perform an exchange transfusion

    (E) initiate a transfusion of packed red blood cells

Questions 114 through 116
A 21-day-old male infant is admitted because of vomiting for 12 days. Birth weight was 2925 g. The child had been normal at birth and did well for the first 9 days of life. He was initially begun on breastfeeding only, but on the eighth day of life, supplemental feeding with a commercially prepared cow milk formula was added. Vomiting began on the tenth day of life and persisted despite discontinuation of the prepared formula. On the twenty-first day of life, the child was hospitalized. Diarrhea had never been present. Several days prior to admission, the stools had become hard and infrequent. On admission, the anterior fontanel is sunken, the mucous membranes are dry, and skin turgor is poor. The diaper is dry and the mother cannot recall when the child last urinated. The child appears poorly nourished. Wt 2850 g, HR 152 bpm, RR 12 times/min, T 37.5°C. Pulses and color are good. No abnormalities are palpated on examination.

114. The best diagnostic test for this condition is

    (A) an unprepped barium enema

    (B) a sweat test

(C) an abdominal ultrasound

(D) chromosomal analysis

(E) stool for *Giardia* antigen

115. One would expect the initial laboratory data to reveal

(A) mixed metabolic and respiratory acidosis

(B) mixed metabolic and respiratory alkalosis

(C) normal acid-base status

(D) primary metabolic acidosis

(E) primary metabolic alkalosis

116. Which of the following intravenous solutions would be most appropriate as the initial hydrating fluid?

(A) 5% dextrose in water

(B) normal saline

(C) 140 meq/L of Na, 120 meq/L of Cl, 20 meq/L of bicarbonate

(D) 5% glucose, 40 meq/L of Na, 40 meq/L of K, 80 meq/L of Cl

(E) 3% dextrose plus 140 meq/L of Na, 115 meq/L of Cl, 20 meq/L of bicarbonate, and 5 meq/L of K

Questions 117 through 119

A 15-year-old male presents with a 2-day history of fever, chills, and cough. He complains of aching muscles. Today he noticed his urine was red. Examination revealed a tired-appearing adolescent with fever, pharyngitis, nasal congestion, and tender calf muscles.

117. Urinalysis reveals a positive test for hemoglobin with no red blood cells seen on microscopic examination. Which of the following is most likely to reveal the source of the red urine?

(A) detailed dietary history

(B) renal ultrasound

(C) intravenous pyelogram

(D) immunoglobulin levels

(E) serum creatine kinase

118. You obtain the above study and it is markedly abnormal. The most important next step is to

(A) perform a lumbar puncture

(B) initiate intravenous antibiotics

(C) obtain a chest x-ray

(D) order serum electrolytes, BUN, and creatinine

(E) order liver function tests

119. Of the following infectious agents, which is most likely to cause this condition?

(A) influenza

(B) group A *Streptococcus*

(C) group B *Streptococcus*

(D) hepatitis A

(E) *Escherichia coli*

Questions 120 through 122

A 2-year-old child is hospitalized because of fever, cough, and hepatomegaly. The child lives in a poor, crowded home on a small farm. No one else at home is ill. Physical examination reveals a thin child with marked hepatomegaly. The spleen is not palpable and all lymph nodes are within normal limits. There are mild, bilateral rales and wheezes, minimal tachypnea, and retractions. The remainder of the examination is within normal limits. Chest x-ray reveals bilateral scattered densities. White blood cell count is $14,000/mm^3$ with 36% eosinophils.

120. Which of the following would be most likely to establish the diagnosis in this patient?

(A) bone marrow aspiration

(B) stool examination

(C) blood smear

(D) liver biopsy

(E) duodenal aspiration

121. The child most likely acquired the disease by

(A) eating poorly cooked pork

(B) eating dirt

(C) kissing a dog

(D) contact with a sick bird

(E) contact with a sick rodent

122. This condition is

    (A) more prevalent in the United States than in developing countries

    (B) more common in rural areas

    (C) nearly always symptomatic

    (D) most frequently present in school-aged children

    (E) transmitted only by mature dogs

Questions 123 through 125

A 4-month-old girl is admitted because of failure to thrive and persistent pneumonia. The child was well at birth but severe, recurrent diarrhea began at about 6 weeks of age. At 8 weeks the child developed pneumonia which responded only poorly to antibiotic therapy. Recurrent monilial infection of the skin and oral mucosa had been a problem. Physical examination reveals a small, poorly nourished child with moderate respiratory distress. There are bilateral rales, oral thrush, and a monilial-appearing rash in the diaper area. The remainder of the examination is within normal limits. The total white blood cell count is 5200/mm^3 with 87% polymorphonuclear cells, 12% lymphocytes, and 1% eosinophils. Serum immunoglobulin levels are: IgA not detectable; IgG 280 mg/dL; IgM <5 mg/dL.

123. Which of the following diagnoses best explains the clinical picture?

    (A) pediatric AIDS

    (B) Wiskott-Aldrich syndrome

    (C) hereditary agammaglobulinemia

    (D) severe combined immunodeficiency

    (E) transient hypogammaglobulinemia of infancy

124. On further evaluation one would also expect to find

    (A) increased numbers of plasma cells on bone marrow examination

    (B) enlarged superficial lymph nodes

    (C) absent thymic shadow on chest roentgenogram

    (D) positive intradermal reaction to Candida antigen

    (E) Western blot positive for HIV

125. Chest roentgenogram reveals bilateral patchy consolidations and diffuse granular densities with an almost ground-glass appearance to the lungs. The most likely cause of these x-ray findings is

    (A) pneumococcal pneumonia

    (B) *Pneumocystis carinii* pneumonia

    (C) pulmonary hemorrhage

    (D) pulmonary lymphangiectasia

    (E) miliary tuberculosis

Questions 126 through 128

A 4-month-old boy had been well until 4 weeks prior to admission, when vomiting and poor appetite were noted. Psychomotor development had been normal. The child was being fed whole cow milk and strained foods. Stools were normal. On the morning of admission, the child had a generalized convulsion and was brought to the emergency room where the seizure was controlled with intravenous medication. A second seizure occurred about 1 hour later and again responded to intravenous medication. Physical examination revealed a pale, listless infant, poorly nourished, but in no acute distress. The height was at the 25th percentile, the weight at the 3rd percentile, and the head circumference over the 97th percentile on a standard growth curve. T 38°C, RR 16 times/min, HR 110 bpm, BP 76/50 mmHg. The anterior fontanel was full, but not bulging. There were no focal neurologic signs. The remainder of the examination was within normal limits.

126. Which of the following diagnoses is most likely?

    (A) tuberculous meningitis

    (B) mastoiditis

    (C) subdural hematoma

    (D) congenital toxoplasmosis

    (E) pseudotumor cerebri

127. A funduscopic examination performed after one pupil is dilated with atropine reveals diffuse retinal hemorrhages. The most likely diagnosis now is

    (A) tuberculous meningitis

    (B) mastoiditis

    (C) subdural hematoma

(D) congenital toxoplasmosis

(E) pseudotumor cerebri

128. Of the following, the next most important step in diagnosis and management is

(A) lumbar puncture

(B) electroencephalography

(C) CT scan of the head

(D) bone marrow examination

(E) conjunctival biopsy

DIRECTIONS (Questions 129 through 162): Each set of matching questions in this section consists of a list of 4–26 lettered options followed by several numbered items. For each numbered item select the ONE lettered option with which it is most closely associated. Each lettered option may be selected once, more than once, or not at all.

Questions 129 through 137

(A) acetylcysteine

(B) atropine

(C) ammonium chloride

(D) calcium chloride

(E) deferoxamine

(F) digoxin

(G) EDTA

(H) ethanol

(I) fresh frozen plasma

(J) furosemide

(K) glucagons

(L) methionine

(M) methyldopa

(N) methylene blue

(O) naloxone

(P) nitroprusside

(Q) oxygen

(R) phenobarbital

(S) phenylephrine

(T) physostigmine

(U) potassium chloride

(V) potassium citrate

(W) propranolol

(X) sodium bicarbonate

(Y) sodium chloride

(Z) sodium nitrite

For each drug or poison, select the most specific and most important antidote.

129. Lead

130. Iron

131. Acetaminophen

132. Organophosphate

133. Jimson weed

134. Ethylene glycol

135. Morphine

136. Cyclic antidepressants

137. Carbon monoxide

Questions 138 through 144

(A) 2 months

(B) 4 months

(C) 6 months

(D) 9 months

(E) 12 months

(F) 18 months

(G) 2 years

(H) 3–4 years

(I) 5 years

For each description of developmental accomplishments, select the earliest most appropriate age.

138. Walks if led and is able to take a few steps unsupported, demonstrates a good pincer grip, drinks from a cup

139. Copies a circle, hops on one foot, recognizes colors

140. Smiles responsively, follows a moving object or face with turning of the head

141. Kicks a ball, builds a tower of six 1-in cubes, combines two different words

142. Sits without support, pulls to a stand, babbles loudly and happily, grabs a block with the entire hand

143. Startles at sudden noise

144. Draws a triangle, uses past and future tense in language

Questions 145 through 149

    (A) atrioventricular septal defect

    (B) mitral valve prolapse

    (C) supravalvular aortic stenosis

    (D) coarctation of the aorta

    (E) pulmonary stenosis

Choose the cardiovascular anomaly most closely associated with the condition below

145. Down syndrome

146. Williams syndrome

147. Marfan syndrome

148. Turner syndrome

149. Noonan syndrome

Questions 150 through 154

    (A) tongue fasciculations

    (B) Gower sign

    (C) heliotrope sign

    (D) nonthrombocytopenic purpura

    (E) thrombocytopenic purpura

For each of the conditions below, choose the most closely associated finding from the list above.

150. Dermatomyositis

151. Werdnig-Hoffmann disease

152. Hemolytic uremic syndrome

153. Muscular dystrophy

154. Henoch-Schönlein purpura

Questions 155 through 160

    (A) adenovirus

    (B) *Borrelia burgdorferi*

    (C) *Ehrlichia chaffeensis*

    (D) *Eikenella corrodens*

    (E) *Escherichia coli*

    (F) group A coxsackievirus

    (G) human herpesvirus 6

    (H) *Pasturella multocida*

    (I) parainfluenza virus

    (J) *Shigella*

    (K) *Spirillum minus*

For each of the following clinical scenarios, choose the most likely etiologic agent from the list above.

155. A 3-year-old presents 2 days after a cat bite to her face. She is febrile but not toxic and has three tubular shaped areas of induration approximately 1×3 cm each with surrounding warmth and erythema. The infected areas are very painful to touch.

156. A 4-year-old child presents in Missouri in late summer with a 3-day history of progressive vomiting and abdominal pain, fever, and petechial rash. He is obtunded and has multiple insect bites. He has leukopenia, elevated liver enzymes, and evidence of DIC on laboratory evaluation.

157. A 6-year-old presents with "pink eye," sore throat, and fever in the summer. His mother tells you that three or four of his friends have similar symptoms. Examination reveals pharyngitis with large tonsils and bilaterally erythematous conjunctiva.

158. A 6-month-old female presents with a 3-day history of fevers 39.5–40.0°C. On the fourth day, she developed an erythematous maculopapular rash and the fever resolved.

159. An 8-month-old with severe inspiratory stridor, fever, and a barking cough is admitted to the hospital for treatment with aerosolized racemic epinephrine and corticosteroids.

160. A 4-week-old presents with fever. She has a history of being well until 1 week prior when she was found screaming in her bed. Her mom noted she had a bite wound on her neck and suspected a rat to be the perpetrator. She watched the infant, who seemed to be doing well, until the past 24 h when she developed fever. On examination, the infant is irritable and has mild erythema surrounding the bite wound.

Questions 161 through 162

   (A) tuberous sclerosis

   (B) neurofibromatosis type 1

   (C) Sturge-Weber disease

   (D) von Hippel-Lindau disease

   (E) Albright syndrome

161. Facial port wine stain and intracranial angiomatosis

162. Axillary freckling, long arm of chromosome 17, autosomal dominant with 50% of cases associated with new mutation

Answers and Explanations

1. **(C)** Both Turner syndrome and Pierre Robin sequence are associated with short stature; however, Turner syndrome is also associated with gonadal dysgenesis and infertility. Children with Klinefelter syndrome and Marfan syndrome typically have long extremities, and children with Beckwith-Wiedemann syndrome typically have gigantism. *(Rudolph CD:745, 2087–2091)*

2. **(A)** Multicystic dysplastic kidney is one type of renal dysplasia, a group of disorders characterized by developmental abnormalities of kidney structure and differentiation. The entity is *not* related to polycystic kidney disease. Bilateral multicystic kidneys are rapidly fatal in the newborn period. The unilateral multicystic kidney usually presents in infancy as an abdominal mass. Hypertension has been noted, but is rare. In unilateral cases, renal function is preserved by the opposite normal kidney. *(Rudolph CD: 1704)*

3. **(B)** The term Fanconi syndrome currently is used to indicate a complex dysfunction of the proximal tubules, characterized by glycosuria, amino aciduria, and phosphaturia. Blood glucose as well as urea and creatinine levels usually are normal. It may be seen as an isolated finding (primary Fanconi syndrome) or secondary to disorders such as cystinosis or tyrosinemia. [*Note*: Fanconi syndrome is not related to Fanconi anemia, an autosomal recessive disorder characterized by pancytopenia and hypoplastic thumb and radius.] *(Rudolph CD:1709–1710)*

4. **(E)** The defect in proximal renal tubular acidosis is renal loss of bicarbonate due to an abnormally low threshold. Serum chloride is elevated and serum bicarbonate is low. Therefore, choices (A), (C), and (D) can be eliminated. A distinctive feature of these patients is their unimpaired ability to excrete adequate amounts of titratable acid and thereby lower urinary pH. The urine pH usually is acidic in these patients when the serum bicarbonate level is low. However, if they are given an infusion of bicarbonate to raise the serum level, urine pH will be alkaline during the infusion. *(Rudolph CD:1710)*

5. **(E)** The presence of bilateral renal masses and a midline suprapubic mass (the distended bladder) in a newborn infant is congenital urethral or bladder neck obstruction until proven otherwise. Posterior urethral valves are an especially important cause of such obstruction in the male infant. Early diagnosis is critical, as the renal parenchyma eventually will be destroyed by the resultant hydronephrosis. *(Rudolph CD:1641)*

6. **(A)** An abdominal or flank mass is the most common presenting sign in children with Wilms tumor. Often, the mass is discovered on routine examination or during examination for a minor illness. This underscores the importance of a thorough examination at every physician visit. Occasionally, the parents will bring the child to the physician because they note an enlarging abdomen or feel the mass themselves. *(McMillan: 1515–1517)*

7. **(D)** Meconium ileus typically presents within the first 24–48 h of life, and almost always occurs in neonates with cystic fibrosis. Of all children with cystic fibrosis, 10–20% have a history of meconium ileus as a neonate. The usual location of the obstruction is the distal ileum, resulting in a colon of small caliber referred to as a microcolon. Older patients with cystic fibrosis often develop obstruction of the distal ileum (typically in the ileocecal region) secondary to inspissated stool. This obstruction, termed meconium ileus equivalent or distal intestinal pseudo-obstruction syndrome, can be seen in cystic fibrosis patients of any age beyond the newborn period. *(Rudolph CD:1407)*

8. **(E)** Clearly this child's presentation suggests meningitis, a diagnosis which is confirmed by the CSF results. The relatively low number of total white blood cells, the predominance of lymphocytes and the normal glucose and protein values are all suggestive of a viral illness. Therefore, the most likely etiologic agent is enterovirus. Both aseptic meningitis and aseptic meningitis due to enterovirus peak in the summer months. *(Rudolph CD:900, 1021; Hay:719)*

9. **(B)** In most regards, chronic ambulatory peritoneal dialysis and chronic cycling peritoneal dialysis compare favorably to other methods of chronic dialysis. However, there is an increased risk of peritonitis. Usually diagnosed by a caretaker who notices cloudy effluent dialysate, the peritonitis most often is due to coagulase-negative staphylococcus and is treated with intraperitoneal antibiotics at home. Frequent episodes of peritonitis may cause the nephrologist or patient to seek another form of dialysis. *(McMillan:1574)*

10. **(B)** In the past, evaluation of hearing was recommended for infants who met high-risk criteria such as birth weight less than 1500 g, family history of sensorineural hearing loss, and presence of congenital infections or craniofacial abnormalities. However, 50% of children with sensorineural deafness (1/1,000 infants in well newborn nurseries) did not meet these criteria for screening at birth. Many states have passed legislation which mandates universal newborn hearing screening programs. The American Academy of Pediatrics and the Joint Commissions on Infant Hearing recommend that the diagnosis of hearing impairment be made before 3 months of age and the infant be receiving intervention services before 6 months of age. *(Hay:227–228; Rudolph CD:477–478)*

11. **(C)** Most cases of minimal-change nephrotic syndrome are diagnosed in children 2–5 years of age with a peak age of onset between 2 and 3 years of age. Older children presenting with nephrotic syndrome are more likely to have an underlying chronic nephritis (membranoproliferative glomerulonephritis, lupus nephritis, etc.) rather than minimal-change nephrotic syndrome. *(Rudolph CD:1678, 1691)*

12. **(E)** A low serum concentration of the C3 component of complement in a child with nephrotic syndrome almost always indicates the presence of membranoproliferative disease (assuming that the child does not have systemic lupus, endocarditis, or a shunt infection). Membranoproliferative glomerulonephritis is very unlikely either to respond to corticosteroids or to remit spontaneously. *(Rudolph CD:1681, 1694–1698)*

13. **(E)** Strict vegans eat exclusively foods of plant origin. Through education, strict vegans can have a diet balanced for most requirements. However, B_{12} is found only in products of animal origin. Therefore, strict vegans are at high risk for B_{12} deficiencies. Breast-fed infants of strict vegan mothers are at marked risk of B_{12} deficiency. In children with B_{12} deficiency, irreversible neurologic damage can occur before the presence of anemia. *(Rudolph CD:1338, 1530)*

14. **(B)** Generalized or diffuse hyperinflation of the lungs, manifested by an increased anteroposterior diameter of the thorax and flattened diaphragms, is the earliest and most frequent roentgenographic abnormality in children with asthma. Infiltrates, atelectasis, and pneumomediastinum are seen occasionally during an acute attack. Bronchiectasis is a rare complication and would suggest the possibility of an underlying disorder such as cystic fibrosis,

immunodeficiency, foreign body, or recurrent aspiration. *(N Engl J Med 309:336, 1983)*

15. **(B)** Achondroplasia, the most common form of short-limbed dwarfism, is an autosomal dominant disorder. Most cases, however, are the result of a sporadic mutation of *FGFR3*. Most patients have an identical missense mutation of codon 380 of *FGFR3* causing an arginine residue to be replaced by glycine. The incidence of achondroplasia is approximately 1 in 26,000 live births. *(Hay:797; Rudolph CD:759)*

16. **(D)** Chronic airway colonization and infection with *Staphylococcus aureus* and *Pseudomonas aeruginosa* is characteristic of patients with cystic fibrosis. Antibiotic therapy occasionally eliminates *Staphylococcus aureus* from the bronchial tree, but almost never eradicates *Pseudomonas aeruginosa* despite in vitro sensitivity to a variety of antibiotics. *(Rudolph CD:1795)*

17. **(B)** Marfan syndrome is a disorder of connective tissue affecting many organs. Affecting 1/5000 individuals without ethnic or gender predilection, this syndrome carries an increased risk of sudden death due to cardiovascular complications, primarily related to progressive dilation of the aortic root and ascending aorta. Ultrasound is a useful tool in diagnosing and following this potentially fatal manifestation of Marfan syndrome. *(Rudolph CD:762–763, 1897)*

18. **(D)** In the congenital abnormality of anomalous origin of the left coronary artery (LCA), the aberrant LCA arises from the pulmonary artery rather than from the aorta. This results in perfusion of the left ventricle by poorly oxygenated blood under low pressure. Myocardial ischemia can be severe. The presenting signs are irritability and congestive heart failure. The age at presentation is related to the degree of collateral circulation between the LCA and RCA. *(McMillan:1386–1387)*

19. **(E)** The findings of cyanosis and blood which is chocolate brown and does not become red upon exposure to air are indicative of methemoglobinemia. One cause of methemoglobinemia is exposure to well water which has

been contaminated with nitrites. In contrast, carbon monoxide poisoning (automobile exhaust) results in carboxyhemoglobin which binds oxygen so tightly that it cannot be released to the tissues. In this situation the blood would be bright red, rather than dark brown. Fava beans are a cause of hemolysis in patients with G-6-PD deficiency, but are not a cause of methemoglobinemia. *(Rudolph CD:371–371, 1544–1545)*

20. **(C)** Peak height velocity occurs typically during SMR 2–3 for girls, and during SMR 4 for boys. *(Rudolph CD:223–224)*

21. **(A)** Night terrors are partial arousals that occur during stage 4 non-REM sleep to near arousal transitions which typically first present in the preschool-aged child. The child appears awake, but does not respond to surroundings, including the family members attempting to calm the child. Amnesia of the event is another one of the events distinguishing these from nightmares. Night terrors persist into adolescence in about one-third of the cases. *(Rudolph CD:418)*

22. **(C)** The primary lesion in acne is plugging of the duct of the sebaceous gland by dried or excessive sebum and keratin. The obstructed gland (comedo) eventually becomes inflamed. The relative roles of fatty acids, bacteria such as *Propionibacterium acnes* and *Staphylococcus epidermidis*, and the immunologic response in determining this inflammatory reaction are uncertain. [*Note*: The question asked for the *primary* lesion in acne. Infection of the gland, which is an important factor in many cases, is a *secondary* rather than a primary lesion.] *(McMillan:729)*

23. **(B)** Although all the diseases listed can cause nasal obstruction and discharge, allergic rhinitis is by far the most common and the most likely in this child. Bilateral choanal atresia causes respiratory distress in the neonatal period; unilateral atresia causes persistent unilateral, purulent discharge. Immunodeficiency is most likely to cause chronic sinusitis and purulent discharge. Cystic fibrosis is much less common than allergy, and a defect in the cribriform plate is extremely rare. *(McMillan: 2064–2065)*

24. **(D)** Atopic dermatitis (eczema) is characterized by exudation, pruritus, and lichenification. Involvement in infancy is common, although the distribution and other features may be somewhat different than in older children. The classical adult distribution with predilection for popliteal and antecubital areas usually is not seen in infancy. Involvement of the face is common. Most patients have *elevated* serum IgE levels and normal levels of the other immunoglobulins. *(McMillan:2059–2060)*

25. **(B)** The copperhead is a member of the group of poisonous snakes known as pit vipers or *Crotalids*. This group also includes the rattlesnake and the cottonmouth (water moccasin). All members of the group share similar toxins, the effects of which include local tissue injury and necrosis, neurologic manifestations, generalized bleeding, and shock. The severity of the reaction is related to the amount of venom injected (size of snake) and size of the victim. Local reactions are most common and are seen in almost all significant envenomations. Systemic reactions are less frequent and generally are seen only with severe envenomations. *(Rudolph CD:397–398)*

26. **(E)** The major concern for children with chronic otitis media with effusion (chronic OME) is that the associated conductive hearing loss will interfere with speech and language development during the critical early years of life. *(Rudolph CD:1253)*

27. **(D)** The most common indication for repair of pectus excavatum is to improve the appearance of the chest wall. *(Rudolph CD:2001)*

28. **(E)** Nasal polyps are uncommon in childhood. The two leading causes are allergy (allergic rhinitis) and cystic fibrosis. Although allergy is more common, any child with nasal polyps probably should have a sweat test, since allergic manifestations are not uncommon in children with cystic fibrosis. Benign (hemangioma, fibroma) and malignant (rhabdomyosarcoma, esthesioneuroblastoma) lesions are rare and can be mistaken for polyps. *(McMillan:1245)*

29. **(C)** Unlike the situation in older children and adults, in infants the most frequent target organ of alpha$_1$-antitrypsin deficiency is the liver. This may take the form of prolonged neonatal cholestasis and/or cirrhosis and portal hypertension. Obstructive lung disease can be seen in older children, but is rare in infancy. *(Rudolph CD:1490–1491)*

30. **(A)** Cushing syndrome (glucocorticoid excess) should be considered in any child with the combination of weight gain and growth arrest. In children younger than 7 years of age, glucocorticoid excess (noniatrogenic) is most often secondary to an adrenal tumor. In older children, the most common noniatrogenic cause of Cushing syndrome is true Cushing disease, adrenal hyperplasia caused by hypersecretion of pituitary ACTH. Over 80% of these older children have surgically identifiable pituitary microadenoma. *(Rudolph CD:2045–2046)*

31. **(B)** The most common tumor to cause destruction of the anterior pituitary gland in childhood is the craniopharyngioma. The diabetes insipidus that occurs as a result of the pituitary destruction can be very challenging to manage. The chromophobe adenoma is the most common destructive lesion in adults, but is rare in childhood. *(McMillan:1780)*

32. **(A)** Acute chest syndrome is a well described and potentially life-threatening complication of sickle cell disease. Early recognition and treatment are essential. Patients with acute chest syndrome can deteriorate rapidly and therefore require keen observation. *(Pediatrics 109:526–535, 2002)*

33. **(E)** Splenic sequestration is characterized by an acutely enlarging spleen and a decreasing (or decreased) hemoglobin, and frequently is associated with thrombocytopenia. Prompt recognition and treatment is necessary because some of the severe cases will rapidly progress to shock and death. Most of these acute splenic sequestration crises occur during infancy and early childhood and are uncommon after the fourth or fifth birthday, by which time autosplenectomy (due to recurrent infarctions) has

occurred. In patients with sickle-C disease or sickle-thalassemia, however, the spleen may remain large and sequestration crises can occur into the teens and adulthood. *(Behrman:1480; Pediatrics 109:526–535, 2002)*

34. **(A)** Since 1992 the American Academy of Pediatrics has recommended infants be placed on their backs to sleep in order to decrease the risk of SIDS. It has been called "The Back to Sleep" campaign, and has been very successful in helping to decrease SIDS by >40%. Yet SIDS remains the leading cause of death in infants beyond the neonatal period. *(Pediatrics 105: 650–656, 2000)*

35. **(E)** Modifiable risk factors for SIDS that have been documented thus far include prone sleeping, soft sleep surfaces and loose bedding, overheating, maternal smoking during pregnancy, bed sharing (especially if the adults sharing the bed are smokers), and preterm birth and low birth weight. The factor most strongly associated with protection against SIDS is supine sleeping. Interestingly, studies recently have shown a substantially lower incidence of SIDS among pacifier-using infants compared to infants not using pacifiers. However, there is no proof that pacifier use *prevents* SIDS, and the use of pacifiers has other negative consequences. Therefore, a specific recommendation regarding pacifier use in SIDS prevention has not been made by the AAP. *(Pediatrics 105:650–656, 2000)*

36. **(B)** Although some cases of encopresis may be secondary to organic causes (spina bifida, Hirschsprung disease), the majority are psychologic or behavioral in nature. In contrast, the majority of cases of enuresis are most often due to a disturbance of bladder physiology or sleep mechanism, and generally are not considered to represent an emotional or behavioral disorder. If a child has been dry, then becomes enuretic (secondary enuresis), emotional factors may be involved in the process. Secondary enuresis may indicate sexual abuse. *(McMillan: 518:1559, 1563, 1566–1568)*

37. **(B)** This child probably has cyclic neutropenia, a defect in the production of granulocyte-

macrophage colony-stimulating factor (GM-CSF). In these patients GM-CSF is produced in a cyclic rather than continuous manner. Episodes of neutropenia, often accompanied by fever, aphthous stomatitis, and cervical lymphadenitis recur at *regular* intervals, usually every 21–42 days. Few other conditions have such a remarkable periodicity. Schwachman-Diamond syndrome is the association of neutropenia with exocrine pancreatic insufficiency. Chediak-Higashi syndrome is an autosomal recessive disorder characterized by morphologically abnormal neutrophils, recurrent infections, partial albinism, mental retardation, and eventual pancytopenia. *(McMillan:1462)*

38. **(C)** Random eye movements, ataxia, developmental delay, and abnormal behavior are found in the opsoclonus-myoclonus syndrome (otherwise called "dancing eyes, dancing feet" syndrome). This syndrome is associated with neuroblastoma. Though the associated tumors typically are small and resected, neurologic symptoms may persist. There may be an immune mechanism for these neurologic symptoms. *(McMillan:1518)*

39. **(B)** Infantile botulism should be considered in any infant with a history of progressive weakness, poor feeding, and constipation. Except for the insidious development of symptoms, the infants can be confused with those with sepsis or hypoglycemia. Their alertness with weakness resembles that seen in Werdnig-Hoffmann disease. However, infants with Werdnig-Hoffmann disease typically present before 6 months of age, lack lower limb deep tendon reflexes, and have very expressive faces. *(Rudolph CD:917–918, 2002, 2280)*

40. **(B)** Snoring is the hallmark of chronic upper airway obstruction from enlarged adenoids and tonsils in children. An infrequent but important complication of this is pulmonary hypertension with cor pulmonale. These children appear to hypoventilate, especially when asleep. The hypoxemia which results from the hypoventilation causes pulmonary arteriolar vasoconstriction, and this in turn results in cor pulmonale. *(Rudolph CD:1270)*

41. **(C)** Essentially all febrile seizures occur in children between 6 months and 5 years of age. Indeed, most authors incorporate this age range into the definition of febrile convulsions while some broaden the definition to between 3 months and 6 years. The peak age clearly is between 6 months and 3 years. In one study, the mean age was 23 months. (*Rudolph CD:330, 2270–2271*)

42. **(C)** The clinical picture described is extremely suggestive of a brain tumor. Head tilt in these cases can be due to several mechanisms, including cranial nerve involvement with acute strabismus and secondary compensation by tilting the head. Head tilt is particularly common with posterior fossa tumors. Central nervous system tumors are now the most common neoplasms of childhood, accounting for 20%. The incidence of brain tumors is evenly distributed throughout childhood and adolescence. (*Rudolph CD:2207–2211*)

43. **(C)** Hartnup disease is an autosomal recessive disorder with a single defect in the transport of monoamino-monocarboxylic amino acids by the renal tubules and intestinal mucosa. There is increased loss of the involved amino acids (neutral amino acids). Most children remain asymptomatic, and the major clinical manifestation is cutaneous photosensitivity. Some children with this disorder will have attacks of cerebellar ataxia, which resolve spontaneously but also can be reversed by the administration of nicotinic acid. None of the other conditions listed are associated with ataxia. (*Behrman:353*)

44. **(C)** The rash described is that of a contact dermatitis, most likely due to poison ivy. The lesions, papules, and vesicles, are intensely pruritic. Restriction of the rash to the legs also is characteristic of poison ivy. Although the rash of Henoch-Schönlein purpura is usually restricted to below the waist, it is purpuric rather than pruritic. (*Rudolph CD:1180*)

45. **(A)** Bilious vomiting in the neonate can represent any gastrointestinal obstruction distal to the entry of the common duct into the duodenum and requires immediate evaluation and treatment. In this case, the "bird beak" appearance of the distal duodenum is diagnostic of midgut volvulus probably secondary to malrotation. The resultant strangulation of the superior mesenteric artery can lead to total destruction of the jejunoileum. (*Klaus:185; Rudolph CD:1376*)

46. **(D)** Annular pancreas is a congenital malformation in which the pancreas encircles the duodenum. The condition may be asymptomatic or may cause partial or complete duodenal obstruction. The most frequent presenting complaint is vomiting. (*Rudolph CD:1002*)

47. **(C)** The classical radiologic finding in duodenal atresia is dilatation of the stomach and of the proximal duodenum—the so-called "double bubble" sign. The double bubble sign can also be seen with annular pancreas, and occasionally malrotation. Remember, 40% of all neonates with duodenal atresia have trisomy 21. (*Klaus:185; Rudolph CD:1403*)

48. **(B)** During the first year of life, the average infant grows about 25 cm (10 in). That is, they grow from about 51 cm (20 in) at birth to about 75 cm (30 in) at the first birthday. Another way to phrase this is that by the end of the first year, birth length increases by 50%. (*Rudolph CD:5*)

49. **(C)** Infants typically double their birth weight by approximately 4 months of age, and triple their birth weight by approximately 12 months of age. Contrast this with height. A child doubles their birth length by 4 years of age and triples their birth length by 13 years of age. (*Rudolph CD:5*)

50. **(B)** The picture described is most suggestive of the X-linked recessive disorder of end-organ insensitivity to androgenic hormones (testicular feminization). Although the 20, 22-desmolase deficiency does cause male pseudohermaphrodism, the associated adrenal insufficiency is quickly fatal in infancy, unless diagnosed and treated. All other forms of congenital adrenal hyperplasia are virilizing rather than feminizing. True hermaphrodism is very rare and requires that both testicular and ovarian tissue

be present. No evidence for this is presented in this case. *(Rudolph CD:2011, 2085)*

51. **(C)** At birth, the average hemoglobin is 17 g/dL in term babies. It then falls rapidly over the next 2–3 months to a low of about 11 g/dL. Hemoglobin values then gradually rise and eventually equal adult normal values in the early teen years. *(Rudolph CD:1519–1521)*

52. **(E)** Breath-holding spells always terminate spontaneously and are never fatal; they have no known relationship to sudden infant death syndrome. Breath-holding spells are common in early childhood, have a peak incidence between 12 and 18 months and usually disappear by about 5 years of age. The exact mechanism or etiology is not known. Although many youngsters will hold their breath to the point of cyanosis and syncope or seizure, there is nothing to suggest that breath-holding is a type of epilepsy. Rather, the syncope and seizure are secondary to cerebral hypoxia. *(Behrman: 1829–1830)*

53. **(D)** The major manifestation of pinworm (*Enterobius vermicularis*) infection is rectal or perirectal itching. The female worms leave the rectum at night to lay their eggs in the perineal area and die shortly thereafter. Eggs remain viable and infective for 2–3 weeks in indoor environments. *(Red Book:486–487)*

54. **(D)** Although all the conditions listed as possible answers are associated with bullous lesions, epidermolysis bullosa (EB) is the best fit and should be highest on the differential diagnosis. There are at least 15 known forms of EB, varying in severity and age of presentation. Many present in the newborn period, with lesions mostly at areas of friction or trauma as described in this patient. Both drug-induced toxic epidermal necrolysis (rare in neonates) and staphylococcal-scalded skin syndrome (common in neonates) are associated with more generalized erythema and lesions than described in this patient. Neither the lesions of bullous impetigo nor the lesions of congenital syphilis are related to areas of trauma; the latter have a special predilection for the palms and soles. *(Rudolph CD:1173, 1187)*

55. **(C)** Juvenile polyps are most commonly found in the rectum. These are hamartomas with inflammatory infiltration. They are not adenomatous polyps and are neither malignant nor premalignant. They generally present in the first 5 years of life with the passage of red blood streaking on the stool. *(Rudolph CD:1453–1455)*

56. **(D)** The elevated white blood cell count and low glucose in the cerebrospinal fluid are most suggestive of a bacterial pathogen, of which group B *Streptococcus* would be the most likely. Though a Gram stain of CSF provides presumptive evidence in the evaluation of meningitis, it frequently is misleading. The gold standard for diagnosis of a bacterial pathogen is the culture of the spinal fluid. *(Red Book:585–586; Hay:719)*

57. **(E)** Cow milk and human milk have many differences in composition. Cow milk has a higher protein content (32 vs. 10.6 g/L) and human milk has a higher fat (45 vs. 38 g/L) and carbohydrate (71 vs. 47 g/L) content. Cow milk also has higher sodium and calcium content. Except for colostrum—milk produced during the first few days following delivery of the baby—human milk has more calories (747 kcal/L) than does cow milk (701 kcal/L). *(Behrman:156)*

58. **(E)** Umbilical hernias are quite common, especially in premature and in Black infants. Although there is an increased incidence of umbilical hernias in infants with a variety of syndromes (e.g., Beckwith-Wiedemann) and diseases (e.g., hypothyroidism), the great majority occur in otherwise normal infants. Most resolve spontaneously and no therapy is required except for the rare case that incarcerates. An abdominal ultrasound examination should be done *only* if there is clinical evidence of an abdominal mass or ascites. Strapping or taping are ineffective and irritating and should not be advised. *(Behrman:528)*

59. **(B)** Chylous ascites is characterized by a high concentration of lipids in the ascitic fluid. Most

cases in infancy are due to congenital malformation of lymph channels; occasional cases are due to obstruction of the thoracic duct, tumor, inflammation, or intestinal obstruction. Loss of albumin, gammaglobulin, and lymphocytes in the ascitic fluid leads to depletion of these elements from the blood. The prognosis is guarded, even with treatment. Spontaneous resolution has been reported, but is the exception rather than the rule. (*Rudolph:1497, 1515*)

60. **(A)** The clinical picture described is typical of acute pancreatitis, and can be the result of each condition listed. However, of these, blunt abdominal trauma (including child abuse) would be the most common cause. (*McMillan: 1711*)

61. **(D)** Although idiopathic scoliosis can present at any stage of growth, it is most commonly manifest during, or shortly before, adolescence. It is considerably more frequent in girls than in boys. These children are mentally and intellectually normal. The condition is never painful and is usually detected on routine physical examination. The diagnosis is made on clinical grounds using physical examination and an inclinometer. When the scoliosis exceeds 6 or 7 degrees with the use of the inclinometer, x-rays will be used for a more precise assessment. (*McMillan:2118*)

62. **(A)** The Wiskott-Aldrich syndrome, an X-linked disorder, typically presents during the first 6 months of life with recurrent infections or bleeding episodes. The unusual aspect of the thrombocytopenia is that the thrombocytes are very small and thus called microthrombocytes. These small platelets are not common in any other thrombocytopenic disease. The treatment of choice is with HLA-matched bone marrow transplantation. (*McMillan:2098*)

63. **(B)** Testicular torsion actually is torsion of the spermatic cord and is a true surgical emergency because irreversible change can occur in testes within 4–6 h, and after 24 h, infarction is the rule. This condition occurs in 1 in 4000 males 25 years of age and younger, with peak

occurrence in the preadolescent age group. (*Rudolph CD:1740*)

64. **(B)** The minute structures attached to the hair are most likely nits, the eggs of the scalp louse (*pediculosis capitis*). The safest and most effective treatment of scalp lice is the topical application of a 1% permethrin cream rinse. Griseofulvin is useful for certain fungal infections such as tinea capitis, but is not effective against pediculosis. (*Red Book:464*)

65. **(B)** Chemical pneumonitis is the most common clinical manifestation of poisoning with hydrocarbons such as kerosene and may result from the aspiration of even minute amounts. Central nervous system changes are less common but can be seen. (*Rudolph CD:366–367, 1988*)

66. **(B)** Congenital hypothyroidism may be associated with prolonged neonatal hyperbilirubinemia, either indirect or mixed. The indirect hyperbilirubinemia is due to impaired hepatic glucuronidation of bilirubin and to enhanced enterohepatic circulation of bilirubin secondary to decreased intestinal motility. The mechanism of the mixed hyperbilirubinemia is uncertain. Hypothyroidism also can be associated with anemia and impaired renal function, but these are mild. (*Klaus:334*)

67. **(B)** Laryngomalacia is a condition of excessive compliance, or softness, of the cartilage of the larynx. It is presumed to be a problem of maturation rather than a congenital abnormality and is the most common cause of persistent inspiratory stridor in the young infant. Symptoms usually begin in the first month of life; are worse with agitation and in the supine position; and eventually resolve, usually by a year or so. Foreign body aspiration is an important cause of persistent stridor in the older infant and toddler but would be very unusual at this age. (*Rudolph CD:1271*)

68. **(B)** Hypercalciuria has been found in a very significant number of children with otherwise unexplained gross or microscopic hematuria. In most cases, the hematuria is not associated with

renal stones or precedes the formation of stones by many years. The serum level of calcium is normal in these patients. *(Rudolph:1663)*

69. **(B)** The chest roentgenogram reveals air trapping of the left lung with a shift of the heart and mediastinum to the right. This is most suggestive of a foreign body in the left mainstem bronchus. In the case of infantile lobar emphysema, the findings would be present in the first few months of life and would not cause the sudden onset of wheezing at 4 years of age. Also, in this condition, one lobe rather than an entire lung would be overdistended. Asthma is associated with bilateral, rather than unilateral, air-trapping. *(McMillan:570–571)*

70. **(B)** The unequal leg length and asymmetry of the inguinal (anterior) and thigh (posterior) skin creases are indicative of severe developmental dysplasia of the hip. Neither tibial torsion nor equinovarus deformity affect leg length or inguinal skin creases. Arthrogryposis is associated with severe joint contractures. *(Rudolph CD:2434–2436)*

71. **(E)** Any child with uveitis involving primarily the *anterior* structures of the eye should be suspected of having juvenile rheumatoid arthritis (JRA). This association is strongest in girls with the pauciarticular form of JRA, especially those who are antinuclear antibody positive. Toxoplasmosis and toxocara are more likely to be associated with *posterior* uveitis. Neither leukemia nor hypoparathyroidism are associated with uveitis. *(Rudolph CD:837, 2382)*

72. **(E)** Intoeing is a very common pediatric issue and in most cases represents a developmental process which is self-limited. Femoral anteversion is seen in preschoolers and typically resolves around the age of 8 years. Tibial torsion typically is present in toddlers and is diagnosed with the toddler in a sitting position with legs dangling from the table at 90 degrees. Metatarsus adductus is seen more commonly in infants, and involves the foot. *(Rudolph CD:2422–2425)*

73. **(E)** There are many factors to be considered in the decision to obtain throat swab specimens for testing of GAS. Testing is not recommended in children with signs and symptoms such as coryza, conjunctivitis, hoarseness, anterior stomatitis, diarrhea, and discrete ulcerative lesions which are highly suggestive of viral syndromes. Testing generally is not recommended in children younger than 3 years of age because the risk of rheumatic fever is so remote. Testing is recommended only for symptomatic household contacts of patients with documented GAS pharyngitis, but is recommended for all household contacts of patients with documented rheumatic fever or poststreptococcal glomerulonephritis. *(Red Book:577)*

74. **(A)** Lymphocytic thyroiditis (Hashimoto thyroiditis) is an autoimmune disorder and circulating antithyroid antibodies can be demonstrated in most patients. However, other autoimmune disorders, including diabetes mellitus, adrenal insufficiency, hypoparathyroidism, and pernicious anemia, occur in only a *minority* of patients. The thyroid gland is *invariably enlarged*, often irregularly so. Most patients are euthyroid, some are hypothyroid, and a few are hyperthyroid. *(Rudolph CD:1811)*

75. **(B)** Before the 1970s, zinc deficiency was not known to be the cause of this devastating condition called acrodermatitis enteropathica. Breast-fed infants are at risk of zinc deficiency when the maternal levels are low and vegetarians are at risk of zinc deficiency because the bioavailability of zinc in plant sources is low. Therefore, this infant was at risk. Patients receiving TPN also are prone to this condition, and should receive supplementation and monitoring. *(Rudolph CD:1338; McMillan:708)*

76. **(E)** Primary pulmonary hemosiderosis is an uncommon disease of unknown origin characterized by repeated pulmonary hemorrhages. The clinical picture of recurrent episodes of fever, cough, and radiographic infiltrates is frequently misinterpreted as recurrent pneumonia, especially in infants and young children who do not expectorate and in whom hemoptysis may go undetected. The first clue often is

a severe iron deficiency anemia. Some of these infants or children have improvement in pulmonary manifestations when cow milk is eliminated from their diet. Diffuse pulmonary hemangiomatosis and extramedullary pulmonary erythropoiesis are nonentities. *(Rudolph CD:1997–1998)*

77. **(B)** Chondromalacia patellae (also called patellofemoral pain and patellar compression syndrome) is a repetitive stress injury resulting from rubbing between the femoral groove and patella associated with high forces generated through sports and jumping. As with other conditions suffered from overuse or repetition, the pain remits with rest. Night pain or unremitting pain in this situation should always prompt further evaluation. *(Rudolph CD:2432–2433)*

78. **(D)** The anterior fontanalle normally closes between 9 and 18 months of age. Each of the choices, except for craniosynostosis, is associated with *delayed* closure of the anterior fontanelle. Craniosynostosis is the premature fusion of skull sutures which results in abnormalities of calvarial shape and occurs in about 1 in 2000 live births. The most common form of single suture fusion is sagital synostosis. Although most cases of craniosynostosis are diagnosed in the newborn period, early closure of the fontanelles should raise suspicion for this diagnosis, and with careful examination you should be able to palpate the ridging of the prematurely fused suture. *(Hay:5; Behrman:455; Rudolph CD:755)*

79. **(E)** The rash described in this question sounds like urticaria, for which there are many causes. Although allergy to foods, drugs, or chemicals is high on the list, in most cases, no specific cause can be found. A few cases are associated with infections caused by hepatitis viruses or group A *Streptococcus*. A very few cases are due to collage vascular disease or malignancy. Hereditary deficiency of C1-esterase inhibitor (extremely rare) is usually associated with angioedema rather than urticaria. *(Rudolph: 1195)*

80. **(C)** The XYY karyotype is relatively common, occurring in about 1 in 1000 males. Patients with this karyotype generally are tall. It is debatable whether or not the XYY karyotype is associated with an increased risk of impulsivity, antisocial behavior, and psychopathic personality. But whether or not this is true, *most* XYY individuals are behaviorally normal, although IQ and language development tend to be low normal. *(Jones:70–71, 707)*

81. **(A)** Thrombocytopenia with giant platelets in an otherwise well-appearing newborn most likely represents platelet destruction secondary to transplacental transmission of maternal antiplatelet IgG autoantibodies. Maternal thrombocytopenia would be expected if this were the case. If the maternal thrombocytes were normal and she had no history of autoimmune disease, alloimmune thrombocytopenia is the likely diagnosis. This would result from transplacental passage of a maternal antibody that specifically recognized an antigen on baby's platelets that baby inherited from the father. *(Klaus:475)*

82. **(C)** Pertussis is most deadly for young infants. Complications include pneumonia, seizures, encephalopathy, and apnea. The case fatality rate in the United States is 1% for those infants less than 2 months of age. In adolescents, the illness more likely is only a persistent cough. For those in between these age groups, the more classic picture is seen: paroxysms of 10–30 uninterrupted staccato coughs followed by a long loud gasping inspiration known as a "whoop," accompanied by an absolute lymphocytosis. *(Red Book:472–475)*

83. **(A)** The abnormality in pseudohypoparathyroidism is a defect in end-organ (kidney and bone) response to parathyroid hormone. Serum levels of parathyroid hormone are normal or elevated. Short stature and skeletal abnormalities, including demineralization, are common. Fingers are short and broad (brachymetacarpals). *(Rudolph CD:2001)*

84. **(B)** Also called pseudohemophilia, von Willebrand disease is characterized by a prolonged bleeding time. There is a *variable* deficiency or molecular abnormality of factor VIII, giving rise to a *variably* abnormal PTT. The

platelet count, factor XII level and prothrombin time are all normal. The location for the encoding of the von Willebrand factor is on chromosome 12. Most commonly, children with von Willebrand disease will present with a history of nosebleeds and easy bruising. *(Rudolph CD:200)*

85. **(A)** Dysgenesis (aplasia, dysplasia, hypoplasia) of the thyroid gland is the most common cause of congenital hypothyroidism. Inborn metabolic errors of thyroid synthesis are much less frequent. Maternal ingestion of iodides (as in expectorants) is a recognized cause of neonatal hypothyroidism but is rare today. *(Rudolph CD:2066, 2068–2069)*

86. **(E)** Cysticercosis is a condition of generalized tissue invasion by the larva of *T. solium* and results from the ingestion of *T. solium* eggs which have contaminated food or cooking utensils. Eating undercooked infected pork results in ingestion of an encysted worm which causes an intestinal tapeworm infestation, not cysticercosis. Cysticercosis is endemic in Mexico and is one of the most common causes of seizures in children in that population. In the United States it is seen primarily in areas with large Latin American immigrant populations. The central nervous system is the most common target organ and seizures are the most frequent presenting complaint. *(Feigin:2526; Red Book:608–609)*

87. **(E)** Approximately 40% of adults with cystic fibrosis have diabetes mellitus. It is thought to result from chronic obstruction of ductal flow from inspissated secretions which results in pancreatic fibrosis and beta cell destruction. It behaves like maturity onset diabetes, with little tendency to ketoacidosis. Diabetes should always be considered when an older child with cystic fibrosis loses weight. *(Rudolph CD:2114)*

88. **(A)** Elevated sweat chloride concentration is an almost universal finding in patients with cystic fibrosis (CF). Even in this era of molecular diagnostics, the diagnosis of cystic fibrosis most often involves a sweat test. Normal children have sweat chloride concentrations less than 40 meq/L while CF patients have concentrations greater than 60 meq/L. It is strongly recommended that sweat tests be performed only in established CF centers because tests performed outside these centers have unacceptably high rates of false positive and false negative results. *(Rudolph CD:1972)*

89. **(D)** Acute otitis media (AOM) resolves spontaneously in about 80% of cases. And, 60% of children are pain free in 24 h, with or without antibiotic treatment. However, in the United States it is the standard of care to treat symptomatic children with AOM with antibiotics in order to relieve symptoms and to decrease the incidence of complications such as mastoiditis and hearing loss. To choose the antibiotic, you must know the etiologic agents and their susceptibility to antibiotics. The bacteria most commonly involved in acute otitis media in childhood in the United States are *Streptococcus pneumoniae* (causes 40% of AOM, 40% are resistant to penicillin), *Haemophilus influenzae* (causes 25% of AOM, 25% are beta-lactamase producers), and *Moraxella catarrhalis* (causes 12% of AOM, 100% are beta-lactamase producers). Most experts agree that amoxicillin remains the initial drug of choice, and that an increased dose (80 mg/kg per day) is indicated given the resistance patterns above. *(Rudolph CD:1249–1252)*

90. **(A)** Inguinal hernias are not at all rare in female infants, and the great majority of these infants are genetically female and otherwise normal. Such hernias may contain intestine or an ovary, either of which can incarcerate. Prompt surgical correction is indicated. Most inguinal hernias in infants, males or females, are indirect. *(Rudolph CD:1742; McMillan: 1640–1642)*

91. **(B)** Large ventricular septal defects (VSD) usually are associated with left deviation of the electrical axis and evidence of left ventricular hypertrophy on electrocardiogram, although signs of combined ventricular hypertrophy are not uncommon. An enlarged heart is common, but the pulmonary vasculature is increased, not decreased. The murmur of a VSD is systolic, rather than continuous. With large left-to-right shunts and a high pulmonary flow, there

also may be a mid-diastolic rumble, but still not a continuous murmur. *(Rudolph CD:1354–1356)*

92. **(C)** All of the choices listed are manifestations of hypoparathyroidism, the hallmark of which is hypocalcemia and hyperphosphatemia with resultant neuromuscular instability. The most common presentation is seizure. *(Rudolph CD:1768)*

93. **(D)** Nearly 60% of adolescent women will experience dysmenorrhea. It is the leading cause of school absenteeism among these young women. Most cases are primary dysmenorrhea (painful menses without pelvic pathology), and are associated with high levels of prostaglandins which correlate with the severity of the symptoms. For these young women, nonsteroidal anti-inflammatory agents are generally very effective. Oral contraceptives often are a good therapeutic option because they successfully treat the dysmenorrhea in 80–90%. *(McMillan:541–542)*

94. **(D)** This child meets diagnostic criteria for Kawasaki disease. To establish the diagnosis the patient must have fever for at least 5 days, then have at least four of the following five criteria: (1) bilateral bulbar conjunctival injection without exudates; (2) changes in oral mucosa including erythematous mouth and pharynx, strawberry tongue, and red, cracked lips; (3) rash that is polymorphous, generalized, morbilliform, maculopapular or scarlatiniform or erythema multiforme-like; (4) changes in peripheral extremities consisting of induration of hands and feet, palmoplantar erythema, or periungual desquamation; (5) acute, nonsuppurative cervical adenopathy with at least one node measuring 1.5 cm. The complication of coronary artery aneurysms occurs in about 25% of untreated patients. This declines to about 3–6% with intravenous gammaglobulin treatment. Treatment should be initiated as soon as the diagnosis is made. *(Red Book:392–393; Rudolph CD:844–845)*

95. **(A)** Fanconi syndrome is a proximal tubule transport disorder which leads to hypophosphatemia, hypokalemia, and a hyperchloremic metabolic acidosis. The most common inherited cause in children is cystinosis, a disorder in which cystine accumulates in the lysosomes eventually leading to cell dysfunction. Children with this disorder typically are healthy for the first few months of life, then develop the symptoms described. Two other choices, tyrosinemia and glycogen storage disease also are associated with Fanconi syndrome. *(Rudolph CD:1708)*

96. **(A)** Pityriasis rosea (PR) is a common dermatosis. It is characterized by a progressive eruption of dozens of 2–10 mm salmon colored flat patches with a scaly perimeter. Lesions may be intensely pruritic. Characteristically the lesions follow skin lines and on the back create the so-called "Christmas tree" pattern. This generalized rash may be preceded by several weeks by a herald patch, a larger well-circumscribed lesion on the extremities or trunk. In any patient who also has palmoplantar or mucous membrane lesions or who is sexually active, serologic testing for syphilis is indicated. Epidemiologic evidence has long supported the idea this has an infectious etiology. Recently, PR has been described in patients with active human herpesvirus 6 and human herpesvirus 7 infection. *(Rudolph CD:1181; J Investig Dermatol 119:779–780, 2002)*

97. **(B)** The presenting sign in over 60% of patients with retinoblastoma is leukocoria, or white pupil. Often, this is noted during a well-child examination. This patient represents the average age at diagnosis, 18 months. In 30–35% of patients, tumors occur bilaterally. There is a 90% survival rate for patients with small, unilateral, promptly-treated tumors. *(Rudolph CD:2396)*

98. **(C)** A grave disparity regarding neonatal and infant mortality rates exists between African American babies and babies of other races. Though preterm births are more common among African American mothers, this does not completely explain the nearly double rates for infant and neonatal mortality as compared to Whites. *(Rudolph CD:57)*

99. **(D)** Children with constitutional growth delay have no endocrine disease but lag behind their peers in both growth and physiologic maturation. Such children are small for their age. Bone age also is delayed and, therefore, is commensurate with height. Puberty is delayed, and, consequently, growth continues for a longer than normal period of time, resulting in ultimate adult height which is normal. *(Rudolph CD:2103)*

100. **(B)** The most common form of systemic vasculitis in childhood is Henoch-Schönlein purpura. The most consistent sign is the presence of the purpuric rash on the lower extremities. Unfortunately, this rash does not necessarily develop at the beginning of the illness. Frequently a child is evaluated for arthritis or abdominal pain for 1–2 days before the onset of the rash makes the diagnosis apparent. The renal disease associated with HSP typically is variable, with most children having complete recovery. However, 3–4% of children will develop end-stage renal disease. *(Rudolph CD:842, 1689)*

101. **(B)** This child most likely has transient synovitis of the hip, an acute inflammatory process that is generally self-limited. It is most important for this to be distinguished from a septic hip, which typically presents in younger patients and is accompanied by fever and laboratory evidence such as increased white blood cell count, increased platelets, or increased erythrocyte sedimentation rate. And, follow-up is your friend. This child should be closely observed and examined again within 24 h; sooner if there are any parental concerns or worsening symptoms. *(Hay:807)*

102. **(B)** The selective disturbance of skeletal growth in achondroplasia results in disproportionately short extremities. In the extremities the proximal bones are further disproportionately shortened in relation to the distal bones. The fingers are short and stubby. Hydrocephalus is seen occasionally, possibly related to a small foramen magnum. Overall height, of course, is markedly decreased. These patients characteristically have a relatively large head, bulging forehead, and depressed nasal bridge. The diagnosis is confirmed by skeletal radiographs. Most cases arise from a new mutation at *FGFR3* codon 380 to normal parents. However, achondroplasia, when inherited, behaves as an autosomal dominant trait. *(Lissauer:288)*

103. **(D)** Goat milk, compared to human milk and cow milk, is low in folate and iron. Babies exclusively fed goat milk are susceptible to megaloblastic anemia from folate and B_{12} deficiency. Additionally, if the goat milk is fresh and not boiled, the infants are at risk of brucellosis. *(Behrman:156–157)*

104. **(E)** Rotavirus is the most common cause of winter diarrhea in the United States and is a leading cause of death among children in developing countries. Clearly, the development of a safe, oral vaccine is ideal, and is ongoing. Hypernatremic dehydration (serum sodium >150 meq/L with dehydration) is frequently seen in hospitalized infants with rotavirus infection. *(Red Book:534–537)*

105. **(A)** Motor vehicle accidents lead to approximately 5500 adolescent deaths each year in the United States. Homicide and legal intervention result in the death of nearly 3000 adolescents per year, making this the second most common cause of death in this age group. Of these 3000 deaths, 2500 are associated with firearms. The importance of firearms in these deaths is evident. An additional 1200 suicidal deaths are associated with firearms each year. *(McMillan:9)*

106. **(E)** Despite the devastating effect congenital infection with cytomegalovirus can have on the fetus and newborn, most congenital infections are asymptomatic. If however, symptoms of infection are present at birth, most will have severe neurodevelopmental disabilities such as cerebral palsy, epilepsy, sensorineural hearing loss, and learning difficulties. Most severe effects are seen in infants whose fetal infection occurred during the first half of pregnancy. *(Lissauer: 73–74; McMillan:449–430)*

107. **(D)** The syndrome of inappropriate secretion of antidiuretic hormone (SIADH) is a common complication of a variety of central nervous system problems, including bacterial meningitis. Usually the SIADH resolves as the meningitis is treated, even if a subdural effusion is present. *(McMillan:857, 861, 2207)*

108. **(B)** Theoretically, the syndrome of inappropriate ADH secretion would be most accurately diagnosed by measurement of serum ADH levels. However, the assay for antidiuretic hormone is not readily available. Therefore, the diagnosis usually is confirmed by demonstrating a low urine output and inappropriate high urine osmolality in the presence of low serum osmolality. *(McMillan:857, 861, 2207)*

109. **(D)** Patients with inappropriate secretion of ADH have a decreased urine output and are hypervolemic. They are neither hypotensive nor alkalotic. High urine specific gravity is one of the criteria for the diagnosis of SIADH. *(McMillan:857, 861, 2207)*

110. **(B)** Therapy of inappropriate ADH secretion consists primarily of fluid restriction and, of course, treatment of the underlying condition, in this case, bacterial meningitis. Attempts to correct the hyponatremia by administration of sodium usually result in more retention of water and further hypervolemia and edema. Intravenous administration of hypertonic saline would be indicated only if the hyponatremia were life-threatening. Maintenance amounts of sodium should be administered. Diuretics are not very effective in this condition. *(McMillan:857, 861, 2207)*

111. **(B)** The cerebrospinal fluid findings, especially the xanthochromic appearance after centrifugation, indicate an intracranial hemorrhage. The bleeding is primarily subarachnoid or, at least, there has been extension of the bleeding into the subarachnoid space. Intraventricular hemorrhage is uncommon except in the small, premature infant. Fever is seen in patients with intracranial hemorrhage. *(Rudolph CD:2196, 2238)*

112. (C) Of the abnormalities listed, only cerebral arteriovenous malformation (AVM) and aneurysm predispose to hemorrhagic disasters. In

children, cerebral AVMs are the most common cause of spontaneous intracranial hemorrhage. Unlike the situation in adults, intracranial hemorrhage in children is rarely due to a ruptured aneurysm. *(Rudolph CD:2196, 2238)*

113. **(A)** The most appropriate management at this time would be to perform a CT scan, followed, *if necessary*, by further imaging. It would not have been unreasonable to have performed the CT prior to the lumbar puncture. It is a question of judgment as to the likelihood of meningitis in this child with only a slight fever. Intracranial hemorrhage rarely is associated with volume depletion or the need for transfusion. In the absence of evidence of a bleeding disorder, there is no indication for administration of fresh frozen plasma. *(Rudolph CD:2196, 2238)*

114. **(C)** The clinical picture described is almost pathognomonic for infantile hypertrophic pyloric stenosis, which would best be confirmed with abdominal ultrasound. *(McMillan: 80, 311)*

115. **(E)** Most infants with hypertrophic pyloric stenosis develop a hypochloremic metabolic alkalosis secondary to the loss of hydrogen and chloride ions in the vomitus, which in this condition is essentially pure gastric secretion. Hypochloremic metabolic alkalosis occurs so regularly in this disorder, that it often is used as a diagnostic feature. *(McMillan:80, 311)*

116. **(B)** The physical findings suggest that the child is moderately dehydrated. Glucose and water alone is never the appropriate hydrating or maintenance solution for an infant or a child. Bicarbonate should be withheld from this child who is not described as appearing clinically acidotic and who is very likely to have a metabolic alkalosis secondary to the prolonged vomiting. Indeed, the respiratory rate of 12 is rather slow for an infant of this age and could be explained on the basis of respiratory compensation for a metabolic alkalosis. Although the child might be hypokalemic secondary to prolonged alkalosis, there also is the possibility of hyperkalemia secondary to dehydration and

prerenal azotemia. Normal saline is the most appropriate initial rehydrating fluid until the serum electrolytes are documented. *(Behrman: 1131)*

117. **(E)** In this clinical scenario urine positive for hemoglobin on dipstick but negative for red blood cells on microscopic examination probably represents myoglobinuria. This would be presumptively confirmed with an elevated serum creatine kinase. *(McMillan:1985)*

118. **(D)** Acute myoglobinuria can lead to tubular injury and acute renal failure. Serum electrolytes and renal function should be evaluated. *(McMillan:1985)*

119. **(A)** Acute myoglobinuria is caused by influenza viruses A and B, coxsackievirus B5, echovirus 9, adenovirus 21, herpes simplex virus, and Epstein-Barr virus. This patient most likely has influenza virus infection. *(McMillan: 1985)*

120. **(D)** This child most likely has visceral larva migrans, which in this country usually is caused by *Toxocara canis*, or *Toxocara cati*, the dog and cat ascarids, respectively. Diagnosis can be established by biopsy of an involved organ such as lung or liver. Since the human is an unnatural host, the parasite does not complete its life cycle and ova or worms do not appear in the stool or in duodenal fluid. The diagnosis cannot be established by examination of the bone marrow or a blood smear. Serologic tests are helpful. Most patients, if not blood type AB, have markedly elevated anti-A and anti-B isohemagglutinin antibody titers. Often the diagnosis is made on the basis of the clinical, hematologic, and serologic data, without liver biopsy. [*Note:* The question asked which of the listed procedures would be most likely to establish the diagnosis, not whether or not the procedure was necessary or indicated.] *(Rudolph CD:1110–1111)*

121. **(B)** *Toxocara canis* infection usually is acquired by eating soil contaminated by dog stool. The *T. canis* eggs which are passed in the dog's stool are not directly infective, but in the soil the eggs develop into infective ova containing second stage larva. Infection, therefore, is probably not acquired by direct contact with the animal, but only by contact with infected soil, usually as a result of geophagy. *(Rudolph CD:1110–1111)*

122. **(A)** If you keep a mental picture of preschoolers playing in the dirt around puppies all over the United States, you can begin to remember the epidemiology of this infection. This parasitic infection is more common in the United States than in developing countries and is equally prevalent in urban and rural populations. In humans, this infection is most frequently reported in children of 1–4 years of age. The vast majority of newborn puppies are infected. *(Rudolph CD:1110–1111)*

123. **(D)** The most likely diagnosis is severe combined immunodeficiency syndrome (SCIDS). Both Wiskott-Aldrich syndrome and hereditary agammaglobulinemia are X-linked recessive conditions and, therefore, are unlikely in this female child. Most 3-month-old infants have low, but detectable, levels of IgA and IgM (normal range for 3-month-old: 3–90 and 115–120 mg/dL, respectively). The IgG is maternal. Patients with AIDS usually have elevated levels of immunoglobulins. Also, infants with AIDS are usually not this sick this early; infants with SCIDS often are. Patients with transient hypogammaglobulinemia of infancy usually are not as sick as this patient and infection generally does not start as early as 6 weeks. Of the diagnoses listed, only SCIDS explains all the findings including lymphopenia. *(Rudolph CD:793–796, 799)*

124. **(C)** Severe combined immunodeficiency is associated with an absence or paucity of plasma cells in the bone marrow, absence or paucity of superficial lymphoid tissue, and an absent thymic shadow on chest roentgenogram. Cutaneous reactivity to various common antigens is absent. In an immunologically normal child with Candida infection, one would expect to find a positive reaction to intradermal testing with Candida antigen. In a child with severe combined immunodeficiency, there is global

anergy and all skin tests are nonreactive. (*Rudolph CD:793–796, 799*)

125. **(B)** The roentgenographic picture described is typical of *Pneumocystis carinii* infection, to which these infants are unduly susceptible. Viruses such as cytomegalovirus could produce a similar picture, but it is not listed as a choice. Lymphangiectasia is a congenital lesion of the lung, unrelated to immunologic disorders. Neither pneumococcal pneumonia nor pulmonary hemorrhage is likely to be so protracted or indolent. Miliary tuberculosis is a possibility, but usually does not produce such extensive bilateral disease or a ground-glass appearance radiographically. It also is uncommon in patients this young. (*Rudolph CD:793–796*)

126. **(C)** Of the conditions listed, subdural hematoma is the most likely and would best explain all the clinical findings. Tuberculous meningitis can cause obstructive hydrocephalus and a large head, but fever and cranial nerve abnormalities usually are evident on physical examination. Mastoiditis is generally associated with fever, and, by itself, would not explain the neurologic findings. Pseudotumor cerebri is relatively benign and is not associated with convulsions. All three conditions—tuberculous meningitis, mastoiditis, and pseudotumor are uncommon in the first few months of life. With congenital toxoplasmosis, other findings and delayed psychomotor development would likely be present. (*Rudolph CD:465, 953, 2398*)

127. **(C)** Retinal hemorrhages may be found in up to 40% of cases of subdural hematoma and usually are indicative of the shaking injury as a form of child abuse now termed the shaken baby/impact syndrome. The forceful shaking of the infant creates shearing forces in the brain and retina, resulting in bleeding in both organs. Congenital toxoplasmosis is associated with chorioretinitis rather than hemorrhage. (*Behrman:1937; Rudolph CD:465*)

128. **(C)** The presentation of this infant necessitates CT scan of the head to begin to define the extent of the intracranial injuries. Head injuries

remain the most common cause of death to children who have been abused. (*Rudolph:469*)

129. **(G)** The most important intervention in any child with an elevated lead level is to stop further exposure of the child to the source of the lead. Children with blood lead levels of 45–69 µg/dL should receive chelation therapy. Chelation with oral meso-1,3-dimercapto-succinic acid (DMSA) should be considered for children who have no signs of symptomatic lead poisoning. EDTA is the chelation agent of choice for children with symptomatic lead poisoning or severe lead poisoning involving the central nervous system or any child with a blood lead level of ≥70 µg/dL. (*Rudolph CD:370*)

130. **(E)** Children with either acute iron poisoning or chronic iron overload from repeated transfusions should be treated with the iron chelating agent deferoxamine. For acute ingestion, the drug usually is administered intravenously. (*Rudolph CD:368*)

131. **(A)** If treatment is begun early (ideally within 24 h of ingestion), acetylcysteine may prevent hepatic injury from acetaminophen ingestion. Acetaminophen itself is not hepatotoxic, but some of its metabolites are. These hepatotoxic metabolites ordinarily are inactivated by glutathione as soon as they are formed. Large overdoses of acetaminophen deplete the liver's stores of glutathione, permitting the toxic metabolite to accumulate. Acetylcysteine replenishes hepatic glutathione, protecting the liver from the toxic by-products of acetaminophen metabolism. (*Rudolph CD:360; Hay:341*)

132. **(B)** Atropine is an important part of the treatment of organophosphate poisoning. Although it has little effect on the central nervous system effects of organophosphate, atropine will control respiratory secretions and other cholinergic effects. Pralidoxime, a cholinesterase-regenerating oxime may be needed to reverse muscle weakness. (*Rudolph CD:373–374*)

133. **(T)** Jimson weed is ingested, typically by adolescents, for its hallucinogenic properties. The anticholinergic symptoms this chemical causes include the classic "red as a beet, mad as a hatter, hot as a hare, blind as a bat, and dry as a bone." Physostigmine, which binds competitively to acetylcholinesterase in the synapse, can reverse the anticholinergic symptoms. *(Tobias:424; Rudolph CD:359)*

134. **(H)** Ethylene glycol is the primary component of antifreeze. Organic acids formed by metabolism of ethylene glycol are more toxic than the parent compound and are responsible for most of the major toxicity. Ethanol, an effective antidote, works by competing for the enzyme alcohol dehydrogenase which catalyzes the first step in the metabolism of ethylene glycol. The same enzyme initiates the metabolic pathway for methanol and isopropyl alcohol, and therefore, ethanol is also useful in treating poisoning with these substances. Some prefer fomepizole as an alternative. *(Rudolph CD:359; Tobias:423)*

135. **(O)** Naloxone is a competitive antagonist to the opiates, including morphine. The drug is best administered intravenously. The usual dose is 0.03 mg/kg, but a second larger dose (0.1 mg/kg) may be given if there is no response. Naloxone is not itself a depressant, and is a very safe drug. *(Rudolph CD:359, 372)*

136. **(X)** Cyclic antidepressants remain a leading cause of death from ingestions of pharmaceutical agents. These deaths occur principally in two age groups: toddlers who are unaware and adolescents who are attempting self-harm. The treatment of the cardiovascular toxicity seen in this overdose is the administration of sodium bicarbonate. The therapeutic effect of alkalinization most likely is multifactorial. *(Rogers:1375–1377; Rudolph CD:359)*

137. **(Q)** The most common cause of poisoning death is carbon monoxide inhalation. The sources most often are home fires and exposure to incomplete combustion of carbon fuels. When the source is smoke inhalation, most victims of fatal CO poisoning will die before arrival to the hospital. However, CO poisoning is treated with the antidote 100% oxygen.

Hyperbaric oxygen is used in many centers. *(Rudolph CD:359, 363)*

138. **(E)** Most 1-year-old children are able to perform the tasks described. The pincer grip is developed on average at 10.5 months of age. *(Lissauer:15)*

139. **(H)** Children typically are able to copy a circle at 3 years of age, and copy a cross at 4 years of age. Hopping on one foot generally is accomplished at 4 years of age. *(Lissauer:17)*

140. **(A)** These are expected findings in the evaluation of the supine infant (6–8 weeks of age). An 8-week-old infant who does not demonstrate responsive smiling should be further evaluated. *(Lissauer:14)*

141. **(G)** The 2-year-old is at the end of the mobile toddler phase and is expected to walk will with normal gait, and to be able to kick a ball. Though most 20-month-old toddlers are able to combine two different words, toddlers are more likely closer to 24 months of age before they are able to build a tower of six 1-in cubes. *(Lissauer:16)*

142. **(D)** The sitting child, 6–9 months of age, typically develops the ability to pull to a stand by age of 9 months, and babbles nonspecifically, but quite happily, by 9–10 months. The palmar grasp is predominant at 6 months of age and the pincer grasp develops between 10 and 11 months of age. *(Lissauer:15)*

143. **(A)** Newborns should startle to sudden loud noise, so the best choice is the 2-month-old. *(Lissauer:14)*

144. **(I)** Most 5-year olds are able to copy a triangle. (Remember, most children are able to copy a circle by 3 years of age, a cross by 4 years of age, and a triangle by 5 years of age. The ability to copy a square is demonstrated between 4 and 5 years of age.) Past tense typically is used in language by 4 years of age, and future tense by 5 years of age. *(Lissauer:17; Behrman:43)*

145. **(A)** Among children with Down syndrome and congenital heart disease, 40% will have atrioventricular defect, 30% ventricular septal defect, and 20% atrial septal defect. Approximately 5% will have tetralogy of Fallot. *(Lissauer:174)*

146. **(C)** Williams syndrome, also known as idiopathic infantile hypercalcemia, features growth delay, mental retardation, characteristic facial features, stellate iris, and supravalvular aortic stenosis. A very interesting characteristic of children with Williams syndrome is their unique chatter ability, referred to as "cocktail chatter." *(Rudolph CD:740, 1805)*

147. **(B)** Mitral valve prolapse can be demonstrated by echocardiography in about 80% of patients with Marfan syndrome. The most important cardiovascular manifestation, progressive dilation of the aortic root and ascending aorta, was not listed as a choice. *(Rudolph CD:1797)*

148. **(D)** Turner syndrome (45X) occurs in about 1/2500 live newborns. Clinical features include short stature, neck webbing, ovarian dysgenesis with infertility, cardiac defects, and normal intellectual development. The most common cardiac defect in this syndrome is coarctation of the aorta. One-third of girls with Turner syndrome have bicuspid aortic valves. *(Lissauer:56; Rudolph CD:1781)*

149. **(E)** Children with Noonan syndrome have a high incidence of valvular pulmonary stenosis. *(Smith:122; Rudolph CD:1810)*

150. **(C)** The heliotrope sign is a purplish discoloration of the periorbital skin which is frequently found in children (typically school-aged children) with dermatomyositis. Dermatomyositis is a chronic inflammatory disease affecting primarily the skin and skeletal muscles. *(Rudolph CD:1109)*

151. **(A)** Profound muscle weakness, hypotonia, tongue fasciculations, and swallowing dysfunction are characteristic of Werdnig-Hoffmann disease, or spinal muscular atrophy type 1. This disease *typically* presents before 6 months of age and is fatal by 2 years of age. The infants involved are of normal intelligence and normal social ability, making their slow demise all the more difficult for the loved ones involved. *(Rudolph CD:2002, 2279)*

152. **(E)** Hemolytic uremic syndrome is diagnosed by the presence of microangiopathic hemolytic anemia, thrombocytopenia, and renal insufficiency. Most affected children will have a preceding gastrointestinal infection with *Escherichia coli* that produces a *Shigella*-like toxin. *(Rudolph CD:1696)*

153. **(B)** Gower sign, or Gower maneuver, reflects hip-girdle weakness and most commonly is associated with Duchenne muscular dystrophy, although it can also be seen in spinal muscular atrophy and in some cases of dermatomyositis. The Gower maneuver enables children with proximal muscle weakness to move from a prone to standing position and involves first moving the feet close to the hands, then walking hands up the legs to push the trunk upright. *(Rudolph CD:2278, 2289)*

154. **(D)** The most common form of systemic vasculitis in children is HSP. Nearly 100% of children with this disorder will develop purpura with a normal platelet count. *(Rudolph CD:842)*

155. **(H)** This scenario most likely represents bacterial infection following the cat bite. Cat bites are particularly prone to infection because the very long narrow teeth of the cat inoculate the cat's oral flora deep into the tissue. Of the choices given, the most likely causative agent is *Pasteurella multocida*. The drug of choice for treatment is penicillin. However, because of the possibility of a polymicrobial infection including *Staphylococcus aureus*, the drug most often chosen in this scenario is oral amoxicillin-clavulanate or intravenous ampicillin-sulbactam sodium. *(Red Book:462)*

156. **(C)** This clinical picture is most consistent with human monocytic ehrlichiosis, most commonly seen in the southeastern and south central United States. The clinical findings closely resemble Rocky Mountain spotted fever, another

tickborne infection. Both are treated with doxy-cycline. *(Red Book:266–268)*

157. **(A)** Pharyngoconjunctival fever is an acute viral illness typically seen in summer-time pool outbreaks and manifests with fever, conjunctivitis, and pharyngitis. The most likely etiologic agent is adenovirus. *(McMillan:1318)*

158. **(G)** Roseola (sixth disease) typically presents in children less than 24 months of age. Fever is characteristically high and persists 3–6 days. Frequently, the fever abates with the onset of the rash. Febrile seizures occur in 10–15% of cases. *(Red Book:356–357)*

159. **(I)** Most cases of croup (laryngotracheobronchitis) are due to infection with parainfluenza. Among other viruses, adenovirus, influezna virus, and measles virus infections can also cause croup. *(Red Book:454–455)*

160. **(K)** Rat bite fever is caused by *Streptobacillus moniliformis* or *Spirillum minus*. Typically the fever does not begin at the time of the bite but develops a few days later as the wounds appear to be healing. *(Red Book:520–521)*

161. **(C)** Sturge-Weber disease, also called encephalofacial angiomatosis, is the most unique of the neurocutaneous conditions listed. It does not have a clear inheritance pattern, lacks cutaneous pigmentation, and does not carry an increased risk of tumors. It is a progressive disorder and may be associated with mental retardation, seizures, hemiparesis, and visual problems. For children less severely affected, deterioration after age of 5 years is unusual, but learning difficulties and seizures may persist. The nevus flammeus (port wine) generally is in the distribution of the trigeminal nerve. *(McMillan:2025; Lissauer:310)*

162. **(B)** Neurofibromatosis type 1 (Von Recklinghausen disease) is an autosomal dominant neurocutaneous condition with cafe au lait spots as the hallmark. Typically, the cafe au lait spots develop during the first year of life and increase in size and number for the first few years of life. Axillary freckling is closely associated with neurofibromatosis. Cutaneous neurofibromas often are not apparent until puberty. Though inheritance is autosomal dominant, one-half of all cases are the result of new mutation. *(McMillan:2019–2021)*

BIBLIOGRAPHY

American Academy of Pediatrics Committee on Infectious Diseases. *2003 Red Book, Report of the Committee on Infectious Diseases*, 26th ed. Elk Grove, IL: American Academy of Pediatrics, 2003.

American Academy of Pediatrics Section on Hematology/Oncology, Committee on Genetics. Health supervision for children with sickle cell disease. *Pediatrics* 2002;109:526–535.

American Academy of Pediatrics Task Force on Sleep Position and Sudden Infant Death Syndrome. Changing concepts of sudden infant death syndrome. *Pediatrics* 2000;105:650–656.

Behrman RE, Kliegman RM, Arvin AM. *Nelson Textbook of Pediatrics*, 16th ed. Philadelphia, PA: W.B. Saunders, 1999.

Feigin RD, Cherry JD. *Textbook of Pediatric Infectious Diseases*, 4th ed. Philadelphia, PA: W.B. Saunders, 1998.

Gershel JD, Goldman HS, Stein RE, et al. The usefulness of chest radiographs in first asthma attacks. *N Engl J Med* 1983;309:336–339.

Hay WW, Hayward AR, Levin MJ, Sondheimer JM. *Current Pediatric Diagnosis & Treatment*, 16th ed. New York, NY: McGraw-Hill, 2003.

Jones K. *Smith's Recognizable Patterns of Human Malformations*, 5th ed. Philadelphia, PA: W.B. Saunders, 1997.

Klaus MH, Fanaroff AA. *Care of the High-risk Neonate*, 5th ed. Philadelphia, PA: W.B. Saunders, 2001.

Lissauer T, Clayden G. *Illustrated Textbook of Pediatrics*. London, England: Times Mirror International Publishers Ltd., 1997.

McMillan JA, DeAngelis CD, Feigin RD, Warshaw JB. *Oski's Pediatrics: Principles and Practice*, 3rd ed. Philadelphia, PA: JB Lippincott, 1999.

Rogers MC. *Textbook of Pediatric Intensive Care*, 3rd ed. Baltimore, MD: Williams & Wilkins, 1996.

Rudolph CD, Rudolph AM, Hostetter MK, et al. *Rudolph's Pediatrics*, 21st ed. New York, NY: McGraw-Hill, 2003.

Tobias JD. *Pediatric Critical Care: The Essentials*. Armonk, NY: Futura Publishing Co., 1999.

Watanabe T, Kawamura T, Jacob SE, Aquilino EA, et al. Pityriasis rosea is associated with systemic active infection with both human herpesvirus 7 and human herpesvirus 6. *J Investig Dermatol* 2002;119(4):793–797.

Index